Patient Autonomy and the Ethics of Responsibility

Basic Bioethics

Glenn McGee and Arthur Caplan, editors

Pricing Life: Why It's Time for Health Care Rationing, Peter A. Ubel

Bioethics: Ancient Themes in Contemporary Issues, edited by Mark G. Kuczewski and Ronald Polansky

The Human Embryonic Stem Cell Debate: Science, Ethics, and Public Policy, edited by Suzanne Holland, Karen Lebacqz, and Laurie Zoloth

Engendering International Health: The Challenge of Equity, edited by Gita Sen, Asha George, and Piroska Östlin

Self-Trust and Reproductive Autonomy, Carolyn McLeod

What Genes Can't Do, Lenny Moss

In the Wake of Terror: Medicine and Morality in a Time of Crisis, edited by Jonathan D. Moreno

Pragmatic Bioethics, 2nd edition, edited by Glenn McGee

Case Studies in Biomedical Research Ethics, Timothy F. Murphy

Genetics and Life Insurance: Medical Underwriting and Social Policy, edited by Mark A. Rothstein

Ethics and the Metaphysics of Medicine: Reflections on Health and Beneficence, Kenneth A. Richman

DNA and the Criminal Justice System: The Technology of Justice, edited by David Lazer

Is Human Nature Obsolete? Genetics, Bioengineering, and the Future of the Human Condition, edited by Harold W. Baillie and Timothy K. Casey

End-of-Life Decision Making: A Cross-National Study, edited by Robert H. Blank and Janna C. Merrick

Making Medical Decisions for the Profoundly Mentally Disabled, Norman L. Cantor

Ethics of the Body: Post-Conventional Challenges, edited by Margrit Shildrick and Roxanne Mykitiuk

Patient Autonomy and the Ethics of Responsibility, Alfred I. Tauber

Patient Autonomy and the Ethics of Responsibility

Alfred I. Tauber

The MIT Press
Cambridge, Massachusetts
London, England

MIT Press books may be purchased at special quantity discounts for business or sales promotional use. For information, please e-mail special_sales@mitpress.mit.edu or write to Special Sales Department, The MIT Press, 55 Hayward Street, Cambridge, MA 02142.

This book was set in Sabon by SNP Best-set Typesetter Ltd., Hong Kong. Printed and bound in the United States of America.

Library of Congress Cataloging-in-Publication Data

Tauber, Alfred I.
Patient autonomy and the ethics of responsibility / Alfred I. Tauber.
    p.   cm.—(Basic bioethics)
Includes bibliographical references and index.
ISBN 0-262-20160-7 (hc : alk. paper)—ISBN 0-262-70112-X (pb : alk. paper)
1. Patient participation—United States. 2. Physician and patient—Moral and ethical aspects—United States. 3. Medical ethics—United States. 4. Autonomy (Philosophy)
[DNLM: 1. Patient Care—ethics. 2. Patient Rights—ethics. 3. Ethics, Clinical. 4. Patient Participation. 5. Personal Autonomy. 6. Physician-Patient Relations—ethics. W 85 T222p 2005] I. Title II. Series.
R727.42.T38   2005   174.2—dc22   2005047911

Printed on recycled paper.

10 9 8 7 6 5 4 3 2 1

For Ingrid

The best physician is also a philosopher.
—Galen 1884, 1

Contents

Series Foreword   xi

Acknowledgments   xiii

Prologue   1

1 Medicine as Moral Epistemology   27

2 Shifting Foundations of the Doctor-Patient Relationship   57

3 Defining Autonomy   83

4 Balancing Rights and Responsibilities   125

5 In Search of a Moral Glue   157

6 Reforms and Reconciliations   189

Epilogue: On Praxis and an Ethics of the Ordinary   235

Notes   243

References   277

Index   307

Series Foreword

We are pleased to present the seventeenth book in the series Basic Bioethics. The series presents innovative works in bioethics to a broad audience and introduces seminal scholarly manuscripts, state-of-the-art reference works, and textbooks. Such broad areas as the philosophy of medicine, advancing genetics and biotechnology, end-of-life care, health and social policy, and the empirical study of biomedical life are engaged.

Glenn McGee
Arthur Caplan

Basic Bioethics Series Editorial Board
Tod S. Chambers
Susan Dorr Goold
Mark Kuczewski
Herman Saatkamp

Acknowledgments

I cannot enumerate all those who have contributed to my own thinking about this book, but I gratefully acknowledge critical discussions that I have enjoyed with my colleagues and friends: Henry Allison, George Annas, Gary Belkin, Daniel Callahan, Hal Churchill, Richard Cooper, Dan Dahlstrom, Shimon Glick, Michael Grodin, Amanda Green, Mark Hall, Simon Keller, David Khazdan, Dick Lewontin, Jim Marcum, Margaret Paternek, Diana Post, David Roochnik, and, in particular, the Boston University Medical Ethics Reading Group—Peter Keating, Lydia Mayer, Ken Richman, and Edvin Schei; one could not ask for better interrogators. I especially appreciate the encouragement offered by Daniel Dugan and Peter Schwartz, who each assured me that this project was worthwhile, when I was less sure. Without the able research assistance of Wendy Savage, this book would have been much more difficult to write, and to the various editors of The MIT Press staff, I offer a heartfelt sigh of relief, with special thanks to Clay Morgan for his steady support. And, as always, a smile and a salute to my wife, Paula Fredriksen, who patiently listened to my musings, fussing, and vacillations as I drafted, crafted, and rewrote this text.

Modified selections from several publications have been included in this text, and I hereby acknowledge permission from the publishers for their reproduction: "Historical and Philosophical Reflections on Patient Autonomy," *Health Care Analysis: An International Journal of Health Care Philosophy and Policy* 9:299–319, 2001; "The Quest for Holism in Medicine," in D. Callahan, ed., *The Role of Complementary and Alternative Medicine: Accommodating Pluralism*, 172–189 (Washington, DC: Georgetown University Press, 2002); "Putting Ethics into the

Medical Record," *Annals of Internal Medicine* 136:559–563, 2002; "The Ethical Imperative of Holism in Medicine," in M. H. V. Van Regenmortel and D. L. Hull, eds., *Promises and Limits of Reductionism in the Biomedical Sciences*, 261–278 (West Sussex, UK: Wiley, 2002); "Sick Autonomy," *Perspectives in Biology and Medicine* 46:484–495, 2003; and "Medicine and the Call for a Moral Epistemology," *Perspectives in Biology and Medicine*, 48:42–53, 2005.

Prologue

Practically every development in medicine in the post–World War II period distanced the physician and the hospital from the patient and the community, disrupting personal connection and severing the bonds of trust. (Rothman 1991, 127)

Health care in the United States is going through a period of self-examination, and all signs point to a malady. The debate, of course, swirls around defining the ailment. One component, and the one on which this book is focused, concerns the relationship of doctor and patient. And the prescription, at least that offered by the governing boards of medical education, is an infusion of a newly defined professionalism. Medical schools and residency training programs are increasingly aware of public expectations that physicians exhibit humane qualities in dealing with their patients. A major expansion of competencies beyond technical knowledge is now part of training programs to specifically include interpersonal skills and a professionalism that promotes behaviors designed to scrupulously protect human dignity. Indeed, the signs of a growing awareness that the profession must provide more humane care are, literally, everywhere.

In June 2004, I happened to be walking on the UCLA medical campus and wandered alongside a construction site for an expanded pediatrics hospital. There, on the fence separating the construction from the pedestrian walkway, were various "advertisements" about the new facility. One caught my eye in particular:

The UCLA medical staff and faculty are dedicated to building and sustaining an ethical environment supported by values: respect, honesty, integrity, compassion, fairness, innovation, and stewardship of our resources.

I had a mixed response. On the one hand, I was gratified to see this pronouncement, for I was certain that behind that fence resided an honest intention to fulfill this commitment. On the other hand, I recognized these words as a public relations effort to reassure a disgruntled public. The hospital administration justified the expensive expansion precisely on the promise of humane care, not only on the technological prowess of contemporary clinical science and its products. And well might they remind the professional health-care providers of this ethical dimension of care.

The dual demands of achieving technical proficiency and the unrelenting pressures of managing patients leave doctors in training and their mentors with precious little time to carve out another niche for humane medicine. Indeed, physicians are literally torn between the demands of efficiency and personalized care. The balance is difficult to achieve and remains a symptom of a divided agenda driven by very different values. Howard Spiro (1993, 8–9), a gastroenterologist from Yale, is particularly forthright in his characterization: "During medical education, we first teach the students science, and then we teach them detachment. To these barriers of human understanding, they later add the armor of pride and the fortress of a desk between themselves and their patients. . . . Students begin their medical education with a cargo of empathy, but we teach them to see themselves as experts, to fix what is damaged, and to 'rule-out' disease in their field." In short, the casualty of professional training is lost empathy. Unfortunately, Spiro's observation is amply supported by various studies, which have uniformly shown that as the process of professionalization progresses, sensitivity toward patients decreases (e.g., Self et al. 1993).

Despite the best intentions and attempts to counter these professional lessons, with their attendant loss of humane values, the forces restricting the expression of an enhanced empathy are powerful, and seemingly forbidding. Doctors have learned how to cope with the huge demands on their time and energies, and too often they simply cannot address all of the ethical concerns that arise in the care of their patients. Some blame the system, and others simply defend themselves behind the shield of professionalism. Accordingly, medicine is dedicated to treating disease; physicians are trained experts essentially committed to addressing the biomedical problems at hand; as time allows, as others fill in, the more peripheral concerns of care will be "covered." Is this a "straw man" easily blown away? Yes and no. Health-care providers, by and large, harbor abundant moral sensitivity, but to function effectively in the contemporary environment of health care, they must learn how to deal with schedules that are too busy, comply with administrative details that are too taxing, cope with a reward system that suffers glaring inequalities, and function within an economy that has reduced the hospital and clinic to something like a glorified buttons factory. These are pervasive determinants of how medicine is practiced in the United States. Few are satisfied with the present state of affairs. Indeed, the profession has chafed at its lost autonomy and its inability to modify the practice of medicine in accord with its own aspirations: competency and humane care. All too often professional conduct is defined as efficient in terms set by the market, and under the mask of efficiency, humane intentions are compromised. So while efficiency may define a sense of effectiveness, the ten-minute visit robs physicians of the resources from which they draw their empathy, compassion, and patience.

Unfortunately, there are no simple formulas or prescriptions for how to better balance the demands of corporate medicine and the calls for empathy in a medical marketplace that is driven by economic forces conspiring against a more intimate relationship between doctor and patient. For me, the key challenge in clinical practice is how to capture that intimacy and make it work toward better care—that is, effective (as measured by scientific and economic parameters) and humane. More specifically, I seek the basis for strengthening the *moral intimacy* between doctor and patient. I reject an intrusive attitude, one that many might construe as invasive to personal privacy and misdirected to the doctor becoming a "friend" or "confidant." Instead, I seek the means and justification whereby a physician intimately understands and acknowledges the values and goals of the patient's moral universe.

I suggest the most sympathetic to my orientation are those who find that the most interesting fact about contemporary medical ethics is that it exists at all. These "innocents"—of whom I am proud to be counted— still wonder how and why we face the moral predicament of a strained doctor-patient relationship and then ask why, given the strong sentiment to "fix" the problem, it is so hard to do so. What are the tensions and where do they come from? Of course, we have explanations, but at a deeper level a sense of denial—perhaps a naive moral outrage—turns these questions into rhetorical, ironic dismay.

To begin to unravel these perplexing questions and to find a way they might be answered in terms that offer the hope of change, we must recall the history of bioethics and, in particular, the milieu in which complex social forces demanded medicine's reform about thirty years ago. The initial concerns of bioethics (of which medical ethics is a subset) reflected tumultuous reappraisals, all of which seemed to converge on a newfound suspicion of authority and a reawakened sense of classical Hippocratic ethics (Do no harm!). Regarding the first issue, the Vietnam era was marked by the unsettling of confidence in government, education, business, and medicine, and the activism of the period culminated in the ascendancy of a rights-based culture different from any era preceding our own (Sandel 1996). On this interpretation, although presumably committed to traditional democratic ideals, judicial interpretations were radically altered to reflect a changing political environment and social values. This is clearly appreciated when we examine how clinical medicine itself was caught up in the rights-based movements of the 1960s, which borrowed models of autonomy (drawn by the legal and political claims of the period) to ground its own ethics. The second tributary, alarm over dehumanizing patients and making them subject to an intimidating technology, was easily coupled to suspicions of authority. Together, they combined to create bioethics, a potent antidote that defended patients and placed respect for persons front and center in health care.

Medical ethics thus became the articulation of an ancient moral philosophy governing the doctor-patient relationship, beneficence, and a new demand concerning the respect of patient autonomy in the guise of informed consent. In the explicit elaboration of these principles, their interaction and balance, bioethicists found themselves embroiled in debate as to what, indeed, medicine's ethics might be. Dominant voices advocated patient autonomy, not only because it was the most easily extrapolated from our rights-based politicojudicial culture, but because it offered a plain antidote for a pervasive mistrust. Whereas trust had hitherto been the implicit moral understanding governing physician behavior and patient delegation of authority, in the age of Johnson and Nixon, patient confidence required both new definition and novel substitutes. In short, medical ethics generally, and patient autonomy in particular, filled an ethical lacuna left by the erosion of patient trust, and thus patient autonomy became the sacrosanct principle governing medical ethics.[1]

From this perspective, medical ethics is very much of one piece with the deep moral crisis Americans face in the beginning of the twenty-first century. The balance between individualism and communal concerns is no less than the search for the social glue that ties us together in a highly pluralistic culture. On this view, medical ethics provides a lens by which we may peer into the American moral psyche to refract a pervasive problem besetting a culture that increasingly is alarmed at the loss of social cohesion and social capital. In seeking an ethical medicine, we find many points of stress clearly demarcated in the dramatic setting of illness and death, and the prescriptions for both how to understand and how to address our predicament remain elusive.

The underlying rationale of this book is that if a realignment of patient and caregivers is sought, the profession must revise its own standards and better align itself with more traditional and fundamental values of patient care. Most directly, this book is a reflection on the moral crisis faced by all physicians who are caught in a vise of multiple responsibilities that demand different kinds of responses beyond a focus on the ethics of caring for patients. After all, doctors are accountable not only to their patients but to their employers, managed-care plans and insurance companies, and hospitals and professional associations. Overriding each of these domains, the government monitors professional competence, legal and ethical conduct, and adequacy of access (Emanuel and Emanuel 1996). As if these diverse domains of accountability were not enough, there are at least three models in which these relationships are enacted: a professional model, which answers the demands of professional services to provide patient care (e.g., licensure, certification, malpractice, and so on); an economic model, which defines health care as a commodity with certain performance standards and financial expectations and restrictions; and finally a political model, where policy decisions concerning health-care delivery are made and executed (Emanuel and Emanuel 1996). Situated within the matrices of these interacting systems reside the various components of the intimate doctor-patient relationship. This last domain cannot be circumscribed, as might the others, but instead fills in the spaces between them to hold in place (or cohere) the social, economic, and political influences that so powerfully affect the character of health care.

Each of these contending points of view describes, and ultimately redefines, the doctor's professional identity from one characterized by simple (perhaps naive) responsibility for patient care to one that reflects the complexity of our contemporary health-care system. What has been lost as a result of the growing dominance of the corporate structure of health-care delivery? How do, or should, physicians respond to the mixed responsibilities to their employers or payers on the one hand, and to their patients, on the other hand? With this "splitting" of professional focus, something crucial seems to be missing. The debate swirls and critics abound to address the discord—both patient mistrust arising from perceived physician conflicts of interest (e.g., Mechanic 1996; Mechanic and Schlesinger 1996; Kao et al. 1998b; Shortell et al. 1998; Jacobson and Cahill 2000) and physician behaviors that undermine corporate strictures on care (Kao et al. 1998b; Kao et al. 1998a; Freeman et al. 1999; Wynia et al. 2000). (Conversely, physicians not infrequently deny patients possibly useful choices because their medical insurance does not cover such services or medications (Wynia et al. 2003).) But the managed-care setting presents only the most obvious example of the shifting relationships between patients and their caregivers. I maintain that a more general ambiguity has replaced the traditional trust characterizing the patient-doctor dyad, and the sources of this misalignment lie deeply embedded in contemporary society.[2] To understand the quandaries of health care, we must dig deeper into the shifting sands of identity politics and philosophical notions of personhood.

During the past twenty years, commentators from sociology and psychology have highlighted a contemporary fact of American life: mistrust has assumed greater prevalence in all spheres of our social interactions. Indeed, I regard the quest for patient autonomy as a symptom of the more general realignment of relationships, which reflect a less cohesive society and a more self-protective posture of its citizens. Many factors have conspired to alter the communal character of American life, and in medicine, the commercialization of care has had a particularly powerful disruptive effect on traditional trust. With managed care, a contract model has become prominent at the expense of an older covenant. Contracts define obligations and minimize risk. To the extent they are specified and enforced, the concerned parties are protected. The principal difference from the covenant model of care is this substitution of explicit rules for the implicit expectations governed by an ethics of responsibility. Whereas traditionally, patients might expect to have their best interests protected, when health care is just another commodity, services are specifically limited and the older ethic of care is replaced with a market model of goods and services purchased and provided by defined business arrangements. This rich mulch for patient dissatisfaction allowed mistrust to grow, and bioethics was, in part, a response to new demands for physician accountability.

Most would agree that contemporary medical ethics has successfully offered a scaffold for understanding how ethical decisions are made at the bedside and in the clinic. By using various strands of moral reasoning required for thoughtful decision making and legal case-law precedents, a vibrant partnership between philosophy and the law has improved medical practice, which prior to the age of informed consent, allowed doctors to govern the profession without due regard for the full dimensions of patient autonomy. Their failures gave rise not only to a deepened awareness of professional responsibility on the part of doctors, but in addition, to the adoption of a more reflexive stance toward their own professional behavior. This is the arena in which moral philosophy is contributing to medical practice.[3]

Patient Autonomy and the Ethics of Responsibility probes the underlying ethical implications of shifting professional allegiances and thereby continues the discussions initiated in my *Confessions of a Medicine Man* (1999a), which was also concerned with defining the physician's identity. The earlier book, which portrayed the relational ethics between doctor and patient, elaborated an *ethical metaphysics*; here I am engaged in defining a *moral epistemology*. (Note that this is not the characteristic use of the term; moral epistemology typically addresses the epistemic status and relations of moral judgments and principles—for example, justification of statements or beliefs, in epistemology, or validation of judgments or actions, in ethics.) The difference is telling, but both books reach the same philosophical spot, albeit in very different ways. *Confessions* described the implicit responsibility physicians have for their patients by extending a general ethical position to the domain of clinical medicine. Contemporary medical ethics only tangentially appeared, and instead, the discussion situated itself in the tradition of dialogical philosophy. That project might fairly be characterized as an ethical metaphysics because it argued for the primacy of ethics—that is, medicine was fundamentally ethical and its science and technology were in the employ of its moral agenda.

Perhaps because I ventured into such thin airs, I remained dissatisfied with *Confessions* as everyday concerns continually beckoned to me as a practicing physician and educator. Moreover, one might well want a more direct line from medicine's technical and scientific practice to its ethics. Others (Whitbeck 1981; Porn 1984; Seedhouse 1986; Nordenfelt 1995; Richman 2004) have provided such a rationale, effectively arguing that the criteria of health are inseparable from the goals and values of the patient, and thus for medicine to perform its own technical duties, these human ends require an awareness of the patient's moral universe. On this instrumentalist account, the doctor is committed to forging a link between the science and the ethical concerns of care:

Talking to patients about their goals is an absolutely central part of responsible health care. Medical science and biology may discover the means to reach our personal goals, but they tell us little about what those goals are or should be. For this reason, physicians and other HCPs [health care providers] cannot know what will improve the health of any individual considered as a *person* [emphasis added] without substantial information about that individual's goals [and values]. . . . This is not due to ethical worries about patient autonomy, but to metaphysical issues surrounding what it means to be healthy. (Richman 2004, 57)

I have assumed this instrumentalist position, and I too reject the present dominance of autonomy as the premier principle guiding medical ethics. Much of what follows deals with how the preoccupation with patient autonomy arises from outside medicine and why the ethical basis of care must instead grow from medicine's own philosophical roots. To this extent, I nod to my instrumentalist predecessors as forming a kindred group, but I begin from a different place and follow a different philosophical path.

This book seeks to construct a philosophical portrait of the doctor-patient relationship by starting with medicine's epistemology. By showing the value-laden character of the clinician's knowledge, I argue that the ethics naturally follow; indeed, the moral and the epistemological are inseparable. Thus I adopt the designation *moral epistemology*—moral, because clinical evaluation and care are value-laden, and epistemological, because medicine expresses and employs a form of knowledge. The argument begins with a discussion of medicine's epistemology as a product of dual concerns: establishing facts and applying values. The ideal of separating facts and values into different domains is contested and once the dichotomy is appreciated as false and collapses, clinical epistemology is opened to an expanded view of scientific facts, whose ultimate meanings are determined by the biopsychosocial context of the patient. That diffusion of values into the domain of facts is expressed in every facet of care, and in recognizing the impact of values on therapeutic options, the doctor-patient relationship then may be characterized in a more complete fashion. In short, the ethics governing clinical medicine rests on two pillars: the primacy of responsibility (*Confessions*) and the structuring imposed by a moral epistemology.

Balancing Facts and Values

Because of its multifarious activities, conceptual approaches, and moral demands, it seems self-evident that medicine rests on various philosophies. But if one tried to arrive at a singular viewpoint to tie the various elements and approaches together, I submit the answer is not to be found only in medicine's epistemology, its forms of knowledge and manner of understanding, but rather in some synthesis that must include its moral philosophy as well. If we expand the idea of knowledge and form a synthesis between two branches of philosophical discourse—the moral and the epistemological—provocative alternatives appear. Although epistemology and moral philosophy are generally regarded as separate subdisciplines of philosophy, I combine them: any form of knowledge, no matter how objective and divorced from subjective bias, is still imbued with value. And here, value is construed as moral.

Morality is not simply about good and evil, but is more generally concerned with values—that is, how values are used to judge choices and actions. Values presuppose judgment, and in this sense ethics is based on structures of values. Even objective science is ordered by its own values: objectivity, coherence, predictability, comprehensiveness, simplicity, and so on (Putnam 1990, 2002). At least since the 1840s, these values, have given a particular cast to scientific knowledge, a form of positivism, which assumes that objective facts are freed of bias, subjectivity, and value. Positivists would not deny the utility of such values, and consequently the door is left ajar for considering how facts and values may be linked. But they do restrict the kind of value allowed to participate in the scientific endeavor: objectivity divorced from personal value is embraced precisely because such knowledge is regarded as making facts universal. Indeed, it is the universality and impartiality of scientific knowledge that confer its authority.

I would hardly argue against science's successes, and indeed, who could quarrel with the triumphs of such an approach? To be sure, science is governed by its own values, and these have served medicine well. However, these values, while necessary, are insufficient for clinical medicine. For the view from nowhere, the absent perspective, is not only inappropriate for medicine, it is unattainable as well. Indeed, medicine's epistemology is thoroughly embedded in *nonpositivist* values and these competing values reflect a moral structure that ultimately orders and defines clinical science. Clinical science scrutinizes and treats the disease and the doctor treats the person; this difference is what makes medicine more than a natural science, for its practitioners must synthesize the various strands of its faculties in the service of the patient. In short, I maintain that the glue holding together the various epistemological strands of contemporary medicine is of a *personal* moral character, and what we seek is a better understanding of medicine's moral epistemology as it is guided by responsibility, namely, an ethics of care. What this means is the subject of this book.

Two components are intertwined here. The first is the ethical thesis that, simply stated, argues that the practice of medicine employs certain tools—scientific and technological—to fulfill its moral mandate, the care of the person. That entity—the person—defines an ethical response, as opposed to only a strict attention to the *disease*. The second component concerns scientific practice and scrutiny, which highlights the integrative character of clinical science. After all, the organism as an integrated, functioning entity frames all approaches to the patient. Clinical science is, by its very character, holistic in orientation, endeavoring to address all systems at once and to enable the full function of each. This requires a global view of function, from molecule to intact organism. So we witness a synthesis supporting a unified vision of the patient: the orthodox moral calling—the responsibility of care—and the character of clinical science both point to a holistic medicine.

Neither position goes uncontested. The drive toward molecularization has dominated recent biomedicine, and the power of that approach is indisputable. But the trend toward a reductive biochemical and genetic characterization of disease often eschews the problems of complex organization and regulation. As I discuss in later chapters, reductionism requires hybridization with a science that is able to effectively put the components back together into functioning systems. New advances in bioinformatics, modeling of the nervous and immune systems, and ambitious programs to decipher metabolic and genetic organization herald a new science focused on regulation of complex systems. Medicine will be the beneficiary of the expected advances in this new field of "systems biology."

The moral character of medicine is also disputed. Consider these radically different views from respected medical academicians:

I believe medicine is inherently a moral profession. . . . The practice of medicine—caring for the sick—takes what are presumed to be facts about the body and disease and on the basis of that technical knowledge does something for a person. In that sense it can be seen in the same light as any moral behavior—moral because it has to do with the good and welfare of others. (Cassell 1976, 87)

Is medicine a "moral enterprise"? I doubt it, any more than plumbing or auto repair is. Physicians rarely cure or save lives, and spend most of their time trying to provide some comfort, relieve symptoms and perhaps prolong life. The moral issues seldom come up in situations that constitute physicians' practice. The dramatic life and death issues . . . are difficult, but relatively uncommon occurrences of the typical physician. (Lasagna 1977, 44)

For Eric Cassell, even the ordinary acts of medicine are fraught with ethical import; physicians, self-consciously aware or not, are engaged in a profound moral enterprise; and the values governing their behavior are demanding and extraordinary. Louis Lasagna takes a more relaxed approach in seeing physicians as engaged in an ordinary profession. I side with Cassell's view of health-care providers. While it is true some situations are agonizingly complex and others reasonably simply, *all* clinical encounters are value-laden and reflect an array of moral choices.

The implications of assuming this ethical attitude are far-reaching. The most fundamental question asks, How morally reflexive should a physician be? The answer, not surprisingly, is that it depends on the context. Scenarios range widely: vexing end-of-life decisions; clinical rationing of scarce resources; fidelity to patients' self-interest, and so on. Obviously, most encounters are ethically "neutral" or ordinary, while others are demanding, if not excruciating. Much depends on the clinical setting in which care is delivered, the therapeutic options available, the contingencies of personal histories, and so forth, but what strikes me as glaringly obvious is the *depth* of the moral challenge beyond the ordinary identification of ethical issues.

The reified model of disease is aligned with the conversion of patients to consumers, to clients, to covered lives. Each is, in different ways, "objective," but now defined by statistics or a bureaucratic designation instead of by molecules or genes or laboratory data. I believe that in making complex choices from among conflicting data and value judgments, health-care policymakers face challenges similar to those faced by physicians in advocating particular options for the care of individual patients. The dimensions are different and the terms of choice are clearly disparate, but the underlying negotiation of facts and values remains constant, albeit on different coordinates: policymakers factor quality (value) elements into the complex calculus of care, just as physicians do in following clinical strategies. Consequently, health care that forfeits moral self-consciousness, whether regarded from the abstract reaches of public policy or the immediacy of the individual patient, is incomplete.

We *know* this moral fact, but a deep tension remains between our aspirations for an objectivity and efficiency and the demands for humane care. Why are these so difficult to reconcile? Part of the answer is that these goals call on different justifications, which are too often in conflict with one another. To simultaneously observe the patient objectively, *as well as* empathetically, calls on two attitudes that at present are too often regarded as conflicting: one persona peers out, dissociated and removed, while the other looks reflectively within. A physician must do both and become, in effect, a modern Janus.

My vision of an ethical medicine hinges on the free movement of a swinging door that opens easily into two domains: the scientific and the moral. Physicians stand in this portal and with an objective eye place clinical facts within the patient's psychosocial context. The door might close with the practitioners' gaze fixed on the clinical science, and at other times they will be focused on the ethical concerns of the patient, but in the end, a synthesis must occur. Atomistic patients with isolated pathologies, are, in fact, ill persons. Although patients are often reduced to entities, which clinical science defines as disease, malady, disorder, ailment, and pathology, such transfigurations must be "corrected," by putting the findings of a critical science into a larger moral framework.

My organizing question concerns how we are to understand the moral agency of patients in a manner that best protects a humane identity in a factual universe. I pose two contrasting possibilities: the first (presented in more detail below), and the one dominant in contemporary America, is the atomistic model. From that understanding of persons as self-reliant, self-governing, and fundamentally alone, individualistic autonomy arises. In the world of clinical medicine, this conception involves situating persons in a world of neutral fact. Concern with multidimensional identity is moot and even inimical to the positivist approach to disease: as isolated entities, the objective stare is unencumbered by psychosocial complexities, and the physician may proceed with her scientific gaze and technological tools oblivious to the personal context that remains dormant or hidden from such consideration. In short, autonomy as configured in its individualistic stance facilitates the isolation required for positivism to operate freely. As an alternative formulation, a relational understanding of persons permits the doctor and patient to engage on a larger playing field: with such an orientation, disease becomes illness and a cooperative venture replaces the social and psychological dissociations arising from clinical scrutiny. The desired outcome is to shift patients from their dissociated state (induced by organic dysfunction and social designation of sickness) to one in which integrated participation supports trust.

At the heart, then, of what I am calling a moral epistemology is the quest for an elusive synthesis of the "personal" and the "objective"—a search for their common foundation (Tauber 1996, 2001). By showing the interplay of facts and values, we might regard medicine as a crucible in which their enigmatic and elusive synthesis is being forged with particularly intriguing consequences. And perhaps more saliently, the health-care crisis is shown to include a moral quandary that regards the economic and political issues currently dominating public debate from a different perspective, one that shifts those dollar-dominated choices into a different currency (Tauber 2003c). The conclusion: we require a medical philosophy that throws its net wider than to cover the "thin" debates currently dominating the discourse of medical ethics (Evans 2002). Pursuing "thicker" concerns will bring renewed attention to philosophy's contributions and better fulfill the ethicists' original promise.[4]

Sick Autonomy

To the trained eye, every patient presents an ethical problem.
—Frost 1976, 3

The desire for autonomy is a powerful antidote to the threats to personhood that result from being ill, by offsetting the power of those who define identity by defining disease. Physicians achieved power by tapping into two large reservoirs of belief. The first is the primordial human concern with illness and death. The mystifying power of the shaman (and doctor) over life forces evokes an entire universe of primitive fears and hopes. To be subject to forces beyond normal control places the individual in a highly charged, dependent position. Technology powerfully transforms patients into objects of a science with a new authority to define the normal and the pathological (Canguilhem [1966] 1989). The second array of beliefs arise from the application of this biological template to the self-assessment of who we are and what we might do by conferring identity in terms of health and disease. This occurs in both obvious and more obscure ways. Consider how physical fitness is regarded as a source of fulfillment. Ordinary health confers energy levels for work and play; youth and vigor are championed; extraordinary physical abilities are rewarded as heroic from the sandlot to the professional athletic arena. Americans, obese and underexercised, denigrate themselves for their laxity and feel they have fallen short precisely to the extent that they fail to meet cultural health norms. By any standards, health is an ideal that comprehensively defines cultural status. And correspondingly, in western culture the ill, those with disabilities, and the elderly are compromised precisely because of their physical ailments and dysfunctions. Maintaining autonomy allows people to claim control and retain choices in the face of the medicalization of personal identity—in other words, to resist being reduced from persons to patients.

Within this context, protecting patient autonomy has been at the heart of medical ethics in the United States since the late 1960s as a consequence of the dual assaults of an unleashed technology and a mass-market medicine, each of which dehumanizes and manipulates patients. Indeed, according to virtually all students of the discipline, "autonomy" has dominated the debate on the moral foundations of clinical practice and research. Whether presented as the basic ethical principle or one of several, the recurrent questions seem always to be, Where and how does patient autonomy fit into the framework of bioethics? I take this question as central to my own investigation.

To understand the crucial role of autonomy in medical ethics, we must decipher the other roles it might be playing on the stage of biomedicine and within the even vaster drama of Western moral philosophy and culture. After all, clinical medicine is not an isolated enclave but is practiced in our social midst, and the rules of governance apply there as in every other domain of the community. I think it no accident that the moral philosophy that informs and directs American liberal, democratic society, where respect for the individual dominates judicial and political precepts, was so readily transferred to the medical arena. But I maintain that this extrapolation is exactly that, an extension from one domain to another—one, despite its power and importance for our political and social life, that still may not be altogether appropriate.

The cultural preoccupation with individual autonomy is a distinctly post–World War II social phenomenon, and medicine has been caught in a massive social realignment that reflects this increasingly important personal value (Sandel 1996). Contemporary American bioethics developed in that milieu (Jonsen 1998). The early founders of the discipline, Joseph Fletcher (1954) and Paul Ramsey (1970), held the sanctity of life and the dignity of persons paramount and autonomy thereby became a derivative principle, which reflected their basic humanitarianism as theologians. Indeed, autonomy had little philosophical support in their writings, and by not delineating how this principle competed with other moral tenets, these early discussions obscured the complexity of medicine's moral universe.

Indisputably, autonomy serves a vital judicial-legal function in our system of medical law, and this may account for its continued importance, but it is more likely that the pervasiveness of our respect for persons reflects a deeper commitment to Western religious roots (Thomasma 1984; Engelhardt 1996). Our care of the ill is based on a metaphysical response to the other, a reaction that generates *responseibility* (Tauber 1999a), or put differently, "respect for the person" (Ramsey 1970). For theologians as well as nonbelievers, the sanctity of life—essentially a religious principle—remains paramount even as it has been secularized into the political principle of autonomy (Callahan 1969; Jonsen 1998, 337ff.).

Ironically, theologians, poised and ready to engage in a discourse they had already developed for their own purposes, soon found themselves on the outside looking in as the secular philosophers articulated moral principles shorn of their religious trappings. The theological insights (and ideologies) of a rich intellectual and religious heritage (Lammers and Verhey 1987; Verhey and Lammers 1993; Camenisch 1994) did influence the development of contemporary judicial and philosophical medical ethics, but the calculus had shifted: instead of social justice and communal caring serving as the dominant orienting principles, autonomy assumed supremacy. Medical ethics moved from being an ethics dominated by religious and medical traditions to one increasingly shaped by philosophical and legal concepts. The consequence has been a model of public discourse that emphasizes secular themes: universal rights, individual self-direction, procedural justice, and a systematic denial of either a common good or a transcendent individual good (Callahan 1990, 2). Yet despite this secularization, a deep commitment to care underlies recent medical developments, and we could regard clinical medicine's interpersonal ethical commitment as an unquestioned presupposition.[5]

But if we probe a bit, we will see that although autonomy carries the ancient banner of life's sanctity, its secularized meaning and applications have made new allegiances. So when this political and judicial principle is extended to medical ethics, the law accompanies the ill to the clinic and hospital to protect *citizens*. Due to this legal extrapolation, the traditional basis of the doctor-patient relationship must accommodate an orientation different in kind and purpose from the older ethic of caring. I have previously argued that bioethics functions too often as applied jurisprudence, reflecting a parallel legal ethos rather than effectively asserting its own agenda (Tauber 1999a). This is hardly a novel observation; while some see this as a problem, others remain unapologetic.[6]

The "moral space" in which patients reside is not necessarily coincident with that of autonomous *citizens*. While their respective moral identities overlap, they nonetheless are distinct because patients, while carrying their rights as citizens into the clinic, exercise those rights by essentially delegating them. The patient, at least in the autonomy model, receives medical attention only to the extent that his or her rights as an autonomous citizen are respected. This is problematic in as much as autonomy is a product of the milieu of advocacy and conflict, dynamics foreign to medicine (O'Neill 2002, 25). In the medical setting such a construction is at odds with the moral concerns of caring. Let us now delve into this issue.

Balancing Rights and Responsibilities

In facing the growth of patient autonomy, clinical medicine is confronted with a reexamination of its moral foundation, for "autonomy" is an interloper, a new principle that has encroached on the doctor-patient engagement, which is based on trust. At least traditionally, clinical care has been built on trust (the expectation that the patient's best interests would be ministered to) and trustworthiness (the commitment of physicians to achieve those ends). Accordingly, doctors and nurses have a primary ethical obligation to be beneficent (Pellegrino and Thomasma 1988) or, from a different standpoint, to be responsible (Tauber 1999a). And thus the two ethical approaches may clash.[7]

Autonomy is inadequate, by itself, to account for medicine's moral calling because of two failings. First, from the patient's perspective, autonomy is frequently diminished in the clinical setting (Schneider 1998; O'Neill 2002). Patients necessarily relinquish their autonomy to experts, and in this regard, they cannot make truly autonomous, that is, self-reliant, fully informed decisions, and must instead rely on the competence and goodwill of their health-care providers to promote their best interests. Second, autonomy as a construct cannot account for the ethical responsibilities of the caregiver (Pellegrino and Thomasma 1988; Tauber 1999a). The sense of responsibility exhibited by physicians and nurses arises from their sense of care for others, not primarily from a set of rules designed to protect patient autonomy. Respect for the person in this setting is implicit in their professional role, a role characterized by a profound sense of commitment to their charge. This ethic of care regards autonomy as only one of a number of moral principles governing the doctor-patient relationship, and it finds in beneficence a more resonant expression of clinical medicine's fundamental ethos. In short, we require a better balance of patient rights and physician responsibilities.

Intimate trust, the product of a relational ethics, permits patients to exercise their autonomy by relinquishing some decision-making power to those with the expertise to care for them. Physicians then act as entrusted fiduciaries. While I reject a return to paternalism, I do believe that physicians may, and should, assume more active advocacy for their patients' interests by helping them identify not only the clinical choices but also the moral issues they face. While time-consuming and often at odds with current rewards for professional effort, I regard such efforts as the most viable local responses to a medical crisis engendered by a distortion of personhood in the name of science on the one hand, and sociopolitical atomism, on the other.

Several conceptualizations of this relationship have been proposed. Perhaps the best known is Edmund Pellegrino and David Thomasma's notion of "beneficence-in-trust" (1988, 55–58). In their construction, medical care is ethically based primarily on physician beneficence, which seeks to protect patient autonomy and, indeed, advocate for the patient's best interests. Beneficence in their view, and mine, is not in conflict with autonomy (paternalism is, however), but rather is a powerful means of supporting autonomy and preserving the dignity of patients.

I enthusiastically join those promoting beneficence-based ethics, which struggles to reorient professional attitudes, to define those new obligations, and then to offer a way to fulfill them. This endeavor is not an "either-or" choice—autonomy or beneficence. The principles "sit" in a weblike structure, where one principle may pull the others toward its concerns in a particular case, and a different principle achieves dominance in another (Kenneth Richman, personal communication, 2004). No principle stands alone, but each must adjust to the demands of the others (analogous to Quine's holistic "web of beliefs"). Indeed, on this view, patient autonomy can become an integral part of an ethics of responsibility when we better balance its claims against those of beneficence. In short, medical ethics must align facts and values, and rights and responsibilities, on coordinates that have been configured by an ethics of care. Although responsibility and beneficence have lost ground as medicine's guiding principles,[8] I propose how they may be reasserted *in alignment with the claims of patient autonomy.*

Plan of the Book

I begin in chapter 1 with a historical survey of how the values governing science have competed with the values of patient care. When allopathic medicine assumed the mantle of the natural sciences, and thereby achieved a legitimacy that set it apart from all other contenders for health-care dominance, it did so at considerable cost. Pretensions to radical objectivity compromised clinical care by allowing a powerful scientism to obscure medicine's older ethical heritage. Specifically, a science concerned exclusively with facts shrank from the messier realm of values. Notwithstanding the protests of a few stalwart humanistic physicians, the profession marched forward with little concern for the ethics of care and was only brought up short by the birth of medical ethics and a new public fury in the form of malpractice suits in the early 1970s. The

history of the fact-value distinction, which underlies this social development, begins with the origin of positivism in nineteenth-century science
and its philosophical sources in the eighteenth century. Chapter 1 surveys
the conceptual issues underlying medicine's scientific epistemology and
shows how and why medicine continues to be only in part a scientific
enterprise.

Chapter 2 explores how the ethical thread of care is inextricably
woven into medicine's epistemological project with a historical review of
the doctor-patient relationship and the attendant patient rights movement. Underlying this social-legal history are shifting understandings and
assumptions about personhood, which strongly influence patient identity. The discussion then delves more deeply into the historical layers of
the concepts of autonomy, selfhood, and individualism. Most saliently,
this historical overview shows how medicine's own ethics reflect the
underlying philosophical and social tenets of interpersonal relationships,
with their attendant obligations and rights. Analysis of the past offers a
perspective on our own rapidly changing culture and the difficulties we
encounter in an increasingly pluralistic society.

Chapter 3 develops a "topology" of autonomy by considering how
underlying notions of selfhood shape various understandings of autonomy, and how "reason" plays its role in distinguishing autonomous
choices and behaviors from heteronomous ones. From Locke to Kant,
from Hume to Mill, the overview presented here describes how autonomy has been contested and, more saliently, provides the groundwork
for the application of this moral principle to patients. We seek a definition of patient autonomy that is appropriate to the moral universe of the
sick, whose needs and expectations are not necessarily the same as those
of citizens in other settings. In short, we must preserve autonomy and at
the same time find a means for its best expression in a setting that challenges the very notion of self-governance.

This historically oriented discussion frames the question, What role
does autonomy play in the care of the patient? This question is addressed
in chapter 4, where I explore various ways autonomy might be preserved
in the challenging setting of the hospital or clinic. Once I have presented
a philosophical strategy for protecting autonomy, I will be in position to
directly address the problematic status of freedom of choice in the clin-

ical setting. My goal is to contribute a response to the basic challenge American medical ethics faces: how to conceptualize autonomy and trust so that they are mutually supporting.

Chapter 5 considers how physician beneficence and patient autonomy need not compete but rather may converge toward the same ethical ideal, the preservation of the personal dignity of the patient. To accomplish this task, we need to heal a weakened social bond. I argue for what some would say is a quixotic ideal: medicine must reassert its covenant with the patient, albeit in the face of powerful social and economic forces impeding that effort. Arising from the ethics of care, autonomy might recede from its defensive posture if physicians are to reclaim their identification as trustworthy and thus avoid the corruption of relationships so prevalent in our era. Admittedly, the tenor of this essay moves against a social reality that has made too many patients angry and defensive. My arguments may seem hollow to those who have suffered or know others who have been mistreated because of the insensitivity or incompetence of their doctors. I have sprinkled through the text several case studies from my own experience to illustrate both the variety of interpretations autonomy lends itself to and perhaps to remind myself, and my readers, that the physician-advocacy model presented here is not necessarily appropriate and may easily be misapplied. Consequently, my attempt to place more responsibility on the physician, when so much evidence points to the need for patients to remain vigilant with respect to their own interests, requires support beyond slogans and general pronouncements.

The concluding chapter charts a strategy by offering practical ways that trust might be better established between physician and patient. An ethics of trust requires a patient-centered approach that takes into account the complex experience of illness and thus factors in relevant social and psychological issues. Seeking to account for the psychosocial dimension in patient care is not to abandon the power and effectiveness of current reductive strategies of biomedicine, but rather to expand clinical care to more effectively include humane concerns as well. So, while medicine prides itself on its scientific character and technical virtuosity, physicians must always synthesize a reductionist approach to disease with a holistic one that regards the patient not only as an organic entity but also as a person with psychological, social, and historical natures besides the strictly organic. Ultimately, if we seek to balance the moral principles vying for dominance, the care of the patient must be informed and guided by complex values—both those of the ill and those of the physician.

A patient-centered medicine directs clinical attention beyond the scientific and technocratic aspects of treating disease to a more comprehensive psychosocial appreciation of illness. This has become an often-cited slogan for reform, and few would oppose such an ideal, but the obstacles for its implementation are formidable. I believe much resistance may be attributed to the power of a philosophical misunderstanding: the radical separation of facts from values. If facts and values are deliberately integrated and seen as influencing each other, a more comprehensive clinical epistemology beckons. If the values of human suffering are deliberately included in the program of care, a more comprehensive medicine would result. This is the purported aspiration of contemporary medicine, but the resistance is strong. One strategy is to understand how an integrated fact-value epistemology may be adopted as a legitimate basis for medicine, and so we bring the beginning and concluding chapters into juxtaposition.

To achieve this goal, I consider how medical education might be expanded from its narrow scientific focus to a more expansive humanism or, more specifically, propose a program that trains doctors to be morally self-reflexive. Again, this discussion brings us back to the earlier consideration of the fact-value relationship in clinical medicine. To embrace their intimate connection, we have to engage the unity of medicine's science and its ethics. But the debate regarding the place of medical ethics training is still unresolved. Can the teaching of ethics and other humanities subjects revive the compassion that too often is displaced because of the demands of time and because of resistant professional attitudes? Given the subjective nature of this goal, how can success even be measured? Are reformers aiming at the proper target, and which arrows should be chosen? There are no clear answers to these questions, but it seems self-evident that classroom pedagogy is not sufficient to offset the professional ethos that champions the aloof technocrat and the time constraints of a corporate medical system. Moral attitudes are ingrained in professional practice. Despite new directives from various medical education governing boards, the failure to adequately address ethics education or moral issues continues to plague clinical practice despite repeated calls for reform over the past three decades. These issues are reviewed here.

Reflecting my own impatience, I am proposing a new addition to medical record keeping, which, in effect, is a reflection of physician reasoning. An *Ethical Concerns* section of the medical record would provide for a synthesis of personal, social, and ethical matters related to patient care. There, physicians would self-consciously address problems that range from decision making in crisis to the mundane details of support for the ill during the hospital stay and after discharge. In making deliberate efforts to identify such questions, the doctor effectively addresses those concerns often closest to the patient's own experience of illness. More than a scientific and legal document, the medical record might then become a more comprehensive construction of a person's illness, and perhaps more to the ethical point, the physician, in composing this narrative, must critically evaluate her own values and negotiate them with the patient. In this way, a moral dialogue is initiated and sustained.

Overview and Final Comment on Method

I seek an ethical ideal by showing how a renewed commitment to expanded responsibility might be achieved. As philosophy, the analysis of autonomy, responsibility, and trust is shown to illustrate the nodal points of medicine's conceptual framework (e.g., the formulation of selfhood as a foundation for notions of individual autonomy or the understanding of the fact-value distinction and how it plays into medicine's epistemology and ethics). But more than an academic exercise, the reconfiguration of autonomy and responsibility points toward an ethical reform, toward what I call an "ethics of responsibility." In this sense, the idealistic moral portrait of the physician serves as a sketch of what ought to be, not what necessarily is. I am not daunted by protestations that my position is impractical or that its expectations are exaggerated. I reply that the philosophical exercise is to identify the weaknesses of the conceptual apparatus that supports current practice; to argue for reformulations that allow reform; to present a moral compass to find our way in a social system of extraordinary complexity. Defending medicine's deepest moral commitments against the competing demands and power of current economic and political forces requires such a philosophy. To settle for less is to misconstrue what philosophical discourse is about. This last issue is addressed in the epilogue and represents my reiteration of Galen's (1884, 1) admonition: "The best physician is also a philosopher."

This book, at first glance, reflects two general attitudes, one philosophical, the other practical. But the point of my exercise is, in fact, to show how these attitudes are inseparable. In framing the practicalities of the clinical encounter by moral reflections, the reader might feel somewhat pitched and tossed—moving from epistemology, to historical surveys, to ethics, to sociology, to education. I plead guilty. But I remain unrepentant. The issues require no less. With its subject matter refracted from various perspectives, and synthesized by an overarching moral vision, I can only hope this eclectic book, which has drawn on several literatures and employs several modes of analysis, offers the reader a sense of medicine's multilayered philosophy. Indeed, the physician cannot be guided by a single point of view. Instead, she practices at the nexus of many different sociologies and epistemologies and thus confusion will reign without a clear understanding of goals and priorities. To see clearly, we must don our moral spectacles, wipe off the smudges and dust, and peer around with keen sight and heightened awareness. If we fail to do so, already-entrenched developments will become irretrievable: health care will become just another commodity; patients will become consumers; and providers, business entrepreneurs . . . a sorry state for a society that champions the individual.

One last comment on method: while I am very sympathetic to the case made by casuists (Jonsen and Toulmin 1988) and even to a Wittgensteinian abandonment of formal medical ethics (Elliott 1999), the discussion adopted here is one framed by a principle-based discourse (Beauchamp and Childress 2001). I am not altogether pleased with the ground rules so applied for two main reasons: First, in structuring my argument on a tension between "autonomy" and "beneficence," I am in danger of being accused of remaining within the confines of what is often regarded as an oversimplified dichotomy. But I am concerned with beneficence in the service of autonomy, for the true obstacle to autonomy is paternalism (Pellegrino and Thomasma 1988, 57). As we define the various conceptions of selfhood and moral agency, as well as probe the philosophical problem of trust in the doctor-patient dyad, these distinctions will become apparent and crucial in transforming the apparent opposition of autonomy and beneficence into a pattern of mutual support. Second, hidden within the principles approach is a formalism that supports a legalistic construction of medical ethics, and this most readily favors a rights-based philosophy extrapolated from our legal system. But principlism has become the preferred theoretical structure of medical ethics, and while I am not necessarily satisfied with this construction, I have organized my own argument with the aid of this template.⁹ I do so because, if "autonomy" is the focus of debate, then the issue becomes, How is "autonomy" understood?

The strategy employed here is to move the rights-dominated arguments into a different framework, where moral relations between atomistic individuals are configured not as the rights of those in conflict but rather as the responsibilities of persons in mutually supporting relationships. Thus, utilitarian, feminist, communitarian, and virtue ethics figure prominently in this account, which would replace the ethical scenario of parties in competition with one based on a covenant. Such an ethics of care better captures the obligations of physicians to their patients and thereby protects the moral intimacy of the doctor-patient relationship. This is the ethics I, like many others, seek to promote.

1

Medicine as Moral Epistemology

Our whole life is startlingly moral.
—Thoreau [1854] 1971, 218

The historical development of Western medicine as it became a product of the scientific ethos of the mid-nineteenth century is well known. At that time, two philosophies of science—positivism and reductionism—emerged, which decisively shifted the character of medicine toward a new scientific ideal. Neither was a totally novel philosophical strategy; indeed each has a venerable history dating to at least the early modern period. But by the 1850s they were articulated within a new context and were joined to set a new agenda for clinical medicine. By the end of the nineteenth century, medical training had been transformed and the application of a laboratory-based approach to therapeutics had established revolutionary aspirations for medical practice. While there are strong social and political reasons for this shift (Foucault [1963] 1973; Starr 1983), I wish to emphasize the reification of the patient as a consequence of positivism, and highlight the moral consequences of that approach. In doing so, I endeavor to show that a set of values—objectivity, dispassion, neutrality—have governed the clinician's scientific persona, and have displaced another set of values—empathy, moral self-consciousness—that should have an equal claim on the doctor's professional attitudes and character. The profession utilizes a complex "typography" of values, an array of orientations that address the various demands of caring for the ill. This chapter presents the historical and philosophical outlines of these contrasting values and begins the argument for embracing the entire spectrum of moral attitudes they represent.

Before we delve into these issues, allow me to briefly define this spectrum. At one end, the more ancient and primary locus, resides medicine as a caring art. The ministration of aid, the compassionate concern for another, the commitment to *humanitas* encircle a set of values that, for convenience, I will call "empathy." This moral attitude and the skills that accompany it have no special attendant technical expertise, and, indeed, the ethics of care falls into a humane domain that only assumes a professional identity because of another set of skills and values. These represent, in this very simple schema, the other end of the spectrum, which I will designate the "scientific" ethos of medicine. Diagnosis and treatment on the basis of scientific expertise and method have become the essence of contemporary medicine's ideal. Indeed, given the attention to teaching scientific knowledge and logic in the medical school curriculum, medicine's stature rests on its identification with modern science. Consequently, the physician is assumed to possess complementary values: one set aligns her with the subjective call from another; the other set places her in the laboratory, where objectivity rules. By encompassing the values associated with both domains, clinical practice is thought to reflect a mosaic of values. Howard Brody (1992, 262) has dubbed this amalgam of moral and intellectual virtues "empathetic curiosity," a label that aptly describes the modes of professional behavior that limit physician power (the paternalistic danger), promote empathetic care, and facilitate the "constant will of a man trying to recognize."

While the need to achieve empathetic care is widely acknowledged, a major thesis of this book is that the values stretching between the subjective and objective poles of clinical practice are inadequately knitted together. The older ethic of empathy has not been forgotten, but in the tremulous balance between the ethos of science and the ethos of compassion, the former usually trumps the latter as a governing orientation. The scientific ethos of our educational system and the technical demands of the hospital reflect a set of values that place the humane concerns of empathy in a subordinate position. When ethics is addressed, the typical setting is crisis management and the skills allocated are designated as "touchy, feely." This disparagement of medical ethics—either as a curricular item or a component of the clinic—is widely recognized, and increasingly, the profession and the public seek redress, as attested by the growing emphasis placed on medical ethics training and on training in related areas of the behavioral and social sciences (Cuff and Vanselow 2004).

While a consensus seems to be gaining momentum that more attention is required to support the humane character of clinical practice, I maintain that the difficulty in finding a better balance between the values governing medicine rests in large measure on an inability to find a way of synthesizing them. In pursuing this problem, I will first examine the value structure on which medicine's scientific ethos rests, and in doing so, I hope to reveal an objectivity tempered by uncertainty and a positivism tainted by humane values. Balancing the values orienting physician practice requires an acknowledgment that the scientific ideals of objectivity are in fact a conceit and hardly operative in the clinical setting. Once the fulcrum's "set point" is reconfigured, a new balance must be sought, and in the process a rationale for a more humane medicine will emerge. A heady prospect, yet achievable.

Medicine's Disputed Scientific Character

Since the Flexner Report of 1910, medicine has formally embraced a scientific curriculum and a scientific ideal to govern its pursuits (Tauber 1992). And that scientific ideal is positivism, which ultimately purports to describe the world in nonpersonal terms (Simon 1963; Kolakowski 1968). Positivism has several meanings and is notoriously difficult to define, yet certain precepts may be identified, especially as positivism was espoused in its nineteenth-century form. Above all, it championed a new form of objectivity, one that radically removed the personal and emphasized facts and perspectives thought to be universally accessible. On this view, to be "true" and "real," knowledge must be attested to by a community of observers. The trend away from the private sphere of experience toward a communal one had begun at the dawn of modern science, but in the mid-nineteenth century this ideal of truth became clearly enunciated as a scientific principle. Thus positivism sought a collection of rules and evaluative criteria to regulate how we use such terms as *knowledge, science, cognition,* and *information.* And values, at least subjective values, were expunged.

As developed in the 1850s, positivism came to be understood as a philosophical approach that held that the methods of natural science offer the only viable way of thinking about human affairs (Tauber 2001, 105ff.). Accordingly, because of a self-conscious fear of subjective contamination, empirical experience came to serve as the basis of all knowledge. Facts, the products of sensory experience, and, by extrapolation, the data derived from machines and instruments built as extensions of human perception, were first ascertained, then classified. Positivism contrasted with, indeed, was constructed in opposition to the romantic view of the world by denying any cognitive value to subjective judgments. Experience, positivists maintained, contains no such qualities of people or events as "noble," "good," "evil," or "beautiful." In a radical reaction to the romantics, positivists sought to objectify nature, banishing human prejudice from scientific judgment (ironically failing to recognize that "objectivity" was itself a value with its own historical contingencies!).

Undoubtedly, purging subjective prejudice from scientific study was a triumph that yielded an explosive growth in the knowledge of and technical mastery of nature. And by subjecting human affairs to scientific scrutiny, the human sciences (anthropology, sociology, and psychology) optimistically promised to make social policy rational (Smith 1997). Not to gainsay or denigrate those hopes and hard-won achievements, but a mistake was committed by those who hoped to apply positivism's methods to the assessment of *all* knowledge. According to their radical aspirations, valid knowledge might only be attained by the total separation of the observer from the object of observation. This epistemological ideal reinforced the positivist disavowal of value as part of the process of observation. One might interpret, but such evaluative judgments had no scientific (i.e., objective) standing. Simply put, where the romantics privileged human interpretation (exemplified by artistic imagination and emotional involvement), the positivists championed mechanical objectivity (e.g., thermometer, voltmeter, chemical analysis) (Daston 2000).

While the positivist dream seems at least dormant among contemporary philosophers, its influence remains potent beyond this critical circle. For medicine, positivism's influence remains far-reaching. The ideal physician of the twentieth century assumed the positivist stance as his own *professional* posture. The extent to which a deeper humanity governed by empathy and personal attachment influenced doctor-patient relations remained idiosyncratic to the individual practitioner. The distinction is important: professional ideals increasingly became positivist at the expense of an older humanitarianism. In a sense, this newly adopted scientific ethos seemed to require the expulsion of the subjective. One might well wonder why.

Part of the answer lies in denial. Medicine's scientific stature has always been contested. For reasons detailed below, the extreme positivism of the laboratory is extrapolated to the clinic with great difficulty, primarily because of the interpretative, or hermeutical character of clinical medicine. Facts are hardly "naked," and they are clothed in two kinds of garments. The first is what I will call the "epistemological" character of clinical data, which fall on a complex continuum of "normality"—both in terms of how *normal* is defined and also because of individual or idiosyncratic parameters, which in turn require judgment to assess their significance. The "framing" of the normal—that is, as distributive value—is itself a matter of choice that must be determined by varying standards of function and individual context (Boorse 1977; Dowie and Elstein 1988; Murphy 1997).

But a deeper issue can derail the positivist aspirations of clinicians, namely, the social constructive character of illness *and* disease, which I will refer to as the "social" definition of the pathological. In observing that "there is no fact which is normal or pathological *in itself*," George Canguilhem ([1966] 1989, 144; emphasis added) showed the ever-changing nature of the normal and the pathological as constructs. He was concerned not only with the distributive, scientific context in which the pathological was defined, but also the context of personal experience of illness as determined by the social mores of suffering and the very definition of dysfunction.

The experience of the ill is not solely "physiological" in some essentialist sense, but is deeply embedded in a rich cultural and personal context. When Canguilhem ([1966] 1989, 88) asked, "What is a symptom without context or background?", he sharply drew in the reins of a scientist medicine, or some might say, freed physicians from false expectations. Medicine both exists in, and helps create, the categories of disease and illness, which are defined and treated as part of a complex web of *human* values. I will flesh out this claim in detail below, but suffice it to note here that recent scholarship has emphasized how social values play into the understanding of disease, whether viewed from the perspective of psychic influences (e.g., Shorter 1988), in terms of the formulation of gender identity (e.g., Ehrenreich and English 1979; Brook 1999), as determined by cultural standards (Kleinman 1980; Good 1994), or as supported by implicit epistemological (Foucault it [1963] 1973) and metaphysical assumptions (Kirmayer 1988; Fadiman 1997). Each of these literatures highlights an anthropological and philosophical truism: disease is defined within a complex of epistemological, social, and metaphysical claims that differ between cultures (i.e., at the macrolevel), and illness manifests among a given culture's individuals (i.e., microlevel) with variables difficult to predict or quantify with any accuracy. This means that while disease has certain characteristics from the perspective of contemporary positivist data and supporting theories, other systems of understanding may determine a patient's experience of illness and even the effectiveness of therapy (Callahan 2002). Indeed, biomedical approaches themselves vary among Western societies (Payer 1988), and when we consider the controversies within orthodox allopatric practice in the United States, we clearly see that *interpretation* is basic to the clinical arts. Indeed, in some respects we might characterize medicine as a hermeneutical discipline. I will repeatedly return to this point; however, for now, I will focus on the way medicine accepts the mantle of science.

To begin, let us try to break out of an archaic mindset: rather than impose nineteenth-century standards on twenty-first century medicine, we must delineate medicine's claims to being a rational endeavor on its own terms. In so doing, we seek a meeting place where medicine may still incorporate scientific ideals and yet distance itself from an inapplicable positivist ideal. Clinical medicine *is* scientific, but it possesses a character that distinguishes itself from physics or chemistry. As detailed below, the value structure of clinical data is simply different from the controlled setting of the laboratory experiment, and while scientific data is used in evaluation, the gulf between laboratory and bedside requires conceptual bridges created by other concerns and contingencies than those governing a controlled experiment. The key factor is the need to balance choices within the particular context of an *individual* patient. While general scientific laws apply, the individuality of disease and the constraints of the personal setting undermine the application of a positivist ideal that operates only within the universal.

Scientific theories generally fall into two camps. Some are simply descriptive with no judgments as to optimal or suboptimal states. Such theories, which characterize the natural sciences—for example, Newtonian mechanics or general relativity—are value-neutral (i.e., they are neutral relative to human or subjective values). Of course, they are *not* value-free. They are judged and governed by their own hierarchy of values—these theories are objective, universal, parsimonious, "aesthetically elegant," simple, and so on. Other kinds of theories embed different social or personal values in their descriptive structure that are necessarily derived from human experience, and, accordingly account for conditions on a *normative* spectrum of values. Physics is not evaluative in this way, because there is no value judgment as to whether an eclipse of the moon is itself good or bad (at least not in Western secular society). Needless to say, the effects of such phenomena on human life are valued, but the phenomena themselves, at least in their descriptions, are neutral and only elicit a normative judgment relative to how that phenomenon or theory affects human well-being.

Physicians use normative theories of health—heavily normative—and they do so by defining the *normal* and the *pathological* in a human context. Thus, simply of necessity, their descriptions are subject to relative and subjective factors so that standards of *function* reflect normative peremeters. Because function is so overdetermined by human evaluations and judgments about those functions—that is, within the context of social and psychological factors—the criteria of "normal" must remain flexible. And herein lies the rub: some critics (Canguilhem [1966] 1989; Szasz 1961; Boorse 1977; Caplan 1993) dismiss normative theories as failing the criteria of "science," because they maintain that the very incorporation of *values* cuts against objectivity and the capture of reality in neutral terms. But to dismiss normative sciences such as medicine as nonscientific is both unnecessary and misconceived. Support for that claim has been richly developed by others (Murphy 1997; Richman 2004), so rather than rehearse those arguments here, I will show that medicine, as a normative science, must acknowledge that its scientific standards are fundamentally different from those of physics precisely because the clinician embraces *different* kinds of value as a governing element of her pursuits. The issue is not that medicine has values and physics does not. Objectivity in the natural sciences occurs in a context-free universe devoid of *human* values; because medicine is circumscribed by human functions and goals, its objectivity is situated in a normative context. An important distinction is that objectivity may, in some sense, coexist in physics and medicine, but whereas physics embraces neutrality in its assessments, clinical science does not (Proctor 1991). Indeed, as I will discuss in detail, there is no neutrality at the bedside. These distinctions are crucial, not only in distinguishing normative from nonnormative sciences, but in highlighting that the difference between physics and medicine is not in value per se, but rather in that the standards of value employed by each group of theories markedly differ.

The most obvious difference is in perspective. Because physics is governed by a certain kind of neutrality (context-free and nonteleological), it employs universal—that is, nonperspectival—objectivity. The clinician is always oriented by the patient, who provides a unique perspective, and thus she operates with a more ambiguous objectivity, one determined by the needs and goals of the patient, or, in other words, a normative structure. Each clinical case determines the meaning of the facts, and thus meaning is conferred within a *specific* context, not a universal one. Thus the difference between physician and physicist resides not only in the standards that must be met, but more fundamentally, in the context in which those standards are arrived at.

The second difference pertains to the goal-directed quality of medicine. Biomedicine is directed toward restoring, optimizing, or maintaining health, which is itself a value relative to some goal or function (Richman 2004, 13–17). The physicist sees no teleological basis for the phenomena she investigates; the physician's science is employed for a *human goal*. These goals are determined on a case-by-case basis. With this agenda, how can a value-neutral evaluation be achieved? Indeed, what is health? Answers may only be formulated in normative terms and determined for the individual patient. The positivist project breaks apart on these shoals. So, rather than dismissing medicine as nonscientific, I am satisfied to acknowledge that it is not positivist. For my purposes, that is enough. I am not alone.

Increasingly, critics are allowing expanded criteria for the scientific enterprise, and with regard to medicine specifically, richer formulations are beginning to appear as the complex kinds of knowledge composing the clinician's practice become better understood. For instance, Paul Thagard (1999), in formulating disease as a confluence of multiple inter-related factors, draws on deductive, statistical, narrative, and hermen-eutical tools to define the locus of physician activity. This so-called causal-network description utilizes the languages of physics, chemistry, genetics, environmental science, sociology, psychology, and ethics to reflect the myriad factors that play a role in defining illness. Thagard has attempted to formalize these various conceptual tools as a network, and in this regard the older, stiffer as it were, definitions of science are sup-planted by one in which many kinds of languages with their particular grammars are acknowledged as playing operative roles. But the argu-ment lingers and cuts two ways, because no matter how pluralistic the network becomes, science remains at its core: science still adjudicates evi-dence and therefore determines what qualifies as knowledge. So the ques-tion now is, To what extent do positivist criteria continue to influence medicine's agenda and its execution?

As already outlined, if the positivist successfully asserts his definition of science, the normative character of medicine places health care, even in the guise of biomedicine, outside the confines of science. The simple rejoinder: medicine cannot attain the status of a natural science, nor should it. Instead, allow biomedicine to establish its own scientific ethos. That should, and must, suffice. But a dilemma remains: if medicine is not scientific by positivist criteria, what are its standards? What are its claims to rationality and validity? If medicine settles for its own prag-matic achievements, its approximations to some objective ideal, and fluctuating notions of evidence, isn't it deviating from a more "ideal" positivist state?

While many have formulated responses to this challenge (e.g., Boorse 1977; Nordenfelt 1995; Richman 2004), an inner tension remains as physicians are forced to reconcile the demands of a positivist posture with a normative one. Indeed, I would go further: this conflict over medicine's basic character demands a dual allegiance that remains too often out of balance. Ultimately, because of vast historical and social forces, physicians (by and large) remain oriented toward an unattainable and inappropriate positivist ideal, and thereby severely compromise the clinician's own moral agenda. This choice—encouraged by the professionalization process—largely explains why medical ethics plays such a minor role in medical education; why complaints of medicine's dehumanization are rampant; why myriad studies, surveys, and testimonies attest to the lack of physician empathy. Indeed, if medicine aspires to an objective, positivist ideal at the expense of its unique value-laden agenda, the profession will be hounded by complaints that it has forsaken its ancient calling for a Faustian pact.

How this state of affairs arose must be sought in its history, and with that background we will be able to explore how the reification of the patient supports an autonomy-based medical ethics. Our objective is to understand how such an ethics inadvertently subverts a more comprehensive ethics of care, and in that analysis, we seek to better balance medicine's competing values.

Positivism and the Fact-Value Distinction

The positivist perspective stems from Francis Bacon's inductive method of scientific inquiry and was extended by the British empiricists (John Locke, George Berkeley, and David Hume), who claimed objective observation as the métier of scientific pursuits. The positivists' position formally originated with Hume's famous proclamation that one cannot infer an "ought" from an "is." This means that a moral case cannot be deduced from a natural fact. The critique is sometimes referred to as *Hume's law* and is introduced in his *A Treatise of Human Nature* (book III, part 1, section I), where he is attacking the apparent rationality of various ethical or religious positions:

I have always remark'd, that the author proceeds for some time in the ordinary way of reasoning, and establishes the being of God, or makes observations concerning human affairs; when of a sudden I am surpriz'd to find, that instead of the usual copulations of propositions, *is*, and *is not*, I meet with no proposition that is not connected with an *ought*, or an *ought not*. This change is imperceptible; but is, however, of the last consequence. For as this *ought*, or *ought not*, expresses some new relation or affirmation, 'tis necessary that it shou'd be observ'd and explain'd; and at the same time that a reason should be given, for what seems altogether inconceivable, how this new relation can be a deduction from others, which are entirely different from it. But as authors do not commonly use this precaution, I shall presume to recommend it to the readers; and am persuaded, that this small attention wou'd subvert all the vulgar systems of morality, and let us see, that the distinction of vice and virtue is not founded merely on the relations of objects, nor is perceiv'd by reason. (Hume [1739] 1978, 469–470)

Thus the fact-value distinction originated in an argument against the illogical deduction of religious belief from natural facts, and of morality from similar constructions derived from natural law or other supposedly rational systems (Putnam 2002). Hume argued instead that ethics are grounded in human need, emotion, and caprice that are rationalized into moral justifications (Lindley 1986; a more nuanced and unorthodox interpretation has been offered by Spector 2003). The ethical dimensions of Hume's position will again be considered in chapter 3, but the salient point for now is that Hume's philosophy supported scientific aspirations toward objectivity—that is, facts divorced from contaminating personal values. This trend was more fully developed in the nineteenth century by the positivists.

But already at the end of the eighteenth century, Goethe, resisting the allure of a radically objective science, appreciated that "facts" do not reside independent of a theory or hypothesis that must "support" them (a point extensively developed in twentieth-century philosophy of science). Goethe's precept that "everything factual is already theory" (Tauber 1993) was offered as a warning about the epistemological complexity of supposedly objective knowledge. He understood the potential danger of subjective contamination of scientific observation, and more to the point, the tenuous grounds of any objective "fact" that relied in any way on interpretation. "Interpretation" stretches from inference to direct observation, for any perception must ultimately be processed to fit into a larger picture of nature and must cohere with previous experience.

The synthetic project of building a worldview thus begins by placing "facts" within their supporting theory, and continues with integrating that scientific picture within the broader and less obvious intellectual and cultural forces in which science itself is situated. Thus "facts" as independent products of sensory experience are *always* processed—by being interpreted and placed into some overarching hypothesis or theory. In short, observations assume their meanings within a particular context, for facts are not just products of sensation or measurement as the positivists averred, but rather they reside within a conceptual framework, which "locates" the fact in an intelligible picture of the world.

To varying degrees, this constructivist interpretation was denied by the positivists. A world built from their principles would appear essentially the same to all viewers, because "facts" for them have independent standing and universal accessibility, so that irrespective of individual knowers, facts constitute shared knowledge. The romantics placed important caveats on that approach to nature, on epistemological grounds as well as on metaphysical ones. From their perspective, each inviolate observer held a privileged vantage point, and the vision so obtained was jealously protected.

The conflict between the "objectified" world of scientific facts and the private domain of personalized experience of those facts dates from the very origins of science, which aspired to discover facts "out there" divorced from a subjective projection of the mind on nature. Francis Bacon, René Descartes, and John Locke were the key architects of the newly defined science, which in separating mind and body, split the "I" and the "world." In this view, humans are subject to an irreducible duality: the mind, *res cogitans*, surveys the world, *res extensa*. This division, irreparable and absolute, framed epistemology for the last four centuries, and, in the context of a positivist-inclined science, studying natural phenomena demanded a dissociated self: to see "objectively" disallowed projection of the self, a contamination of attaining neutral knowledge. (Again, the ethical implications of this position will be discussed in chapter 3.) But this dualism bequeathed the challenge of rendering whole that which was broken in the division between self and world. The Cartesian reductive method imparts an irresolvable anxiety: after dissecting the world into parts, how are those elements to be reintegrated (Tauber 1996)? Cartesianism itself offers no solution. Further, the epistemological standing of the observer is ambiguous: How indeed does the observer *know*?

The positivist movement was a response to this problem. If facts could be universalized, the "private" mind could be "opened" to public discourse. Objectivity at its most basic calling is the attempt to solve the imbroglio of unifying minds that are not only separated from the world, but also dangerously isolated from each other. So the Cartesian mind-world split resurfaces in the public and private scientific experience of "fact." Specifically, in a community of distinct knowers, Who "knows" facts? How are facts used? What do they mean? Although the discovery—or more precisely, the construction—of a fact is intimately linked to the observer, the dynamics of the fact can hardly be limited to the private domain of the observer's experience. Others have a claim to a fact, which is often shared in the narrow proprietary sense, but *always* as the expected outcome of the scientific process. A scientific fact is fundamentally public, for a hidden fact is useless to the community of investigators; discourse demands scrutiny. Scientific objectivity focuses on the discovery or creation of facts and the public debates surrounding them. Scientific facts acquire the status of public entities as they become objectified, circulated, and finally identified increasingly less with the subjective, private report of the scientist. Critical to the development of modern science was precisely this process by which *shared* experience was universalized among scientific practitioners. Within this domain "objectivity" is attained.

Yet there remains a second, private sphere of the fact, which arises from the scientist's identity as an autonomous epistemological agent. The integrity of the scientist as a private, knowing agent remains an implicit and critical characteristic of scientific activity. To know the world remains a fundamental individual aspiration in the age of the Self (Tauber 1994, 141ff.), and while I emphasize the social aspects of science as a cultural activity, the scientist remains that Cartesian agent who experiences the world independently. Scientific knowledge thus has strong commitments to Cartesian dualism, especially to its concept of a universalized corpus of fact and theory, which arises as the product of individual experience. We are left with a complex dialectic between the observer's "personal" relations to those facts as the product of his autonomous personhood and the need for entering that experience into the public sector.

From the positivist standpoint, this independence of the known "fact" rests on its correspondence to a reality, which any objective observer might know. This assumes both a universal perspective—that "view from nowhere"—*and* a correspondence theory of truth. But the subjective components cannot be entirely eliminated, and as stubborn as the positivists might have been in attempting to stamp out subjective influences, they only succeeded in making them seem disreputable (Daston 2000). There is no escape from the constraints of an observer fixed by his individual perspective, contextualized in some observational setting, and committed to processing information through some interpretative (that is, subjective) schema. Such an observer cannot adhere to a rigid identification of "facts" based on an idealized separation of the knower and the known.[1]

The radical separation of the observing/knowing subject and his object of scrutiny is the single most important characteristic of positivist epistemology (Tauber 2001). Because of this understanding, positivists claimed that science should rest on a foundation of neutral and dispassionate observation. The more careful the design of the experimental conditions, the more precise the characterization of phenomena, the more likely the diminution of subjective contaminants. Thus the strict positivist confined himself to phenomena and their ascertainable relationships through a vigorous mechanical objectivity. In the life sciences, positivism exercised new standards in the study of physiology that applied the objective methodologies of chemistry and physics to organic processes. This approach established physiology as a new discipline and gave birth to biochemistry, whose central tenets held that the fundamental principles of organic and inorganic chemistries were identical, differing only inasmuch as the molecular constituents of living organisms were governed by complex constraints of metabolism. This led to a new declaration for the application of a reductionist strategy to biology and medicine, and, indeed, in positivism's philosophical basin, reductionism was baptized.

Positivism's methodology was intimately linked to the assumption that all of nature was of one piece, and the study of life was, in principle, no different in kind than the study of chemical reactions, the movement of heavenly bodies, or the evolution of mountains. Thus, if all of nature was unified—constituted of the same elements and governed by the same fundamental laws—then the organic world was simply on a continuum with the inorganic. According to this set of beliefs, there was no essential difference between animate and inanimate physics and chemistry, and the organic world was therefore subject to the same kinds of study so successfully applied in physics. On this view, medicine studied the body essentially as a machine, which was governed by uniform chemistry, and thus susceptible to mechanical repair. The new problem was both to reduce the organic to the inorganic—that is, to exhibit the continuity of substance and operation—and concomitantly to understand the distinct character of life processes. To accomplish this twofold agenda, reductionism was coupled with positivism.

The reductionists were initially a group of German physiologists, led by Hermann Helmholtz, who in the 1840s openly declared their manifesto of scientific inquiry (Galaty 1974). They did not argue that certain organic phenomena were not unique, only that all causes must have certain elements in common. They connected biology and physics by equating the ultimate basis of the respective explanations. Reductionism, specifically physical reductionism as opposed to the later development of genetic reductionism, was also a reaction to romanticism's lingering attachment to vitalism, that notion that life possessed a special "life force." The appeal of vitalism was not totally extinguished by mid-century, but certainly a new scientific ethos had taken over the life sciences by 1890. And medicine was radically changed as a result of these developments.

The impact of reductionism was to offer a complementary method to enact the positivists' philosophical program. This dual attitude had a profound influence on the doctor-patient relationship, and even more importantly gave new meaning to illness and the body. The holistic construct of man and the medicine that served him were replaced by a fragmenting clinical science that, in its powerful ability to dissect the body into its molecular components, remained unconcerned with addressing what had traditionally organized the clinical perspective.[2] Further, the normative character of medicine's science was left unacknowledged as the positivist tide gained its full momentum. In the wake of this movement, the concerns of humane clinical care, while still important, were subordinated to a new conceit that would assert medicine's scientific credentials—specifically, the logic governing the natural sciences was to be applied to the clinical setting. Largely disinterested in the contextual concerns governing evaluation and treatment, clinical science powerfully asserted its own agenda.

Positivism's triumph also posted loses. Misunderstanding how clinical science must be mediated by a complex array of values, the proponents of the positivist ethos reframed medicine's ideals. In this brave new world, moral self-reflection rested solely with the individual physician, who drew from a personal reservoir of humane concern. Without explicit guidelines and professional encouragement, the "art of medicine" was left to individual development. The consequences were far-reaching and haunt us today. But (as discussed in chapter 6), a new self-consciousness about the doctor-patient relationship is taking hold as medical students and residents are at long last explicitly taught interviewing skills and the outlines of medical ethics as part of a general consensus that training in the clinical sciences alone is woefully insufficient for the challenges of patient care. In the next section, I explore the underlying epistemological rationale for this shift and summarize its philosophical underpinnings.

The Limits of the Positivist and Reductionist Agenda

The holist rejoinder to reductionist medicine is both epistemolgical and moral. I will consider this moral dimension later. Now I address a recurrent question plaguing a reductionist, positivistic clinical medicine: To what extent can medical objectification (patient reification) be mitigated by counterbalancing factors? To answer this query, we must examine the epistemological counterpoint to reductionism: holism. The logic for understanding the relationship of biomedical reductionism and its complementary orientation takes this form:

1. In any clinical encounter, the experience of the suffering patient and his or her reification as a medical object requires a negotiation between the two points of view.

2. While the successful application of rational, scientific knowledge is expected, this application can only be framed by the particular context of care.

3. This so-called context of care is fundamentally moral in character inasmuch as it is framed by the particular values and needs of the patient.

4. Based on those values, science has been developed to address disease, but the care of illness, the care of the suffering patient, requires more.

5. *Ergo*, effective medicine is humane medicine, and the reductive practice must be regarded, always, as only part of the therapeutic encounter. Note that there is no argument *against* reductionism per se, but there is a complaint lodged against radical positivism, where the patient is regarded as the disease—for example, "The cancer in bed 3," or "the pneumonia in room 506."

Ultimately, the argument between reductionism and holism is hollow. From the epistemological perspective, the organism as an integrated, functioning entity frames all approaches to the patient. Medicine is, by its very character, holistic in orientation, endeavoring to address all systems at once and to effect the full function of each. This requires a global view of function, from molecule to intact organism, which in turn refers to the person in all of his or her dimensions. Disease is an objective account of pathology, but this characterization is only one component of illness, and all those other elements of dysfunction that might arise from disease also require attention. In this sense, the patient cannot be simply regarded as an entity, an organic construct, but also must be seen as a person suffering an illness. If one regards medicine as dealing finally with this larger conception of the patient, then reductionism is a tool, albeit a powerful one when applied to certain questions, but only an instrument in the employ of larger agenda. The demands of clinical medicine simply disallow satisfaction with the positivist stance, either in practice or as an aspiration. To accede to the resulting fragmentation of reductionism is to surrender medicine's ultimate concern, the global care of the patient.

This attitude is best expressed by the biopsychosocial approach to illness, which presupposes that not all ailments are susceptible, in principle, to a biomedical approach. Such psychological and existential crises in life that may lead to illness may be symptomatically alleviated by drug or cognitive therapies, but the personal and social contingencies that have so much to do with the health of persons are, strictly speaking, outside the purview of scientific medicine. Such problems have, to be sure, their own professional specialties committed to understanding and relieving them—for example, psychology and social medicine—but scientific medicine has not traditionally considered itself concerned with such matters. However, the boundaries separating what is amenable to scientific inquiry and therapy, and what is not, remain hotly contested.

So the question remains, how is a balance struck between the holistic—often translated as a humanistic concern for the patient—and the reductionist perspective, which draws on immense resources of technical prowess, and which, because of these successes, has imperialistic designs on what hitherto has been the domain of the social and psychological disciplines? For instance, the "biological imperative" of genetics (readily supported by recent advances in genetic technology and molecular biology) is increasingly regarded as the blueprint of identities by designating to some unknown, but suspected large extent, the physical, cognitive, and emotional characteristics of complex human behavior. This primary level of biological organization is thought then to serve as the foundation for social identities that are made by adding the contingencies of family, social strata, religion, and all the other factors that play in forming character. The growing conviction that genetics lies at the root of complex human behavior belies a more narrow definition of medicine's future, while those more skeptical of genetic determinism argue that these problems, in principle, are not subjects for a reductionist approach (Tauber and Sarkar 1993).

The nature-nurture debate is seemingly never ending, but one conclusion is inescapable: biology is bedrock to our personhood, and while it may be altered or controlled, in the end, biological constitution confers a large, and sometimes overwhelming definition of who we are and what we might do. Genetic determinism powerfully sustains the belief that humans—both their bodily functions and their social behaviors—are ultimately reducible to biochemistry, biophysics, and genes.[3] This is the so-called naturalized view of humans, and the power of its vision has transformed the way we think of ourselves, and to balance this view with an older humanism is a challenge as yet not met.[4] Indeed, the repercussions of this movement away from a holistic approach to one that celebrates the reductive scrutiny leaves medicine with a deep contradiction. Initially designed to address the patient's illness as experienced in an array of meanings directly accessible to the sufferer, disease of a system or organ has become the focus of concern, and contemporary medicine has thereby made a Faustian pact with nonnormative science. Amending and often foregoing integrated care—one that addresses the psychological and spiritual dimensions of illness as well as the pathophysiological—medicine is now accused of losing its deepest commitment to the patient, as a *person*. On this view, the doctor-patient encounter is by its very nature a negotiated attempt to coordinate, if not combine, different frames of reference. Simply put, scientific biomedicine, for all of its authority and promise, still must treat persons, and persons are only in part defined by their biology. A more expansive medicine is required. And here we come to biomedicine's own epistemological crisis.

For all of its power, reductionism has been less successful at building complex systems from its elements than in dissecting physiological processes to their fundamental parts. Philosophers of science are now grappling with redefining the limits of this approach and appreciating that the "unity of science" on which it is built may not yield to our methodologies. If the natural world is seamless, then presumably our scientific approach to its study should also be unified—both epistemologically and metaphysically. But there is growing evidence that the various scientific approaches applied by the different species of scientific inquiry are not easily linked to each other to offer a coherent and seamlessly unified "picture" of the world (Galison and Stump 1996; Cartwright 1999; Schaffner 2002). Glaring rhetorical and cognitive gaps have been highlighted by philosophers, historians, and sociologists of science, who have claimed that the pluralism of methodologies and the diverse kinds of questions posed by different kinds of study point to the inevitability of disunity, which beyond fragmentary knowledge reflects the relative isolation of highly specialized sciences pursuing their own highly specific agendas with their own highly evolved (and therefore peculiar) methodologies. While science continues to pursue a comprehensive and coherent worldview, these critics argue that it is not at all certain that the various strands of scientific pursuit will be unified in any fundamental sense. So in defining the basic elements, from this critical perspective, it remains highly problematic whether parts will effectively be put back together as integrated wholes. Instead, these critics argue that scientific knowledge is assuming a more local character, which in the biological sciences means that one level of explanation may not be easily mounted to understand the next higher one.

Whether these predictions prove correct or not, the disparities currently point to an interesting myopia: we function as if the unified picture exists and thereby rationalize and ratify the metaphysical assumptions leading from the positivist/reductionist program. A more circumspect view may be required—one more critical and less sanguine with the complacency of our success.

Historians might be shocked to hear of those proclaiming the end of science and the dream of final theories. Such optimism has marked many previous ages whose leaders audaciously proclaimed the triumph of their worldview, only to have it, as all the others, evolve into another paradigm a few generations later. While the debate concerning the eventual success or failure of the current reductive program continues, almost all concur that regardless of present strategies and their accompanying aspirations, more comprehensive modes of organizing and resynthesizing complex systems is required to understand complicated physiological function. And from the point of view of this book, positivism's hold on medicine's ideals similarly requires reassessment as other, more comprehensive moral concerns beckon for the care of patients.[5]

Recasting Contemporary Medicine: Seeking a Typology of Facts and Values

In a trivial sense, values direct knowing. For instance, we constantly choose to pay attention to certain elements of our experienced world and ignore the vast majority. Values determine what we study and indeed, as Hilary Putnam (1990) has cogently argued, even the positivist standards or aspirations of science are values, historically arrived at and chosen in everyday practice.[6] In medicine, this view is overwhelmingly self-evident and hardly needs recitation: from the socially based policy decisions of health-care administrators to the attention paid to the individual patient, the care delivered is allocated by a distillation of value choices. Medicine is embedded in a value system, and patients are subject to complex choices, whether declared or not. The ill demand, and expect, that their physician will negotiate the maze of options for them, be their advocate, and protect their interests. For instance, whether an oncologist administers an aggressive chemotherapy to an elderly patient depends on many factors beyond the stage of his cancer, and must include such factors as expected quality of life, support structures, other confounding medical problems, and so on. These are alternatives that must be negotiated with the patient and family. Simply put, medicine is hardly objective in its applications, or in its practices, and doctors must engage the social world of the sufferer, as much as the biophysical and genetic domains of the body. The boundaries are not firmly demarcated. The positivist attitude simply will not suffice in the care of the patient. But more, it is an encumbrance.

The existential state of being a patient forcefully presents the domain of the moral. The loss of autonomy, the fear of the unknown, the dissolution of identity accompanying pain in its multifarious forms, the dehumanization of being subjected to the administrative processes of health care, and the psychological dependence resulting from each of these challenges combine to make patients emotionally dependent on health-care providers. In this setting, individual concerns are paramount, and the most immediate response should be humane. But physicians are trained to be medical scientists, and testaments to the conflict inherent in that orientation are legion. The issue is succinctly stated in a book review about the care of schizophrenics:

Despite their reputation for vanity, many mental health professionals, and medical students in particular, fail to recognize their own importance. They "come and go among patients as if their knowledge and skills were all that counted, their persons not at all." The remark is pertinent, for it points to the underlying vision that

drives the profession. The medical students are not looking for personal engagement with the patient. They don't really want their "person" to make a difference.
That is not the "importance" they are after. Rather they want to learn (why not?)
to heal the patient with a precise and controlled intervention, the exact dosage of
the exact drug chosen after an exact diagnosis based on meticulous and exact
analysis of spinal fluids and brain scans. They are in thrall, that is, to the great
and credible dream of Western medicine. (Parks 2000, 15).

This attitude is well established in the biomedical world, and, to be
fair, the "technocrats" do offer "real" solutions to "real" problems. This
is hardly to be disparaged. But at the same time, the reification of the
patient (the success of the positivist agenda coupled with the time constraints imposed by the economics of health care) competes with the call
for empathy. In later chapters, I will explore the cognitive and moral
reasons for including empathy as a crucial component of clinical care;
here, I only note that a prevalent rationale for relegating these moral and
emotional dimensions of care to a peripheral role is the vacuous claim
that addressing the subjective dimension of the patient putatively dis-
tracts from the true agenda of the clinician, namely, her application of
technical virtuosity and scientific competence. On this view, the science
and technology of diagnostics and therapeutics are the "hard" currencies of the doctor, and the "soft money" used to develop interpersonal
relations and the accompanying humane attentions simply do not purchase what is truly important. Once the ledgers of time and resources
are added up, and one has to choose, the decision seems self-evident:
competency and efficiency trump other softer claims on the physician.
Patients may not agree, and evidence suggests that investment in "soft"
currencies is a more important strategy than previously realized.[7]

But simply on *epistemological* grounds, why must we choose to elevate
one set of priorities over another? The dichotomy between "technocrats"
and "humanists" arises from the sociology of medicine (the way clinical
care is organized, the reward system that promotes certain behaviors
over others, the allocation of resources, and so on), not from medicine's
epistemology, or its morality. There is no compelling *conceptual* reason
why the two orientations must be at odds. Given the moral calling of
medicine, we seek a way to shift from setting hierarchical priorities for
"ethics" and "science" and substitute instead better balance, or even
parity. After all, a medicine that fails to address the elements of person-

hood that have no scientific basis—the social, the emotional, the moral—is ultimately fractional and therefore incomplete. Clinical care demands full attention to both domains—scientific and moral. We are well past the point when medicine could offer little else than consolation. A more global responsibility, which includes empathy, can and should complement a powerful science, and thereby humanize it.

A crucial step in this direction is to recognize the difference between *disease* and *illness*, and reorient care from disease-centered to illness-centered or person-centered medicine (again, a topic explored extensively in chapter 6). Disease is a synthesis and condensation of signs and symptoms, test findings, and a web of sorting categories. Indeed, in the United States, every disease has an international bar code, and if a patient does not have such a code, the doctor does not get paid! Illness, on the other hand, is the experience of disease and thus is a composite of all those elements that conspire to incapacitate a person (Cassell 1976, 1991, 1997; Kleinman 1988). Disease in its biological formulation is optimally based on objective—that is, public—fact. But what, indeed, is the status of objective facts in this setting? First, and foremost, all clinical facts are contextualized at several levels. From the strictly biological perspective, and this, as we will see is already a false depiction, organic dysfunction is witnessed within an array of other integrated elements. No fact resides alone. One of the first lessons medical students must learn is that a laboratory finding or anatomic description is only the beginning of building an integrated clinical picture. What does it mean that a serum sodium level is low? To understand that "fact" is to understand the entire physiology of renal and endocrine regulation of electrolytes; the hormones effecting secretion or retention; the anatomic structures—kidney, intestines, lungs, skin—which are the targets of metabolism—absorption and excretion. And these particulars may only be appropriately understood within the function of the whole organism, in this case, the patient.

For instance, sickle cell anemia has a precise pathophysiological description at the molecular level and the symptom, lethargy, does not. The nature of the fact describing each condition is thus quite different. One might say that sickle cell disease is factual and lethargy is not, because symptoms are subjective, unobservable, and thus unverifiable. But the meaning of the so-called fact of sickle cell disease's etiology and the subjectivity of lethargy is not so easily divided between a factual account and a valued one. Consider how a keenly defined molecular lesion for sickle cell disease is insufficient for understanding the protean manifestations of the illness. Some patients are virtually asymptomatic while others have debilitating pain crises, organ damage, hemolytic anemia, and other comorbid states that lead to a shortened life span. Each sickle cell patient is afflicted with the same "fact"—an abnormal hemoglobin precisely defined. But the molecular abnormality goes only partway in describing an illness that requires individually specified assessment and care due to either compensatory mechanisms or comorbid conditions that complicate the clinical manifestations of the disease. This general observation has important implications for understanding the contextual character of any scientific fact, and how in medical science in particular, each so-called fact exists in a particular context that confers meaning. Perhaps the most striking irony in treating sickle cell patients is the physician's reliance on patients' reports of pain as a principal criterion of pain crisis therapy. To be sure, laboratory data are available (for instance, rate of hemolysis or signs of ischemia), but in the end, the patients' reports of their own suffering guide medical interventions.

Therapeutic recommendations require an integration of diverse modes of interpretation. The cardinal decision in any clinical encounter is to select what should be done diagnostically or therapeutically from among a universe of choices (Pellegrino and Thomasma 1981). In other words, what may be done is narrowed to what should be done, and that winnowing is determined by an array of value-based decisions. For instance, whether to intubate a patient with respiratory failure at the end stage of lung cancer is a judgment governed by values: What is the life expectancy of the patient if the treatment is successful? What are the chances of success? Indeed, what is "success"? What resources must be allocated at the expense of another patient? What is the quality of life to begin with? What are the patient's wishes? Such decisions, usually not as dramatic or as easily formulated, arise in virtually all clinical situations. And beyond this contextualization, the physician must place "disease" within an ever-changing nosography, a system of medical theory and classification that accounts for these facts. Considering the incompleteness of our scientific theory, the social construction of much of it, and the intimate relation of psychological and social factors in defining disease, commentators are increasingly appreciating that the model of clinical medicine based on impersonal "facts" is not only incomplete, it is distorting.

Facts are not simple, inasmuch as relatively little in medical decision making is prescribed by some formula or directed by an algorithm. The literature dealing with this general issue is immense, and here I wish only to sketch in the domain of the logic that guides medical heuristics—the so-called "silent adjudicators of clinical practice" (McDonald 1996). If we simply look at this decision-making process as an epistemological exercise, the intermingling of facts and values is obvious: robust scientific conclusions are too sparse to fully inform clinical decisions for the simple reason that few patients fall exactly into the same criteria of study groups. Physicians routinely must extrapolate from small studies to the general population in which they must situate their particular patient (McDonald 1996). For instance, we treat moderately hypertensive women as we treat men, but the study on which we base this treatment was conducted by the Veterans Administration and no women were included! (Veterans Administration Cooperative Study Group, 1970). Given the increasing concern about gender differences in the natural history of the same disease, this compromise is seen for what it is, a necessary extrapolation for the lack of good data for women. Another example: the evidence that certain antihypertensive medications are life saving has been extrapolated to every new antihypertensive drug regardless of chemical class. Indeed, most practitioners have replaced the older, well-proven agents with newer drugs on the basis of this extrapolation, namely, that because these agents are known to lower blood pressure they must save lives. However, at least in one case, this value-based decision has been proven false (for calcium channel blockers; Psaty et al. 1996). Such extrapolations are unavoidable, and they highlight how medical facts must attain their meaning in a normative context.

While physicians must decide how to interpret a test or treat a patient from a limited set of choices, no test or intervention falls into a clearly defined positive or negative domain (Murphy 1997; Weinstein and Fineberg 1980). Every test result has false positives and false negatives as compared to some gold standard, which in itself may not be absolute. And every drug has toxicities and failure rates that not only vary within subgroups of patients, but more to the point, are unpredictable beyond a frequency figure as determined for a large population. This means that when applied to any given patient, a test result or a therapeutic outcome may only be described as an odds ratio. And when the confounding uncertainty of diagnosis is factored into this complex calculus of therapeutic choices, the degrees of uncertainty seem formidable to the uninitiated. More often than not, the probabilities are inferred, not known, and even when clearly defined, probabilities change the ground rules of what constitutes an objective decision.[8] The choice is made with only certain degrees of certainty, and these depend on variables more often than not untested, and if they have been accounted for, these characteristics may not be applicable because of other confounding factors, whether biological or social. The variation problem is simply beyond the horizon of most factual information in clinical science or the knowledge base of even the most earnest physician. As a result, clinical data are valued, weighed, and sorted, and when formal methods are used to delineate this process, a glaring *fact* appears: likelihood ratios are usually inferred; intuitions are only roughly based on quantitative studies; choices are heavily influenced by the frame of the choices presented. In short, the science of clinical decision making has revealed the normative character of most practice decisions, and thus an unacknowledged intimacy of facts and values marks the doctor's logic.

Yet good clinicians function easily in this climate of uncertainty, because they have internalized methods for dealing with partial data and extrapolations from dissimilar clinical scenarios. They are increasingly aware that the best treatment strategies are largely intuited from experience and involve hidden judgments that are biased in ways usually unrecognized, and as noted, are extrapolated with the aid of measures hardly supported by rigorous analysis. Nevertheless, decisions must be made, and a clinical science that can address issues surrounding the proper development and application of clinical data has been actively pursued. As an extension of the formalized statistical methods introduced in the 1960s (Feinstein 1967), formal decision-analysis programs were inaugurated in the 1970s, in the hope of developing a more rigorous assessment of clinical decision making (Weinstein and Fineberg 1980). (These programs depend on Bayesian inference, a statistical method that includes all previous data to assess likely future outcomes.) Instead of relying on blind intuition, analysts calculate value as a likelihood ratio. But such efforts, despite their obvious utility for measuring cost-benefit ratios in certain well-studied cases, have also pointed to how clinical choices are irreducibly value-laden. Obtaining clinical data is only the beginning of the decision tree of options, exercised or forsaken.

The Imperative of Need

Much has been written on the fact-value distinction in medicine, whether considered as basic to an understanding of causality and explanation in clinical practice or as defining the scientific foundation of medical knowledge (e.g., Engelhardt and Callahan 1980; Delkeskamp-Haycs and Cutter 1993). I have surveyed the status of facts in some detail, but I have proceeded without a definition of value.[9] Consistent with the normative character of clinical medicine, I seek a definition of value in the context of need, which might also be expressed as the *telos* of care determined by the aggregate needs of a patient as expressed in both the biogenic and sociogenic dimensions (Kurtz 1958). So, whether understood as "biogenic" or "sociogenic" in origin, needs are oriented by goals, which in themselves are determined by values. And here I follow the lead of Ruth Ann Putnam (1985), who has argued persuasively how values arise from the context of need. On this view, medical facts are aligned by values and their meaning determined by a system of value-laden options arising from the perceived needs of a particular patient. Given this orientation, perhaps the most direct way of approaching value in the clinical setting is to dissect the concept of need.

Need is both factual (in its various guises) and a value judgment. Or to put it another way, need must be distinguished from want (Hayry 1991). The needs view is framed by scientific or objective standards, while "want" refers to subjective desire. Each has its legitimacy, but from the patient's perspective, wants frame the illness, while a physician is more likely to be cognizant of the needs determined by the disease, a biomedical designation. Thus quality of life (the patient's perspective) may or may not be indexed to need (the physician's professional-scientific perspective), since the criteria governing each domain are different.

In any case, physicians must be aware of potential conflict and ultimately be prepared to seek the resolution of these conflicts if necessary. Beyond this direct ethical demand, we can see how such differing vantage points pose epistemological challenges. For example, Mr. Kramer reports fatigue. Is he depressed, or does he have an underlying disorder that is yet to be defined? The physician assesses the patient's psychological state and remains uncertain. Is the patient lethargic because he lost his job, or did he lose his job because he was physically disabled due to an undiagnosed tumor? Does Mr. Kramer require a thorough evaluation or should further tests be postponed? Or consider the statement, "Mrs. Smith needs antibiotics." Mrs. Smith is recovering from chemotherapy and has a fever. Even if it is uncertain whether she has a bacterial infection, it is perhaps best to treat her proactively and prescribe antibiotics. On the other hand, she more likely has a viral infection, so that the drugs will not be effective and may cause her diarrhea, or worse, a superinfection. She lives alone and has early dementia. What is the best course of action? No single fact is involved, but rather a complex interplay between facts (in this case fever, recent chemotherapy, immune compromise) and values (likelihood of bacterial infection, ability to care for herself, and so on). These examples highlight how need—the category that determines the *techne* of medicine, the ability to do clinical practice—inextricably combines facts and values in a normative domain. The facts assume their respective significance when placed within the context of a person's wants (framed by the social and psychological dimensions). And this raises the moral specter that hovers over the fact-value distinction in medicine.

Conclusion

The aspiration to rigidly distinguish facts from values collapses when faced with the "*ur*-fact," the person, and so the fact-value distinction has a particularly pernicious quality when applied to the ill. Crucial as laboratory data are to the clinician's art, the most important "fact" in medicine is the irreducibility of the patient's *personhood*. In the end, it is this category of moral agency that defines the doctor-patient relationship, determines the physician's epistemology, and frames the ethics of care.

How one functions and what determines one's relationships, choices, and obligations is inseparable from understanding the character of the knowledge framed by personal values. Judgment is not arbitrary or frivolously contingent, but takes its own bearings from the interplay of social and natural realities understood in the context of adaptation and creative growth. The synthetic project of building a worldview begins by placing "facts" within their supporting theory, and continues with integrating that scientific picture with the broader and less obvious intellectual and cultural forces in which science itself is situated. As noted earlier, "facts" as independent products of sensory experience are *always* processed or interpreted. In short, observations assume their meanings within a particular context, for facts are not just products of sensation or measurement as the positivists argued; instead they reside within a conceptual framework, which "places" the fact into an intelligible picture of the world. Inextricable from context, facts must assume their meaning from a universe of other valued facts. In a sense, value is the glue that holds our world together. Thus knowledge is inexorably valued; divorced from the reality of personal choice, it is useless and irrelevant.

Given the general awareness of this point of view, why raise the matter again? On one level, the discussion in medicine is part of the larger issue of how to understand objectivity in scientific discourse. Because medicine so clearly illustrates the intractable, value-laden character of a scientific fact, the clinical scenario becomes important as a case example of science in action. This is not merely an academic exercise, for the use of scientific facts remains a matter of debate as the public continues to scrutinize scientific practice and its application to policy (Tauber 1997, 1999b). Within the confines of medicine's own agenda, the relationships of facts and values raise different kinds of questions. While most discussion has focused on the epistemological status of facts and values, and I have reviewed those issues here, I believe that how we understand this relationship actually reflects a deeper concern about medicine's ethics, both at the bedside and within the community at large.

These issues have also found their way into the public domain. Algorithms and managed-care surveillance (based on "objective facts" of care) are often circumvented by the needs of individual patients (Kao et al. 1998a, 1998b; Freeman et al. 1999; Wynia et al. 2000). Not only have policies derived from research on large patient populations met with resistance at the level of the individual patient, but the tendency to apply such universal directives has encountered serious obstacles, both because the science is imperfect (for lack of data and appropriate assessment tools), and especially because the ethics of care focused on the individual often conflicts with communal interests (see chapter 5). To understand the moral difficulties entailed in assuming an advocacy position for one's patient and at the same time recognizing communal interests, the profession requires a moral compass to orient its practitioners in the bewildering health-care maze, where rationing is becoming an insidious problem (Tauber 2002a; 2003c).[10]

Although others have examined the fact-value distinction, or lack thereof, in discussions framed by the debate about patient self-determination (e.g., Brock 1991)—an issue of great importance to this book—here I follow a different path. I wish to emphasize a key lesson: comprehending the limits of the fact-value distinction in medicine requires that we recognize the role of values in grounding medicine's philosophy. In my view, any viable philosophy of medicine should emphasize the needs of the individual patient and the values surrounding his care. One way of orienting medical practitioners toward this ethical posture is to highlight a "moral epistemology"—that is, to show how clinical science never escapes its moral agenda. If that premise is accepted, then a person-centered clinical science must be adopted and a biopsychosocial medicine (discussed in chapter 6) becomes compelling. In future chapters, I will attempt to strengthen the philosophical underpinnings of those kinds of compelling approaches to clinical practice.

2
Shifting Foundations of the Doctor-Patient Relationship

To treat the patient as a *person*—what does that mean?
—MacIntyre 1979, 83

In the early twenty-first century, clinical medicine is shedding the last vestiges of its historical commitment to paternalism and is adopting a new respect for the autonomy of patients. In this sense, new standards to ensure patient dignity are taking hold—an orientation based on the recognition that physicians should not have the sole responsibility for determining treatment strategies. In this view, collaboration is required, both among health-care personnel and between those professionals and the patient (Balint 1964; Fischbach et al. 1980; Delbanco 1992). This assertion is, of course, an ideal, not a universal precept. Patients in a totally dependent position for reasons of severe physiological or mental compromise, who cannot participate in such dialogue, are obviously exempt from these standards. But putting aside the extreme case, patients now normally expect to participate in collaborative consultation. And contemporary medical ethics has successfully forced a realignment of patient rights—that is, people must be informed of medical decisions affecting their care. This new dynamic has reduced physician power, which hitherto was seemingly sacrosanct (Katz 1984; Brody 1992).

As discussed in chapter 1, moral concerns have always been implicit in medicine. Indeed, the division between science and human values blurs at the bedside. The medical choices made by physicians and their patients must, by their very nature, reflect a complex array of objective and subjective values that determine how the findings of clinical science and their associated technologies are to be applied in the care of the ill. Thus medicine connects clinical science and its object of study and intervention —the person, who becomes the nexus of politicojudicial action, moral agency, scientific scrutiny, and religious sanctification.

The origins of contemporary medical ethics may be traced to the Enlightenment, when the science of morals and the morals of science became the subject of intense deliberation, and from which medical ethics arose as a system of contracts between doctor and patient (Haakonssen 1997). But an even older religious tradition—Catholic (Kelly 1979), Protestant (Fletcher 1954), and Jewish (Jakobovits 1959)— has debated the moral implications of medicine generally, and in particular, since the mid-twentieth century, matters arising from clinical interventions that challenged dogma about life and death, such as abortion, terminal care, genetic counseling, and the like. But medical ethics in its present form—philosophical, secular, legalistic, and professionalized—has had only a brief history. Indeed, writing in 1954, Joseph Fletcher (1954, ix) correctly observed that *medical ethics* commonly referred to "a body of rules to govern the social behavior and graces of physicians," not to the "ethics of medical care" (p. 5), which reflected the deeper philosophical concerns of later periods.

The ethics of medical care burst forth into the political arena amid rapid technological advances that brought new challenges to the very definition of life and death. This in itself would have initiated speculation on how such newfound scientific power should be utilized. And in addition, a massive social realignment, under the auspices of a renewed commitment to civil and human rights, forced the doctor-patient relationship into a new alignment. Focusing on various forms of paternalism, particularly heated debates about informed consent for therapy, protection of subjects enrolled in human research, and recourse to medical malpractice, stimulated both a reexamination of the ethics underlying these issues as well as a more general discussion of medicine's moral philosophy and legal standing (Rothman 1991; Jonsen 1998; Wolpe 1998). Soon, medical ethics was transformed from vague and implicitly understood rules of conduct into a formal discipline, replete with institutes, journals, books, conferences, and professionals.

From a historical perspective, the current crisis in medicine prompted by the hegemony of clinical science over the humanistic concerns of the patient reflects a larger struggle that has been waged for about a century. The establishment of a science-based curriculum as the foundation of legitimate medical practice was won with only qualified assent from such prominent clinicians as William Osler and Francis Peabody. Each was concerned that laboratory-oriented medicine might lead the physician to lose his view of the patient as a person. Peabody (1927, 48) stated the cardinal precept: "The secret of the care of the patient is in caring for the patient." From this perspective, each of the various scientific and technological aspects of medicine is or should be subordinated to this general principle. Thus the patient is neither a scientific entity, nor a technological object, nor a unit of financial value. Indeed, the person bearing a disease should not be mistaken for the disease, and by urging that the patient, rather than the disease, be medicine's primary concern, these early critics voiced a common refrain: if medicine loses its own theory and simply adopts the theories, methods, and tools of its contributing sciences, it will lose its bearings.

I would say that medicine has always had its own theory, its moral philosophy. And physicians must be encouraged and supported in making themselves more morally self-reflective in the care of their patients. Science and technology are in the employ of a wider moral commitment, and it is this larger framework that requires strengthening in the face of challenges that insidiously conspire to alter medicine's most ancient and primary calling (Tauber 1999a).

Medical ethics is the moral response to this challenge, and given the current legal and political culture that is based on the protection of individual rights, patient autonomy became its governing philosophical principle. Autonomy's priority in medical ethics was achieved at the expense of other ethical principles for several reasons:

1. As a result of the erosion of trust between patient and physician, so-called rituals of trust have emerged as substitutes for organic trust (Tauber, 1999a, 50). Informed consent has become the vehicle of such rituals, and they have assumed the legalistic form of a contract (Veatch 1972), whose formulation as a code brings a certain clarity to what had hitherto been an implicit understanding (or covenant (May 1983)) of trust. Thus autonomy, as opposed to beneficence or justice, under the guise of informed consent, is easily applied and codified, and its

directives become comparatively straightforward and uncontroversial (Wolpe 1998, 46).

2. Patient autonomy, rather than being corrosive of professional privilege, may actually reenforce physician authority: autonomy tends to be a negative right (in that a person has the right to refuse treatment) rather than a positive right (a person cannot generally demand a particular treatment). Physicians are translators and filterers of information to their patients, who generally defer to physician recommendations regarding definitions of disease and its treatment (Wolpe 1998, 52). Indeed, physicians have incorporated informed consent into their practice as a means of improving patient satisfaction, and perhaps most importantly, in shifting responsibility to the patient, they offer a potent tactic to combat malpractice suits (Wolpe 1998, 52).

3. A more insidious interpretation maintains that the government and the medical establishment have made autonomous, informed patients into "consumers" and physicians into "providers" as health care has been turned into a commodity. This shift in identification carries a different sense of patient responsibility, and thus avoids difficult reform or critiques of the assumptions underlying health care (Fox 1994).

4. The power of the autonomy principle in medical ethics must also be understood in terms of its prominence as a political solution to the claims of various religious moralities in the American context. Secularized medical ethics is an instrumental, political, and moral response to a basic societal question that the phenomenon of American bioethics poses: How can, and should, an advanced modern, highly individualistic, pluralistic society, like the United States, preserve the separation of church and state and achieve collective and binding consensus about the kinds of bioethical issues now in the public domain? (Fox 1990, 209).[1]

The response: patient autonomy.

Conceptions of the Patient

The priority of autonomy, as opposed to communal-based principles (e.g., justice and beneficence), has effectively taken its place as part of the American political solution to pluralism. But autonomy is not just one of several ethical principles governing medicine; its "template" has overdetermined the ethical discourse through legal and commercial interpretations, one focused on rights, the other on market forces requiring free choice of "purchase." As a result, in this judicial-commercial context, medical ethics is like a lopsided table with four legs: although autonomy, beneficence, justice, and nonmaleficence each claim consideration, autonomy usually trumps other contenders: "For better or for worse . . . autonomy has emerged as the most powerful principle in American bioethics, the basis of much theory and much regulation, and has become the 'default' principle. . . . Indisputably . . ."(Wolpe 1998, 43). This dominance has been widely regarded as both a judicial and philosophical problem.

Alasdair MacIntyre (1979, 83) begins a provocative essay on the experience of being a patient with a keen question: "To treat the patient as a *person*—what does that mean?". That he asks this question and that it resonates with so many people reveal medicine's torment. But this is hardly new. Consider these two rather conflicted views of the physician during what many regard as a more innocent age:

The doctor would enter the home, revered and respected, his every wish and Judgment acquiesced, for his advice and dictation was paramount and the family . . . had all confidence in his ability as a doctor. (S. J. McNeil 1928; quoted by Rothman 1991, 277)

I do not know a single thoughtful and well-informed person who does not feel that the tragedy of illness at present is that it delivers you helplessly into the hands of a profession which you deeply mistrust. . . . As to the honor and conscience of doctors, they have as much as any other class of men, no more and no less. (George Bernard Shaw, preface to *The Doctor's Dilemma*, [1906] 1985, 258–259)

As these examples show, the doctor-patient relationship in modern times has been marked by ambivalence, consisting of a complex mixture of fear and dependency, of mistrust and appreciation, of vulnerability and gratitude. But this ambiguity has been largely replaced by a more defensive posture. Our own contemporary accounts, various surveys, and critics (reviewed in chapter 5) now seem to agree that, on balance, the image of the doctor as trusted provider, and even friend, has been eclipsed by a less intimate picture of someone who is still trusted, but decidedly less than in earlier eras.[2] Indeed, whether the avuncular

Norman Rockwell image of the doctor of the early twentieth century ever existed hardly seems germane to the current popular assumption that patients must be protected from medical harm.

Following this line of thought, MacIntyre answers his own question by delineating three doctor-patient relationships that operate in contemporary America. In his schema, physicians have assumed at least three pseudo-identities: physician as bureaucrat, physician as scientist, and physician as magician. In the first instance, the patient becomes a client; in the second, an object of scientific scrutiny; and in the third, a plaything of forces beyond personal control. A vast literature on the dyadic encounter of doctor and patient reveals a complex relationship that demands contradictory elements of intimacy and efficiency not easily reconciled (e.g., Stoeckle 1987). In the bureaucracy of health care—whether in a private office, a clinic, or a hospital—individuals must conform to procedures of impersonal processing, modes of stylized identification, and rules of governance, often mysterious if not draconian. Persons become "clients" in this setting, and definitions of care are shaped by organizational procedure, not personal need. In the context of physician-as-applied-scientist, patients become "cases" or "diseases," losing their multidimensional identities as "persons."

The imbalance in power, with physicians functioning not as autocrat managers or corporate agents but now as purveyors of knowledge and expertise, immediately reduces persons to dependents. In MacIntyre's third characterization, physician as magus, he draws the portrait of the physician as possessing mysterious (even supernatural) powers to cure and prolong life, and again persons are reduced, in this case to supplicants. Some see such dependency as arising from childhood dynamics (Preston 1981, 67), but irrespective of its psychological heritage, the unequal status of doctors and patients is self-evident.

Dependency needs evolve and other kinds of doctor-patient relationships may emerge in adulthood. Three basic forms are evident: (1) the physician is dominant and active, while the patient is passive; (2) while physician dominance takes precedence, the patient is offered input in managing his care (the "guidance-cooperation" model); and (3) mutual participation exists, in which the doctor and patient are equal partners (Szasz and Hollender 1956). Each of these three possible doctor-patient relationships has its role within particular clinical contexts, but clearly, the guidance model is the most typical. It follows from the disparity in expertise and the consequent compromise of patient autonomy for the sake of regaining health. So in the so-called cooperative mode, guidance dominates to the point where most patients, realistically and appropriately, want the doctor to take responsibility for their health.

The sociological evidence for this description is legion (e.g., Stoeckle 1987). Commentators have often noted how physicians assume control and use professional authority to make decisions for their patients. Intimidation and coercion are not only professionally accepted methods, but are also "taught as a matter of course to medical students" (Preston 1981, 75). Moreover, the patient loses control by just being in the hospital, where he is "clearly on the physician's turf" (p. 75). Patients exchange normal clothes for depersonalizing hospital garb, they relinquish their personal effects, their visitors are restricted, their diet is regulated, their medications are administered by others, and their bodies become subject to procedures alien and at times painful. In various ways, patients are subjected to a medical power they neither fully comprehend nor can control. To be simply informed, in rudimentary terms to be told what is being done with accompanying simplistic explanations as to why, inherently places patients in a subjected position to those who wield medical power. Thus the relationship between patient and doctor may vary from one of total physician authority to one of essentially equal partnership, but the traditional working association of the typical patient with the typical doctor is based on a quid pro quo of an understanding that grants the physician authority to take care of the patient (Preston 1981, 71). In this scenario, the doctor assumes that he possesses superior knowledge and that the patient is incapable of making proper medical decisions, and "it is standard practice for physicians to manipulate information in order to persuade patients to accept recommendations" (p. 73).

This professional posture, despite criticism and reconsideration, remains dominant. The strict hierarchy in teaching hospitals conforms to an acknowledgment of hierarchal knowledge, which translates into professional dominance and power. By a slow and intangible process, the student learns professional discipline. Too often the criterion becomes not what the patient might prefer, but what a well-trained physician should do. This is what is referred to as "professionalization," and it extends from learning a foreign language (the technical language of medicine) to adopting an objective attitude toward the patient. When knowledge is filtered down to the lowest level—the patient—the disparity of expertise and the value structure this expertise carries project an overwhelming disparity of power that simply denies equality of patient and physician. To the extent respect for patient autonomy exists, it must be asserted against this basic sociological structure of knowledge.

Resentment arises from such inequality, and numerous studies (e.g., Starr 1983) have documented a widely held belief that professional self-interest is often confused with service for the public good.[3] Accordingly, knowledge is a commodity, and commodities have costs. In the world of medicine, as in any profession, such costs are the time and effort to learn esoteric knowledge, and then the trials and tribulations of asserting that knowledge through professional scrutiny. These commodities are hard won and their authority not easily relinquished. Again, sharing of commodities, in this case medical knowledge, requires a fundamental reshaping of the doctor's sociology of knowledge, namely, how it is used and to what end.

The assertion of authority is an ancient tradition, since even Hippocrates cautioned his colleagues not to share medical information with patients.[4] But there is a rationale for the unequal doctor-patient relationship, based on psychological and sociological observations. Professional confidence is a critical element for both physician self-esteem (again the professionalism factor) and not unreasonably, for the patient's reassurance that cure is possible or even likely based on the physician's confidence in his power of knowledge. In essence, such confidence is a critical component for both the doctor and the patient, and for similar reasons.

So it is generally acknowledged that doctors err on the side of failing to admit doubt in their field of expertise. This is, of course highly ironic inasmuch as uncertainty in medicine is omnipresent. But that is not the psychologically relevant fact: doubt is perceived to signify a lack of knowledge. Professional competence is widely regarded as a necessary element for the patient's welfare, indeed, confidence in the therapist is a necessary, if not sufficient, element of care. Needless to say, unwavering trust poses a danger, and much of medical ethics over the past twenty-five years has directed itself to correcting this misunderstanding: physicians will work in the best interests of their patients, but doctors cannot act with powers they do not truly possess. The adjudication between what is known, what is possible, and what is best for the patient remains the fundamental moral imbroglio of contemporary medicine (Pellegrino and Thomasma 1981).

This constellation of issues is obviously complex and derives from multiple sources and projects that could take us in many directions. My discussion is focused on what is widely perceived as a fractured doctor-patient relationship, specifically the moral posture assumed by each in this highly charged dyadic relationship. In the end, trust is required for the therapeutic encounter to be successful, and the imposition of impediments can only be counterproductive to what informed consent was ultimately designed as, a freely chosen clinical strategy that promises the best outcome. So, as we review the complex history of informed consent, consider how a deeper dynamic of trust, or mistrust, was being expressed between doctor and patient, how their interaction revealed certain expectations from each party, and how those expectations were challenged and then changed in response to a different social context of twentieth-century American mass society, where ideas of personhood radically shifted. (A detailed discussion of trust in the contemporary setting is deferred until chapter 5.)

Conceptions of the Doctor-Patient Relationship

The history of medical ethics has been written from various moral and historical perspectives. Looking at the paternalism of earlier periods led Jay Katz (1984, 3) to conclude that the doctor-patient relationship was marked by a "stark silence." From this perspective, Katz argued that "disclosure and consent are obligations alien to medical thinking and practice" (p. 1). That interpretation was contested by Martin Pernick (1982, 3; cited by Faden and Beauchamp 1986, 56–59), whose examination of nineteenth-century medical practice concluded that "truth-telling and consent-seeking have long been part of an indigenous medical tradition, based on medical theories that taught that knowledge and autonomy had demonstrably beneficial effects on most patients' health." But he also admitted that both the content and the purpose of nineteenth-century patient-physician dialogue differed from modern conceptions of informed consent. David Rothman (1991, 109ff.) regarded Katz's interpretation as a distortion of the historical record, inasmuch as Katz based his analysis almost exclusively on normative statements, often encapsulated in ethical codes, and failed to regard a broader set of testimonies. These competing views I think are fairly judged by Ruth Faden and Tom Beauchamp (1986, 56–60) in their comprehensive history of informed consent, where they basically agree with Katz. A century ago, doctors spoke with their patients and even informed them of decisions made on their behalf, but the intent of such disclosure was to gain the patient's cooperation, not to permit the full participation of an autonomous agent. Indeed, if one surveys the general social mores of that era, such hierarchy is characteristic of analogous relationships marked by differences in social class, economic power, or other forms of status (e.g. priest-parishioner; teacher-student; employer-employee). That patients exhibited deference to their doctors, and that doctors were condescending to their patients, was simply the accepted social exchange of the era. And no criticism might be leveled without adopting an anachronistic projection of our own values onto the past. Simply put, the beneficence model of care (the doctor acted in the best interest of the patient) had not been challenged by the autonomy model (the basis of fully articulated informed consent) until the twentieth century (Faden and Beauchamp 1986, 60).

The paternalistic attitude is easily traced to ancient medicine, which was dominated by Hippocrates, whose famous oath makes no reference to physicians' obligation to converse with patients (except, perhaps, what is implied in the promise to "keep secret" what the physician learns in the house of the sick). The specified duties were of a different nature, and, as we have seen, Hippocrates expressly warned physicians to avoid disclosure. So while physicians were performing medical duties calmly and adroitly, concealment was considered crucial to the healing process (Katz 1984, 4). The sources consulted from this era are consistent with this orientation; as Katz says, doctor-patient dialogue was not aimed at shared decision making but at creating "trust, obedience and then . . .

cure" (p. 7). Hippocratic ideals continued to influence medicine into the medieval period, but a religious overlay was added, inasmuch as faith was believed to be an important part of healing and led to therapeutic effectiveness. The few available documents from this period fail to reveal "even a remote need to discuss anything with patients that involves their participation in decision making. . . . Conversations with patients served purposes of offering comfort, reassurance and hope, and of inducing patients to take the cure" (p. 7). Three interrelated principles governed the patient-doctor link: (1) patients must honor physicians, for they had received their authority from God; (2) patients must have faith in their doctors as divine agents; and (3) patients must promise obedience. Thus authority was clearly established and free exchange was not part of the doctor-patient relationship.

The first shift in attitude, not unexpectedly, coincides with the emergence of new ideas of personhood and ecclesiastical authority in the early modern period. De Sorbière, a seventeenth-century French physician, priest, and philosopher, in *Advice to a Young Physician Respecting the Way in Which He is to Conduct Himself in the Practice of Medicine, in View of the Indifference of the Public to the Subject, and Considering the Complaints That Are Made about Physicians* (1672), entertained the prospect of full disclosures to patients. This extraordinary suggestion was, however, quickly dismissed as both impractical and counterproductive. Although de Sorbière understood the appeal of disclosure, he rejected his own proposal out of hand, believing that the candor of such relations on the part of the doctor would most likely render patients uneasy and critical of their doctor's capabilities. Rather than engendering trust, such forthrightness would more likely instill mistrust and result in replacement with another physician, perhaps less honest but more willing to play his expected role. De Sorbière was an astute judge of the doctor's craft of his period, arguing that deception, urbanity, flattery, and at times brusqueness were useful interpersonal tools, and that a wise physician should always have "a few doses of nonsense to bestow" (Katz 1984, 11). Notwithstanding this cynical stance, he understood the complexity of decision making, and while some patients might indeed be enlightened enough to actively participate in their care, this would be exceptional.

De Sorbière's radical insight was to reappear before a more sympathetic audience during the next century. Indeed, we might consider the birth of modern medical ethics to be concomitant to the origin of liberal rights more generally. Considering the profound influence John Locke and other liberal political theorists had on eighteenth-century thought concerning citizenship, property rights, religious freedom, and the individual writ large, it should be no surprise that medical ethics might also have undergone profound change in league with these other closely allied issues.[5]

Three late eighteenth-century physicians, John Gregory, Thomas Percival, and Benjamin Rush, are generally regarded as the fathers of Anglo-American medical ethics (to be distinguished from a strong, earlier academic and judicial tradition in France, Italy, and the Germanic principalities (Geyer-Kordesch 1993)). Gregory was a Scot who practiced and taught medicine; Percival, an "English Dissenter," was a physician and a health reformer; Rush, who lived in Philadelphia, was the leading physician in Revolutionary War America. All three were educated at Presbyterian colleges and attended the University of Edinburgh for their medical education. Their clinical training could not be separated from the excitement generated by the Scottish Enlightenment of moral philosophy, and all of these physicians were introduced to, and deeply influenced by, David Hume, Adam Smith, and William Robertson (Baker 1993; McCullough 1993; Pickstone 1993; Haakonssen 1997). This linkage is easily understood when we recall that the separation of the humanities and the sciences was nonexistent in this era. So close was their integration that *scientist*, the term designated to differentiate those who practiced a newly created professional (and technical) science as distinct from an older descriptive natural philosophy, was not even coined until the mid-nineteenth century. (For instance, Charles Darwin referred to himself as a natural philosopher.) Further, even the separation of "natural philosophy" from "moral philosophy" was artificial, because the lines were constantly crossed.[6] So, Gregory, Percival, and Rush, as well-educated gentlemen, were conversant not only with the scientific practices of their day, but also the current philosophical debates, of which a new sensitivity toward the "moral sentiments" was prominent.[7]

Led by Thomas Reid and his circle, these philosophers asserted the integrity of the individual, and espoused how the self might seek moral improvements and cultivated powers.[8] Gregory, Percival, and Rush each embraced these notions of self-improvement as central to their self-image, and to the extent that they identified as part of a profession, they did so with a strong leaning toward individual responsibility for others, toward the community at large, and, of course, toward God. Students of the age concur that no unique code of professional ethics was required for medicine until the end of the eighteenth century, because the code for gentlemanly conduct sufficed (Fissel 1993; Baker, Porter, and Porter 1993).[9]

But in the late eighteenth century, British social structure and its manners were thrown into turmoil when its social code was perceived in crisis as a result of a complex realignment of economic, religious, and political forces. Several factors—including the assertion of a new bourgeois social and political identity, the market and commercial expansion arising from the Industrial Revolution, and the emergence of revolutionary evangelical and republican critiques of the old aristocratic order—had repercussive effects on medicine. In other words, a new social consciousness emerged during this period, and with these demands, a revised code of medical ethics materialized.

Key to this reformulation was the replacement of the unwritten contract of duties of the eighteenth-century physician—traditionally divided into those he owed to God, to himself, and to others—with explicit ethics pertaining to the doctor-patient relationship, one characterized by new reciprocal duties and rights.[10] Sympathy, a crucial organizing element in eighteenth-century moral philosophy, was expressed in medical ethics as a kind of self-reflective modality, whereby the empathy aroused in the physician for another's pleasure or pain evoked a moral assessment of those feelings (see note 7). Indeed, Gregory's *Lectures* of 1772 (Gregory 1998) explicitly built its ethics on the concept of sympathy derived directly from Hume's moral philosophy (albeit not without some reservations (McCullough 1993)), and thereby placed the "primacy of the patient's interests over those of the physician" (Haakonsen 1997, 8–9).

Gregory may be regarded as the father of modern medical ethics, inasmuch as he established the ideal of physician responsibility and "pioneered the idea that the relationship between practitioner and patient is at the center of all medical ethics" (Haakonsen 1997, 3). He suggested that his colleagues must "lay medicine open to the public" and that the study of medicine by disinterested scholars as well as by doctors themselves would provide great benefit. Reason, temperance, secrecy, and candor were key physician virtues, yet the most important quality was sympathy. He thus translated Scottish Enlightenment ideals into the medical scenario: "At the heart of Gregory's medical ethics was a depiction of a medical man who combined the virtues of the 'rational' physician with those of the 'man of feeling'" (Haakansen 1997, 70). Thus sympathy and benevolence were of essential value for physicians, which required linkage to "'reason' informed by the appropriate education and training" (p. 75). Together with secrecy, honor, temperance, sobriety, candor, and discretion, these formed a moral code for patient trust. In short, Gregory espoused a new configuration of the doctor-patient relationship, one built on a more circumspect and modest view of himself as a physician.[11]

Gregory's sensitivity was uncommon, and his contemporaries, notably Percival and Rush, had little concern for weakening the strict dominance of doctor over his charge. Percival was more concerned with professional ethics and how the profession might regulate its own activities. His *Medical Ethics* ([1803] 1927) was dedicated to proper professional conduct by seeking to help resolve professional disputes through the establishment of a code of etiquette. In this era, the guild mentality still played an important role in the practice of medicine, providing doctors with privileges of protection and a strict monopoly in certain goods and services, which Percival encouraged.[12] But a guild mentality does not adequately reflect what was to become a modern profession. Percival's central role is best understood as articulating a shift from codes of gentlemanly (individualistic) honor (Fissell 1993) to the adoption of a code based on collective concerns (Baker 1993).

In the nineteenth century, Anglo-American medical ethics were codified as a collective autonomy of practitioners. As practitioners gave up their individual autonomy, this new professionalism, based on collective self-regulation, was developed into formal codes of medical practice. With an eye toward the patient, these physicians were primarily concerned with establishing the supremacy of their own position, professionally and commercially. Medical ethics was thus initially formulated as self-serving, and precepts respecting patient autonomy were correspondingly subordinated to physician dominance.

None of the pioneers of medical ethics were advocates of patient involvement in decision making. Although they argued that the laity should be educated on medical issues, at the same time they defended the use of deception and secrecy, revealing a greater concern "with manipulating the physician-patient relationship for therapeutic ends than with enlightening patients to share the burdens of decision making" (Katz 1984, 16). This sounds to our own ears as condescending and authoritarian, since our concept of this relationship has been radically altered by what I will call the "autonomy divide"—that political and cultural collective of ideas and events asserting atomistic individuality (described in the next chapter), which fundamentally challenged an older relationship built from a more rigid social hierarchy. I am referring specifically to how respect for individual autonomy (whether called civil rights, individual rights, religious rights, and so on) has become a fundamental precept in our culture.

For our purposes here, it is self-evident, putting aside the philosophical details, that a new ideal of personal autonomy had emerged in nascent form during the nineteenth century, which was to basically alter the relations of individuals in most domains of social life during the twentieth century. This change had different trajectories in various spheres of society, with first one group leading the liberal assault and then another—that is, abolitionists, labor organizers, feminists, civil rights advocates, and so on. The complex connections between social mores, political rights, judicial directives, and intellectual and social innovations have a convoluted history. The details need not concern us here, except to observe that medicine tenaciously held on to an older authoritarian relationship between the doctor and his charge than one might expect, given the centrality of a vision of individualism that gripped the American imagination during this period. Indeed, the dominance physicians held over their patients until well into the twentieth century is a remarkable social fact and attests to the implicit power of the caregiver.

If we place the typical doctor-patient relationship of the nineteenth century within its cultural context, a certain incongruity appears: the U.S. Constitution institutionalized new notions of liberty, equality, democracy, and liberalism, which reached an early climax in Jacksonian politics, a populist movement that was, at its core, an assertion of individualism against widely perceived strictures of an imposing government. Culturally, romanticism celebrated individual freedom in the arts, in religion, in social interactions, and in the irreducibility of autonomous personhood. As I will discuss in chapter 3, this understanding of selfhood was supported by philosophical constructions that were widely accepted. But our contemporary conception of individuality did not extend to an assertion of parity between doctor and patient. Indeed, the domain of choice remained limited to choosing a medical practitioner.[13] Thus autonomy extended to the kind of medical care chosen, but once selected, there is ample evidence that whatever grounding patient trust might have had, the dominant expression of the patient's relationship to the doctor was one that hardly questioned his authority (Rothman 1991).

Thus, despite powerful social forces driving a particular version of individualism, medicine was to prove a bastion of an older social structure, and because of this conservatism, autonomy-based medical ethics was postponed until the twentieth century. The conservatism may be traced back to Percival's *Medical Ethics* ([1803] 1927). While proposing principles and rules to govern physician affairs with colleagues, lawyers, judges, and patients, what we consider essential patients' rights received no notice. Indeed, by emphasizing "urbanity and rectitude," Percival was primarily concerned with establishing public trust in the profession (Jonsen 1998, 7).

Percival's general concerns were extrapolated to the American context in the Code of Medical Ethics adopted by the AMA in 1847 (American Medical Association, [1847] 1977; Duffy 1983), and more specifically, mutual decision making between physicians and patients was as alien to nineteenth-century Americans (not withstanding populist political and social movements) as it was to their English colleagues. The condescension and authority exemplified by these professional self-portraits made patient participation unattainable. The code shared with Percival's *Medical Ethics* a primary concern with protecting and enhancing the professional stature of the orthodox physician. The AMA was, after all, a newly formed professional organization, and it was claiming, like a new suitor, the favors of the public. The benefits accruing to the public, directly and indirectly, from the active and unwearied beneficiaries of the profession, were so numerous and important that physicians were putatively entitled to the utmost consideration and respect from the community (American Medical Association, [1847] 1977, 34). Interestingly, neither the code of 1847 (or 1957, for that matter) acknowledges, or even considers, physicians' duties reciprocally—that is, from those gifts and services that they have received from the community (May 1983, 113). In this view, the doctor has, because of his generous spirit, accepted the mantle of service.

In a close reading, William May observes that the code titles two critical sections, "Obligations of Patients to Their Physicians" and "Duties of Physicians to Their Patients." The shift from *Obligations* to *Duties* may seem slight but, in fact, it reveals a differing source and intensity to moral claim. *Obligation* has the same root as the words *ligaments* and *religion*; it emphasizes a bind, a bond, a tie. The AMA viewed patient and public as bound and indebted to the profession for its services but viewed the profession as accepting *duties* to the patient and public out of a noble conscience rather than a reciprocal sense of indebtedness (May 1983, 113–114). Beyond defining the fundamental relationship between patient and physician, the code attempted to regulate the profession in various respects: it repudiated quackery and advertising, and correspondingly endorsed physicians receptive to modern science. As such, the code defined orthodox medicine by rejecting competing disciplines, such as homeopathy, naturopathy, and hydropathy. So the code was to serve both as the foundation of professional conduct, and as a political tool to enhance a branch of medical practice at the expense of challenges from different traditions (Starr 1983). In a sense, its embrace of esoteric scientific knowledge enhanced the authority of the physician and further strengthened the inequality of the doctor and patient. The code was revised along these lines in 1903 as the *Principles of Medical Ethics* and again modified in 1912 (Duffy 1983, 78). The 1912 *Principles* remained a fair expression of physician attitudes of the period, namely, that "physicians must make decisions for, and not with, patients" (Katz 1984, 20). The *Principles* underwent no major changes until 1957, when the entire code was replaced by an abridged "Principles of Medical Ethics," consisting of a brief preamble and ten short sections (American Medical Association, [1957] 1977).

To be sure, we may find evidence to contradict the equanimity of benign paternalism, but I take my lead from Mark Twain, an astute critic of his own era, who understood that the healing relationship was based on trust, and trust implied faith. His remarks are particularly cogent when placed in the social context of biomedicine's effective dominance over other forms of medical therapies—this is, when biomedicine was invoking science to trump other contenders:

No one doubts—certainly not I—that the mind exercises a powerful influence over the body. From the beginning of time, the sorcerer, the interpreter of dreams, the fortuneteller, the charlatan, the quack, the wild medicine-man, the educated physician, the mesmerist, and the hypnotist, have made use of the client's *imagination* to help them in their work. They have all recognized the potency and availability of that force. Physicians may cure many patients with a bread pill; they know that where the disease is only a fancy, the patient's confidence in the doctor will make the bread pill effective.

Faith in the doctor. Perhaps that is the entire thing. It seems to look like it. (Twain [1899] 1992, 387)

With the promise of science, physician authority became ever more powerful, and consent was regarded as tangential to the obvious benefit of rational therapy.

During this period, only rare, isolated voices questioned this condescending attitude. Most notable perhaps is Richard C. Cabot (1869–1939), a physician well known for his humanistic medical philosophy (Burns 1977). Perhaps the onerous workload—seeing thirty to forty patients in a two-hour session at the Massachusetts General Hospital, most without any examination—inspired Cabot to argue for more humane health care. (Stoeckle 1987, 51–52). In a short article, "Medical Ethics in the Hospital" (Cabot 1931), he called for a patient-centered approach for clinical medicine. He sought to protect patients, who might be exploited for teaching purposes, and advocated that patients be informed of their diagnoses and have their treatments explained. He thus decried deception in physician-patient interactions and identified its negative consequences.

Clinical competence, in Cabot's view, was not a cold, calculating skill. It had to include, not only mastery of science, but also appreciation of the personal and social needs of the patient. He recognized what we now call the humanistic qualities of the physician, not as frivolous, but as intrinsic to clinical competence (Jonsen 1998, 9). But while Cabot (1903) declared that patients can be trusted to hear medical truths, he did not propose that patients and doctors choose treatment strategies together. As empathetic as he might have been, paternalism was still the order of the day.

The erosion of this general attitude may be traced in the history of informed consent, whose scope was to widen and eventually create the moral space for patient autonomy (Faden and Beauchamp 1986; Appelbaum, Lidz, and Meisel 1987). *Schloendorff v. The Society of the New York Hospital* of 1914 is the primary judgment that reaffirmed a citizen-patient's elementary right to be free from offensive (uninvited) contact, a principle found in fifteenth-century common law: "Every human being of adult years and sound mind has a right to determine what shall be done with his own body; and a surgeon who performs an operation without his patient's consent commits an assault, for which he is liable in damages (Justice Cardoza)" (Jonsen 1998, 354). Other cases, such as *Haskins v. Howard* (1929), similarly called for patient participation in decision making, but "the idea that patients had a role to play in medical decision making, beyond a mere right of refusal, rarely surfaced in judicial opinion" (Katz 1984, 53). As late as the 1955 case of *Hunt v. Bradshaw,* judges disregarded both disclosure and consent as governing principles of medical practice, a judgment reaffirmed by the Supreme Court. Informed consent had not yet found judicial articulation or backing.

But consent and disclosure began to play an important role in defining the doctor-patient relationship by the late 1950s. Both the medical profession and judicial rulings became more circumspect about patient rights. In the AMA's *Principles* of 1957, a medical code summed up the patient-physician relationship in one phrase as follows: "The principal objective of the medical profession is to render service to humanity with full respect for the dignity of man" (American Medical Association [1957] 1977, 39). And judges began to consider whether the patient should also decide if an intervention is acceptable in light of its risks.

Punctuated by case law, informed consent most directly emerges from constitutional protections. The doctrine, and expression, "informed consent," arose from the 1957 case, *Salgo v. Leland Stanford Jr. University Board of Trustees*,[14] but did not receive its full articulation until *Canterbury v. Spence* (1972). Mr. Canterbury fell out of bed following a laminectomy and suffered paralysis. He sued his surgeon on the grounds that he was not fully informed of the risk of paralysis following surgery, and the court confirmed that this information was material to the patient's decision to undergo the procedure:

> True consent to what happens to one's self is the informed exercise of a choice, and that entails an opportunity to evaluate knowledgeably the options available and the risks attendant upon each. The average patient has little or no understanding of the medical arts, and ordinarily has only his physician to whom he can look for enlightenment with which to reach an intelligent decision. From these almost axiomatic considerations springs the need, and in turn the requirement, of a reasonable divulgence by physicians to patients to make such a decision possible. (quoted by Jonsen 1998, 355)

Shortly thereafter, a second momentous decision was made by the New Jersey Supreme Court in allowing Karen Quinlan's parents to withdraw life-support measures for their daughter, who lived in a persistent vegetative state following an accident (Filene 1998). The court ruled that Quinlan had a right to terminate treatment grounded in the privacy protected by the federal Constitution (Faden and Beauchamp 1986, 40–41). To guarantee such rights, the "only practical way" to prevent the loss of such privacy due to her incompetency was to allow her guardian and family to decide "whether she would exercise it in these circumstances" (*In re Quinlan* 1976). As David Rothman (2001, 258) observes,

> The event that signals the movement's arrival [autonomy rights], that announces and promotes a fundamental shift in the doctor-patient, or hospital-patient relationship, the point after which there was no going back to the old models of paternalism, comes from the legal forum in the guise of the Karen Ann Quinlan decision. In its aftermath came not only a new insistence on legal forms . . . but a shift in attitude to a "we": "they" patient mentality, as in: don't let them, that is doctors and hospitals, do to me what they did to Karen Ann. Arguably, if one

had to choose just one document to represent the triumph of the autonomy movement, that document would be a court decision, and it would be the Quinlan decision.

The new ascendency of the autonomy ethic was soon firmly established in standards of informed consent set by state statute, and by 1981 the AMA's council addressed the issue in its *Current Opinions of the Judicial Council*:

> The patient's right of self-decision can be effectively exercised only if the patient possesses enough information to enable an intelligent choice. The patient should make his or her own determination on treatment. The physician's obligation is to present the medical facts accurately to the patient or to the individual responsible for the patient's care and to make recommendations for management in accordance with good medical practice. Informed consent is a basic social policy for which exceptions are permitted (1) where the patient is unconscious or otherwise incapable of consenting and the harm from failure to treat is imminent; or (2) when risk-disclosure poses such a serious psychological threat of detriment to the patient as to be medically contraindicated. Social policy does not accept the paternalistic view that the physician may remain silent because divulgence might prompt the patient to forgo needed therapy. Rational, informed patients should not be expected to act uniformly, even under similar circumstances in agreeing to or refusing treatment. (American Medical Association, 1981, paragraph 8.07; 1997, 120)

Note that disclosure is required not by obligation within the medical field, but is based on the exterior force of "social policy." The wording does not provide any parameters on the extent of disclosure, and thus the doctrine is still unclear. There is also some equivocation, inasmuch as the council later seems to retreat from its endorsement of the doctrine by reminding physicians that they must only "properly inform the patient of the nature and purpose of the treatment undertaken or prescribed." It is precisely this ancient minimal-disclosure requirement that judges had found wanting and had tried to expand through their informed-consent doctrine, and critics were quick to point out that full options are also part of the informed-consent ethic (Schultz 1985; Faden and Beauchamp 1986; Appelbaum, Lidz, and Meisel 1987). But under judicial pressure, social demands, and professional retreat from malpractice litigation, by the 1990s it was commonplace that physicians informed their patients about their medical condition and its prognosis, the risks and benefits of any treatment offered, and the options of alternative therapies (Annas

1989). Informed consent became the vehicle for a newfound equilibration of the doctor-patient relationship.[15]

The Contemporary Social Context of the Doctor-Patient Relationship

In protecting the dignity of the patient, the founders of contemporary bioethics responded to two overriding concerns: the legal aspects of informed consent and the ethical challenges of medicine's newfound technical prowess—that is, the novel dilemmas arising from a technology that offered new options for personal health and sexuality, genetic counseling and engineering, life support, and myriad other innovations. These latter concerns arose not so much from the legalistic tradition of protecting patients' rights as from the deeper religious traditions concerned with the sanctity of life and its preservation. But coupled to the judicial character of a newly born medical ethics, the arguments and orientation of these "sanctity of life" concerns shifted from a tradition almost exclusively theological in orientation to one dominated by a secularized approach that was specifically entrusted by the federal government to deal with this new medicine (Evans 2002). In doing so, an extrapolated legalistic orientation, replete with the language of autonomy, rights, and pluralism, was employed to formulate the ethical principles and guidelines to also address this second domain of human dignity. Thus a fascinating history unfolds as one appreciates how the moral discussion moved from the original philosophical and religious strata to a secular, pluralistic discourse dominated by scientists, their interest groups, and professional philosophers dedicated to solving technical problems (Evans 2002). But that history can only be understood within a broader social context, namely, how medical ethics developed as a product of various social movements of the late 1960s (Rothman 1991; Jonsen 1998). I will focus on this latter aspect here.

Beyond judicial rulings and organized medicine's deliberations, contemporary medical ethics may be dated to a series of conferences convened during the 1960s, the establishment of permanent academic forums for the discipline (the Hastings Center, 1969, the Kennedy Institute, 1970, and a theologically oriented Society for Health and Human Values, 1969), and the concomitant appearance of the first systematic presentation of a moral philosophy for medicine. If we seek an *ur*-text for the birth of modern medical ethics, let me nominate Paul Ramsey's *The Patient as Person* (1970), a book Albert Jonsen (1998, 50) rightly calls "the first truly modern study of the new ethics of science and medicine." The text, based on lectures Ramsey delivered at Yale in 1969, was a call to an action-based ethics, a bioethics fully engaged in bedside decisions. He firmly placed medical ethics within the moral ethos of its human community as a special genre of a more general moral philosophy. That philosophy enveloped both the physician and researcher in the same covenants "of moral discourse concerning the claims of persons" (Ramsey 1970, xii), namely, the preservation of their autonomy. Such covenants were moral instruments to protect the freedom and rights of the patient. Ramsey claimed that medical ethics must be committed "to show respect for, protect, preserve and honor the life of fellow man" (p. xiii). Indeed, medicine is a unique setting for the exercise of such moral action.

Ramsey's credo, which converged on a new assertion of patient autonomy in medicine, assumed a new urgency during the social ferment of the era. Within a short period, from the 1968 collapse of the Mondale hearings (called to create a presidential commission on ethical concerns in biomedicine) to the successful Kennedy hearings of 1973 (which resulted in new ethical oversight provisions for federal sponsored research), bioethics was legitimated by congressional mandate. This was the period of social unrest that immediately followed the crested wave of the Great Society and the expansion of civil rights. It witnessed the political birth of feminism and gay rights as assertions of free choice about sexuality; newly affirmed abortion rights extended the legal domain of personal moral choice; insurgency against the Vietnam War attested individual responsibility; radical lifestyles, including new standards in dress, music, and sexual expression, claimed new vistas for private choice. In short, the hegemony of self-determination was forcefully asserted in all domains of American society.

Patient rights grew in this social mulch. Two protective processes worked hand in glove, one proactive, the other reactive. The first was the systematic enunciation of bioethical principles and the formal affirmation of patient rights; the other was the dramatic rise of malpractice suits and resultant awards. The medical establishment quickly assumed a defensive posture, one that has taken a while to equilibrate, but we can look back at the last thirty years with some satisfaction. Bioethics is firmly in place as a crucial part of medical practice and biomedical research, and the hysteria about defensive medicine has calmed, while a significant sensitivity to patient rights has taken hold (Rothman 1991). Let us briefly review these developments.

Certain American moral precepts had become universal after World War II, and cardinal among these was expansive respect for the individual. In the context of medicine, the Nuremberg trials revealed how physicians required vigilant oversight, and while many elements converged, the moral repugnance evoked by the Nazi and Japanese experimental atrocities performed on slave laborers and prisoners of war (Annas and Grodin 1992) heightened the communal sense of the sanctity and the integrity of the patient in the medical setting. Informed consent was extended from bedsides to research facilities, largely due to the groundbreaking revelations by Henry Beecher (1966), a prominent Harvard professor, of unethical human experimentation in medicine's bastions, as well as the outrage evoked by the revelations of the Tuskegee syphilis study (Jones 1981). Thus alerted to the dangers of the supposed good intentions of researchers ethically deaf to the rights of patients, safeguards were soon instituted (*Belmont Report*, 1978).

A complementary but independent moral imperative motivating the medical ethics movement was the general attempt to reclaim humane values from an ever-encroaching technology and debasing material view of the world. This romantic reaction took on renewed vigor in the late 1960s and throughout the rest of the twentieth century. The human body and the environment became contested areas. In medicine, the body as scientific object, analogous to the objective study of nature, was disenchanted and alienated. For Michel Foucault ([1963] 1973), Ivan Illich (1976), Thomas Szasz (1961), and other radical critics, medicine was just another industry or arm of the state, imbued with arrogance and self-aggrandizing power, ignorant or oblivious to the impact of its own encroachment. These critics tapped into a widely felt anxiety stimulated by rapid technical advances in clinical medicine (e.g., the challenges of fetal research, artificial life support, and human experimentation), as well as the specter of new vistas opened by basic research. For these critics, as our bodies were relentlessly reduced to biochemistry and genetics, the disjunction of our material being from our integrated sense of selfhood was epitomized by the objectification of disease.

Another dehumanizing force resulted from the rapid expansion of the corporate character of health care, especially in the form of health maintenance organizations (HMOs). Because of disaffection with depersonalized care and a general appreciation that health care was now driven by a corporate profit structure, patient advocacy assumed new urgency in the 1990s. But I wonder how much current disaffection is focused on an easy target, Big Business. We should note that complaints of friction between doctors and their patients were in abundance well before the rise of HMOs (e.g., Balint 1964; Katz 1984; Brody 1992), and the problems arising from the disparity of power between doctor and patient cannot be reduced to a new corporate mentality or viewed as a result of new constraints imposed by the economies of shortened time and limited resources for clinical care. Nevertheless, two dehumanizing trends seemed to conspire against a nostalgic memory (or fantasy) of a more empathetic moral locus of care: the objectification of illness and the corporate administration of health care.

These moral sentiments—the threatened sanctity of the person, the anxiety of jeopardized patient rights, the perceived encroachment of corporation, state, and technology—each served to raise a collective anxiety about medicine's manipulative power and potentially unchecked restriction of patient autonomy. The complaint identifies both the success and weakness of scientific medicine. Later I will delve into this aspect of the crisis in medicine's self-image, but suffice it to observe here that medical ethics has derived its moral authority as the champion of the rights of patients within the particular context of jeopardized humane values, and the forum of medical ethics has served as an important stage on which the moral character of the human body and our human nature have been debated.

To be sure, I have omitted other critical contributing factors to the upheaval in medicine of which bioethics was one important response. But even with this brief sketch, the sociological point should now be clear. The various components that went into building the bioethics movement had to fall into proper alignment: the Nuremberg trials incubated for twenty years; basic social organs—the military, the corporations, the universities—suffered critical reassessment as a result of heightened mistrust of government, albeit only the latest episode in a series dating to the Revolutionary War (Wills 1999); a period of activism centered on championing individuality became widespread, especially among racial and ethnic minorities, women, and homosexuals; and medicine itself underwent a significant technological revolution. This is not the place to further explore these complex social forces, other than to remind ourselves that autonomy in the medical setting became the articulation of both a deep social preoccupation with free choice and our collective reaction to a world seemingly increasingly hostile to individuality and subjectivity. A renewed assertion of autonomy readily fit a complicated social and political agenda well beyond the confines of medical ethics per se. In short, medicine's current moral philosophy must be seen within its historical context, the larger political and social fabric of American democracy during the cultural upheaval of the late 1960s. As a result of those commanding forces, bioethics assumed its particular cast, namely, as a force to encourage physicians to shed the last vestiges of their historical commitment to paternalism. And, correspondingly, patients asserted new standards of autonomy. To that issue we now turn, namely, what *is* autonomy?

3

Defining Autonomy

Autonomy is like baldness. We know what perfect baldness would consist in, but we use the word "bald" to describe people who have lost a substantial amount of hair. It would be idle to attempt a precise definition of how many hairs, or what proportion of hair, a person must have lost in order to be correctly described as bald.
—Lindley 1986, 69–70

I have reviewed how "autonomy" eventually established itself among the principles of medical ethics as an extrapolation from the political-judicial culture in which it evolved, but I have postponed attempts at defining autonomy. A typical dictionary definition offers "independence" and "freedom," which are hardly explanatory, since the meanings of these synonyms are similarly abstract, context-dependent, and complex concepts with many functions and meanings of their own. Consequently, when one traces autonomy's historical evolution within philosophical, political, or social environments, such narratives provide a variety of interpretations, each dependent on the cultural or conceptual setting in question. But even exhaustive analyses have led some commentators to wry approximations, as illustrated by this chapter's epigraph. Nevertheless, we want criteria for autonomous behaviors (autonomous actions and choices) in order to ground the principle of autonomy. We wish to better understand how *autonomy* is used and understood in everyday parlance, and more specifically, how it is applied in the clinical setting.

To accomplish that end, this chapter is divided into three major sections. The first concerns the understandings of the self, from which conceptions of autonomy follow. I will examine a particular formulation of selfhood, one in which individualism is celebrated and the ostensible ideals of autonomous persons best protected. The middle portion of the chapter considers the role of rationality in establishing the basis for autonomous choice. I focus on Immanuel Kant, and appropriately so, since he is considered the lynchpin of modern moral philosophy, and some would argue the originator of the concept of autonomy (Schneewind 1998). We now appreciate how seventeenth- and eighteenth-century political and ethical theory point toward him, and later developments are seen as reactions to his towering achievements. We live with that legacy, and thus the third area of discussion concerns how to draw the loose boundaries of autonomous acts on a coordinate system that Kant established: one axis ranks rational and emotional claims, and the other axis, individual and communal interests. Where we situate autonomous acts thus represents a balance, or perhaps a composite of these various elements, and in the last section of this chapter, as well as in the next chapter, we will examine how contemporary philosophers have heeded the call for a synthesis of these elements. We will thus consider a broad array of post-Kantian criticisms, ranging from minor refinements to radical revisions of his thinking. My goal is to find a way of preserving autonomy—specifically in a medical context. Among other things, this will entail reformulating it consistent with contemporary conceptions of selfhood.

Thus, I lay the groundwork for a discussion of autonomy by exploring how it might be designated as a characteristic of the self—an attribute of the moral agent, as well as an attribute of moral choice. In short, autonomy cannot be thought of independently of how the self is identified and acts. We seek the conceptual scaffolding of the self that will permit us to assign "autonomous" as one of its attributes. Obviously, many formulations of selfhood have been proposed. It then follows that autonomy—as an attribute of the self, has a particular structure in a Kantian construction and a different one in that portrayed by Hume or Mill, for example, for each configures the self differently. The point is that each philosophy is guided by underlying presuppositions about the nature of the self and the role of rationality, which lead, by the inner logic of those interpretations, to various formulations of autonomy or criteria for autonomous acts.

I can do little more than point to the outlines of this complex story, for today, the characterization of the self seems almost coincident with all of the social sciences, much of historical analysis, psychology, philosophy, and the arts. I will simplify the conundrum of defining personal identity by framing this discussion in terms of two conceptions of personal identity. If the self is defined as atomistic and radically individualistic, autonomy assumes a powerful position in the array of moral principles that both identify the self and empower it to act. Indeed, autonomy assumes a central characteristic of personal identity with this understanding. On the other hand, if the self is understood as a confluence of relationships and social obligations that are constitutive of identity, then autonomy may legitimately be subordinated to other moral principles that determine how the self is governed within a social context. Here, I am following the latter orientation, for I am seeking a construction of selfhood and autonomy that allows for a balance of rights and responsibilities consistent with the deeper moral agenda of an ethics of care.

While medical ethics follows contemporary tenets of autonomy rights consistent with an atomistic definition of personal identity, clinical medicine's own moral code is based on relation and responsibility, where patient autonomy traditionally plays a much reduced function. But as we will see, matters are not so simple, and I will argue that autonomy has a bivalent agenda. On the one hand, the concept accentuates the individuality of personhood, the distinctive and independent character of social identity. And this must be preserved inasmuch as the integrity of autonomy is a key component of how we define ourselves. On the other hand, persons are inseparable from their roles and identities within a social context. And being a patient radically alters the character of personal identity as compared to the normal setting, replacing "independence" with varying degrees of "dependence." The moral task, then, shifts from protecting personal autonomy to preserving personal dignity; in the process of doing the latter, the former also benefits. Differentiating the two categories of personal identity focuses my argument, for I wish to realign autonomy to better fit the particular requirements of the clinical setting. To accomplish this goal, a rather lengthy preamble is required.

Two Modalities of Selfhood

I begin by summarizing competing notions of selfhood—the "social self" and the "atomistic self" (see Sandel 1982 and Taylor 1989 for full descriptions). The proponents of the concept of the social self maintain that we are fundamentally what our social identifications confer on us. To be sure, there is a biological substrate of personality and cognitive abilities, but these are formless until socialization ensues and molds a person's character. From this perspective, it is meaningless to try to dissect away the prevailing social, cultural, historical, and psychological contingencies that make up human experience in order to reveal a core self, an identity that somehow resides separate from experience.

The philosophical tradition supporting this understanding is ancient, dating at least to Aristotle's definition of humans as social creatures. In the twentieth century the idea of personal identity as a social construction became a central theme of American sociology and is most directly linked to George Herbert Mead. In his posthumously published lecture, "A Contrast of Individualistic and Social Theories of the Self," he wrote of how the mind "can never find expression, and could never come into existence at all, except in terms of a social environment" (1934, 223), because of the very construction of self-consciousness:

The existence of private or "subjective" contents of experience does not alter the fact that self-consciousness involves the individual's becoming an object to himself by taking the attitudes of other individuals toward himself within an organized setting of social relationships, and that unless the individual had thus become an object to himself he would not be self-conscious or have a self at all. Apart from his social interactions with other individuals, he would not relate the private or "subjective" contents of his experience to himself, and he could not become aware of himself as such. (Mead 1934, 225–226)[1]

I would be hard-pressed to offer a more succinct and cogent statement of this position.

In contrast, those who advocate an atomistic conception of the self maintain that underlying our social identities is a deeper inner identity, one that is, in a sense, isolated and inviolate. Indeed, modern philosophy is generally acknowledged as commencing with Descartes' assertion that his own self-consciousness, as ultimately and irreducibly a "thinking thing," relieved him from skeptical doubt and allowed for the construction of a world unified and known through a sovereign human knowing faculty. Crucial to this construction is the independent and unmediated mind, which exists in some kind of free-floating cognitive "space." Separated from the universe that it perceives, Descartes' *res cogitans* is "freestanding" and neutral, for to be influenced and potentially prejudiced, or even tricked, by some social construction of knowledge would have crippled his endeavor. Indeed, the entire Enlightenment project built on this idea of individual rationality and independence of knowing.

Acknowledging that persons have complementary identities, individual and social, the distinctiveness of persons emphasizes, and perhaps even confers, the crucial political importance of unique and sovereign citizens as distinct from the roles they play. Because of the high value placed on independent reason and freedom of choice that leads to self-governance, the view of the self as individualistic and atomistic became a basic tenet of Enlightenment philosophy, which offered the conceptual infrastructure for the enlightened political systems based on such citizens. But beyond these political concerns, during the eighteenth century, the individual knower becomes the primary agent for acquiring knowledge, which could only be conceived as a product of private efforts. This individualistic effort was based on notions of scientific inquiry that required investigators to view the world with a dispassionate gaze and judgment. These capacities, in turn, required some *distanced* objectivity. Arising from personal experience, individual facts and opinions would then be pooled and compared in the public domain.

Historians have remarked how the scientific enterprise supported the political legitimization of revised relationships between the monarch and the citizen, and, vice versa, how the cultural notions of personhood supported the authority of science (e.g., Merton [1938] 1970; Jacob 1976). Each subscribed to an atomistic formulation of personhood, for whether engaged in scrutiny of a natural phenomenon (scientific) or deliberating on a political decision, the detached individual was regarded as an exemplar of epistemological and moral agency. The conception of the atomistic self has played a central part in the modern history of philosophy, and arguably has had a greater impact on moral and political philosophies than its erstwhile competitor. Indeed, an inner core identity has been regarded as essential to freedom of moral action. We now review this understanding and its evolution.

The Atomistic Self

Coincident with the English struggle to redefine the relationship of the monarchy with Parliament at the end of the seventeenth century, political theorists attempted to construct the self as an autonomous legal unit to fulfill certain liberal political goals. To do so, John Locke, for instance, extrapolated a new version of citizenship from a philosophical invention of the epistemological agent inspired by modern science (Locke [1700] 1975, 346–348). This neutral, rational, independent, objective "knowing agent" arose from two sources: science and politics. On the one hand, Locke's philosophy was regarded as an important contribution to Newtonian "natural philosophy" (as science was called then), where a radically detached witness might study mechanical nature dispassionately and objectively, and thereby obtain scientific truth. Thus the atomistic (or core) self was part of the early modern scientific conceit that regarded the knowing subject as totally divorced from the world in order to study it. Indeed, the Lockean subject assumes the power to view his objects neutrally, and thereby distance himself "from all the particular features which are objects of potential change" (Taylor 1989, 171). The first-person viewpoint, which demanded disengagement, would ideally become a "view from nowhere" (Nagel 1986)—neutral and universal, that is, no perspective was favored. Indeed, the self would so radically remove himself from the world that the ego would shrink to some "punctual point" and leave undisturbed the scene of scrutiny (Taylor 1989, 159ff.)

On the other hand, this newly conceived knower was usefully extrapolated to the civil world as a political agent. The atomistic citizen fit the liberal political ethos, where self-governance emerged as a new value tempered only to the extent that its exercise might infringe on the freedom of others (Locke [1690] 1980). Thus Locke's epistemological concerns merged with his moral ones—from an autonomous observer the autonomous citizen became the unit of government suspended between its own authority and its subordination to majority judgment.

Self became a forensic term, with new rights and obligations, and the very foundations of regal rule were thereby altered (MacPherson 1962). Locke can hardly be solely credited for this revolution, but he may be recognized as devising a philosophical understanding of the self that ensured its atomism—a separate identity free to think without bias and prejudice (a crucial characteristic of a liberal political understanding of free choice) and to know the world objectively (a critical capacity of a newfound scientific objectivity).

And what then is the self? Locke avoids identifying the self with any material or immaterial substance and thus distances himself from Descartes' "thinking thing," focusing instead on the phenomenology of an independent consciousness. Marked by its rationality, the memory of its thought and action, and its power of knowing the world and giving nature coherence, Locke's formulation configured "a self," albeit a "punctual" self, which recedes to a vanishing point of knowing. Accordingly, the person occupies no special place or unique focus of understanding, for each individual possesses a secure objectivity to survey the world from any perspective, and by tapping into a universal reason, to see that world rationally and objectively as all others would. From this point of view, individual cognitive and moral faculties are ultimately subsumed by natural law to universalize all knowledge and political discourse. These Enlightenment ideals of objectivity and rationality, the key faculties of moral and epistemological agency, became the lynchpins of the Weltanschauung of the period, and they are still very much governing precepts today despite attacks on their claims.

Focusing on the American experience, the indebtedness of the Founding Fathers to Locke has been amply documented (Zuckert 1994; Huyler 1995). Direct references to him in the Declaration of Independence and in the U.S. Constitution clearly exhibit his abiding influence in defining our citizenship, the basis of constitutional authority, the structure of our government, and the centrality of autonomous choice. I will not dwell on these political aspects of Locke's authority, but will rather focus on a second existential domain in which Lockean independence flourished, namely, in the guise of American individualism. It would be simplistic to lay complex notions of American individualism at Locke's doorstep, but he did provide a key conceptual architecture for cultural, religious, and commercial forces that were to find their expression in the frontier spirit of free enterprise, entrepreneurialism, and political freedom in its various social and religious guises. I am referring specifically to the notion of an atomistic self that not only has the characteristics allowing for objectivity, but underlying that neutral stance is the demand for distance and protection from invading interests and bias. In short, independence is a requirement for citizenship, commerce, religious observance, and in the end, psychological health. To be independent, and thereby become "all you can be," was the implicit and then explicit motto for the American dream. The free cowboy, the wild mountain man, the wandering sailor each personified, albeit in different forms, the American ideal. These are iconic instantiations of the autonomous American—a characteristic of the American psyche as much as a precept of citizenship and a powerful determinant of social relationships. In this regard, let us pause to follow the Lockean trajectory into the mid-nineteenth century to suggest how the atomistic self evolved. That cultural moment has continued to define a major component of American identity with incalculable effects on the social fabric of contemporary life.

To do so, I turn to the 1830s, when *individualism* was independently coined by two French commentators, Alexis de Tocqueville and Michel Chevalier, to describe the quaint Americans they encountered (Shain 1994, 90–92; see also 112ff.). Just as they surveyed American culture, Ralph Waldo Emerson was declaring the American Agenda in such essays as "The American Scholar" (1837), "The Divinity School Address" (1838), and "Self Reliance" (1841). But before these essays were conceived, Emerson sought to establish a new metaphysics for himself. In the aftermath of personal crises that resulted in resigning his pulpit in 1832, Emerson followed a complicated series of steps, which ended in his declaration of belief in a newly formed Transcendentalism that had emerged from German romanticism (Richardson 1995). This idealism, refracted by Samuel Taylor Coleridge, lodged itself in New England consciousness as a new form of religiosity in no small measure through Emerson's efforts. The key treatise, *Nature* (1836), presented a core self that eclipsed Locke's own formulation with a stark detachment that declared the inviolability of the individual in no uncertain terms. Indeed, the purity of communion with Nature, as with God, demanded a stark isolation.[2]

When Emerson joined the social domain, he championed a particular form of American individuality that celebrated an unbridled optimism about the potentiality of the American experience (Bellah et al., 1985; Gougeon 1990). Accordingly, the autonomy of the Emersonian self demands that each of us becomes the creator of her own house, of her own personhood. In that creative project, the self is the arbiter of the Good, the source of *poesis*, and the ultimate judge of knowledge. So while the core of our being may remain impenetrable, Emerson moves beyond the metaphysics of personhood to its moral structure: he heralds the potentiality of our personhood, to both define our individual aspirations and achieve them. American optimism is the keynote of his message, so that autonomy becomes both the rationale for mid-nineteenth century individualism, and its authority (see Lukes 1973 for a history of individualism). With such a charge, the ultimate locus of responsibility, both to fulfill personal goals and social obligations, resides squarely with the individual. External authority recedes as autonomy assumes a new lofty position in the hierarchy of values.

Emerson became the nineteenth century's great expositor of this American ideal. In celebrating the splendid primacy of the self, he is rightly regarded as an exemplar of his age. But his construction suffers a compromising ailment, perhaps a debilitating one for formulations of radical autonomy—reliance on the other. The theme I wish to draw out of Emerson's philosophy is perhaps a subtle one: he celebrated the individual; he recognized the social identity of the individual as part of a social community with obligations to that collective, but that involvement rested on a sacrosanct individualism. More specifically, the autonomy of persons was maintained even as identity might be influenced, or even configured, by social relationships. Thus the social did not threaten or compromise Emerson's philosophy of the individual, for he simply extended the boundaries of what the self might call its own.

Emerson's position is close to the political philosophies of Locke and Rousseau, who clearly saw that the state required individuals to subsume their identity, and often their private interests, to a larger collective. In fact, the "social contract" was based on that subordination. After all, inextricable from the independent self is one whose very identity is compromised by a social context. At best, in the formulation of the core self, the individual not only stands putatively alone in his judgment and moral authority (a position we will have occasion to examine later), *but* she also delegates that individual authority to a benevolent state and a community of peers. The moral law is thus balanced between the rights of persons and the needs of the commune, and autonomy as a criterion of the independent self assumes its rightful place only when each parameter is considered fairly.

The limits of this social orientation vis-à-vis Emerson's concept of individuality is dramatically illustrated by his protégé, Henry David Thoreau, who more consistently drew the consequences of Emerson's own metaphysics of selfhood. Thoreau understood that to be a self-reliant individual who must build his own "house," a distancing from the community was required. Such an individual would engage in civil disobedience, espouse solitude, and pursue material and spiritual goals relentlessly determined by his own inner moral compass (Tauber 2001; 2003b).[3] One might easily conjecture that these differing interpretations revealed more about the respective psychologies of the two men, but I believe that beyond the emotional component, Thoreau understood the implications of Emerson's own philosophy better than the master himself did. The reason is not difficult to fathom: Emerson's vision of self-reliance, on which this edifice of identity was built, remained (as discussed below) tethered to an other; Thoreau was free of such encumbrances, and while his political and social morality might appear to us as radical (Tauber 2001, 188–194), and even shocking, it is more consistent with the philosophy of individualism than Emerson's.

Emersonian autonomy has a complex dual allegiance to the independence of the individual and that person's affiliation and responsibility to a greater whole. This self could stand alone only because it partook of the divine. Much as Descartes had done three centuries earlier, Emerson found his relationship to God, and ultimately the character of his own person, inextricably intertwined and made explicit by a self-conscious dependence on God. Emerson's self-reliance, the credo we associate with rugged American individualism, is, in fact, for him not autonomy, but reliance on God: "If he [man] rests at last on the divine soul, I see not how it can be otherwise" ("Circles," [1841] 1979, 182). But not reliance in some passive "so be God's will," but in the recognition that our own freed being is a manifestation of our own divinity. Indeed, Emerson repeatedly asserts that reliance should be placed in that which is his ultimate cause.[4] If man fails to accept this essential dependence, Emerson says alienation follows. The finite human, the experiencing person, is as much a "stranger in nature as we are aliens from God" ("Spirit," in *Nature*, [1836] 1971, 39). The antidote is to recognize the internalization of the Divine.

Given Emerson's strong religious background, this formulation, not surprisingly, remains firmly oriented toward the theological education he received and then promoted as a pulpit minister. Accordingly, while American culture is marked by its pluralism and has come to its particular legacy by combining diverse political and social traditions (Macfarlane 1978; Fischer 1989), its Puritan and nonconforming Protestant religious heritage offer a particularly rich template for defining personal identity with a particular emphasis on self-responsibility. Emersonian self-reliance, self-direction, and authenticity faithfully reflect this religious context. Couple these religious tenets to economic optimism, political meliorism, and psychological perfectability, and we see Emerson seamlessly knitting together his notions of personal identity with threads of various yarns. He thus became a conduit of Protestant theology into a nonsectarian world.[5]

From this historical perspective, autonomy, usually considered as deriving from the political domain, wears a different cloak: in the twenty-first century, the individual attains her sense of autonomy through a complex translation of an abiding religious sensibility of spiritual reunion, but now recast in secular terms. According to this thesis, the fundamental structure of salvation is the same. The ideal self has become a secularized version of Protestant ascetic and mystical visions of the soul's election through human choice, personal effort, and moral action (Kirschner 1996, 95ff.). These depend on a particular understanding of human agency, one in which autonomy—freedom of choice and sanctity of judgment—figures prominently. In this view, contemporary ideals of the self draw on religious wisdom about salvation, albeit in disguised forms of secular theodicy (Weber [1915] 1946, 358–359).

This religious origin of autonomy has been obscured, for the following generation heard Nietzsche's proclamation that "God is dead." (Ironically, Nietzsche had closely read Emerson and found the preambles to *Beyond Good and Evil* and the *Will to Power* in the Transcendentalist's anthem of self-reliance, self-responsibility, and individualism (Stack 1992).) Emerson's formulation seemingly loses its foundations if religion lacks authority, and without the divine making its claims, people are left to fashion belief on other sources of meaning, which is, of course, a risky "wager" (Seligman 2000). But the foundations of this Western sensibility of selfhood are not so easily cast off. The basic structure remains.

With the rise of secularism in the nineteenth century and its dominance in the twentieth (Wilson 1999), the Emersonian vision of Man standing independently with God was eclipsed by others, but the underlying basis of *relationship* as constitutive to identity remained: Marx placed people inextricably in their social milieu—the divine other became "work" or social "class" and thereby defined identity by social context and a new historical interpretation of society's structure and evolution. At least two different moral courses were followed from this position: Some would see humans as alienated and existentially self-defining (à la Nietzsche), while others, following the social lead (per Marx, Mead, and Weber), would construe relationships and social affiliations as constitutive of personal identity. In this latter view, whether couched in terms of social, historical, or psychological determinism, identity assumed various roles inextricable from the social world of other persons.

In summary, if one substitutes *relationship* as a generic term for Emerson's *reliance*, we see that the basic structure of identity has not been so radically challenged in the post-Nietzschean world. Indeed, an interplay of two themes is at work: "individualism" and "relationship" are each derived from a religious sensibility, which remains at the foundation of these more recent secularized conceptions. While one must strive in worldly activities to achieve spiritual election, it is the experience, open to all, of divine contact within one's soul that testifies to the more permanent and definitive salvation to come. According to this interpretation, Emerson presented his concept of individualism and self-reliance as an ironic dependency, which in turn translated a deeper under-standing of personal salvation, albeit from a religious context into a secular one (Tauber 2003b).[6]

In the twentieth century, these ideas continued to exert a powerful influence. With the subordination of the human relationship to God, other kinds of relationship were substituted, a matter discussed below. But for now, suffice it to summarize that on this reading, "autonomy"—generally understood as an expression of individuality and independ-ence—is a complex amalgam of self-reliance and dependency, which thus confers a dual understanding of identity: individual persons are insepa-rable from a constellation of others. So, we oversimplify, if not distort, the concept of autonomy (a concept born with an atomistic under-standing of personal identity) when we fail to recognize the constitutive character of the other. This dualistic construction has profound impli-cations for moral philosophy, a topic that is considered more fully later in this chapter.

The Rational Self: Kant

I must now take a step back and consider a second major tributary con-tributing to our notions of autonomy. Instead of focusing on selfhood as the organizing structure of the discussion, I will turn to the role of ration-ality—that is, its role in conferring moral structure on our behavior. To do so, I will consider two contrasting philosophical visions of moral agency, that of Immanuel Kant and David Hume. In neither case does selfhood per se play a significant role. Neither philosopher gave much credence to the possibility of "knowing" the self. In Kant's case, he argued that there must be some apparatus that perceived the world and organized perceptions according to certain fundamental categories of knowing (e.g., space, time, number, causality). Kant believed that this cognitive apparatus developed concepts and understanding based on some integrative mind function. His "transcendental unity of the apper-ception" provided the cognitive conditions by which the world could be known. And this inner ego was epistemologically equivalent to a natural object, which had important implications. For Kant, the objects found in the natural world could not be known in themselves (they could only be known through our human faculties or mechanical extensions of those faculties), so consequently, the self remained elusive and fundamentally unknowable.[7] In short, comparable to a natural object, "the self" or the ego could not be directly perceived and our self-consciousness then became just another natural object for scrutiny. It had a *noumenal* (the thing-in-itself) nature (unknowable by human faculties) and a *phenomenal* character (as defined by self-consciousness, which employed the same faculties by which we know the world).

Hume gave up the search for a continuous self, a core identity or ego, and settled for a bundle of perceptions, linked by memory as sufficient for the psychological ease of identifying our personhood. Unlike Kant he required no transcendental apparatus, and he skeptically concluded that our self-consciousness was essentially a psychological artifact.[8] For Hume, reason was a derivative function to arbitrate a more fundamental human characteristic, the emotions, or in the vernacular of the day, the "passions." I will consider Hume's views in two contexts: here, in contrast to Kant, and later in regard to the foundation he offers for contemporary critics of strong forms of autonomy. Suffice it now to summarily characterize each of these views of selfhood and move to their central concerns, namely, the role of reason as the mediator or vehicle of judgment. I begin with Kant.

Philosophy both led and followed the momentous political changes of the seventeenth and eighteenth centuries that saw monarchial power eroded, religious authority weakened, and egalitarian rights expanded. In the wake of this drastically altered social and political landscape, moral philosophers struggled to provide a framework by which a new ethics and political philosophy might support and guide the new order. Liberal democracy required a philosophy that effectively extended religious independence (a question of personal belief) to moral independence (a question of private moral authority). In that effort, two looming questions appeared: First, if religion was no longer the source of moral authority, what was to take its place? And second, if morality was an individual responsibility, what would sustain a society of people holding differing interests?

In many ways, an answer to the second question was more readily arrived at than an answer to the first. The new egalitarian moral pluralism supported both a philosophical and a political solution: moral and political deliberation must be based on mutual respect. Morality was reconceived from a dogmatic religious code to one that provided some basic rules by which people could live together despite their differences about ultimate matters. And why would people be mutually respectful? The initial responses: laws were followed either because of fear of punishment or they were adhered to because humans were intrinsically virtuous, seeking either a communal utilitarian end or, as already noted about Scottish Enlightenment teaching, personal perfection.

Kant substituted the notion of rational moral imperative for received religious wisdom in answer to the first question I posed concerning the source of moral order. And to the second question as to why humans are moral, he offered a radical notion of self-governance, one based on his assessment of human rationality. This is a crucial turn, namely, that while the basis of moral law resides beyond human understanding, our rationality nevertheless mediates our ability to know it and follow it. This places moral responsibility firmly on us, enacted by a particular faculty of our human character—the rational mind. So just as our "pure reason" allowed us to construct and thereby know the natural world (Kant [1781, 1787] 1998), so too would our "practical reason" guide us in constructing a human moral universe (Kant [1785] 1996).[9]

Kant radicalized moral philosophy by denying all those philosophies that held, in one form or another, that the ends justified the means. For Kant, morality is neither the pursuit of good results nor obedience to divine will. He argued instead for moral necessity—that is, he thought that we must act in accord with moral principle whether such action was in our supposed best interest or not. He maintained that through the exercise of human reason one might make moral choices that all must follow. Thus for Kant, the idea of "the right" was individually determined, not by personal caprice but by the inviolate ability of humans to interpret a universally accessible moral universe through the exercise of reason. The inner logic is quite simple. To be moral, we must be responsible for our actions. To be responsible, we must be able to choose freely. To choose freely, we must be autonomous. And the tool of human autonomy was human rationality. The free exercise of rationality would lead us to choose, whether to our own benefit or not, a choice applicable to everyone. In short, according to Kant, rationality is the means of exercising our freedom *and* the common moral glue that binds each to the same code of choice unless judgment is clouded. Thus his moral philosophy allowed the free exercise of individual moral reason to self-determine rational conduct. And therein rested the basis of human freedom and autonomy.

For Kant, autonomy characterized the ability of humans to control themselves through their own moral reason, which is independent of subjective wants and needs. Humans might even oppose their own desires because they have a sufficient (rational) imperative to act as they ought in reference to a self-perceived moral understanding. In short, "The Kantian self is literally "auto-nomous," that is, defined by a *self-legislation* that is carried out on itself as well as by itself" (Ameriks 2000, 4). This seems to offer autonomy, as an expression of an individualistic self, an august standing. This last point is of special interest to our own venture, because given the common understanding of autonomy as "independence" (in addition to its connotations of freedom and self-determination), it is telling that Kant would, on the one hand, so firmly place moral decision making in the independent autonomous individual and, at the same time, call on that moral agent to find the common, universal morality to which all rational humans might subscribe. Is there an inconsistency here, or only an inner tension? In other words, how might a Kantian situate a philosophy that currently is invoked by those on the continuum from egalitarianism to libertarianism with an eye toward establishing the social basis for a common morality?

Contemporary American neo-Kantians, whose strongest advocate was John Rawls, have forcefully argued for a social ethical interpretation. In *A Theory of Justice* ([1971] 1999), Rawls, like Kant, builds an ethics on a purely rational moral agent, who makes choices behind a "veil of ignorance" (pp. 118ff.). Rawls uses a hypothetical social contract in which each person is asked to consider options from an impartial point of view, the so-called "original position" (pp. 15–19). Here, all individuals are equally ignorant of the individual characteristics and advantages they posses or might acquire, so by the dictates of the "veil of ignorance," rational choice must be both necessary and sufficient for the selection of public moral principles: "The parties arrive at their choice together as free and equal rational persons knowing only that those circumstances obtain which give rise to the need for principles of justice" (p. 222). Accordingly, individuals must be blind to their individual desires, interests, and objectives, and in such a just society, reason thus dominates selfish desire. Autonomy arises from this common stock of rationality shared by moral agents, because in the original position persons choose and abide by a moral law, which is characteristic of their rational, independent, and disinterested human character. There is a deep social cohesive quality to Rawls's construction, inasmuch as he places a premium on the cooperative nature of morality from which justice must derive, and he thus limits individual autonomy by disallowing even the most conscientious actions if they violate public principles.[10]

Christine Korsgaard extends Rawl's position by observing that one may construct public reasons—that is, reasons that have normative force—starting from the assumption that reasons are private by a rather simple exchange: "If I have reason to take your reasons into account and you have reason to take my reasons into account, then we have reason to share our reasons, and we could just as well call them all *our* reasons: public reasons. So the public character of reasons is as it were *created* by the reciprocal exchange of inherently private reasons, where that in turn is forced on us by the content of the private reasons themselves" (Korsgaard 1996, 133–134; emphasis in original). She thus moves private morality, governed by some private, atomistic individuality, to a public domain in which autonomous individuals buy into public reason and cash out ethical behavior. The emphasis shifts, therefore, from a morality focused on the individual to a morality centered on the individual's abiding relationships to family, community, and the state. Because these relations and the reason that govern them must be factored into the calculus of choice, private reason finds itself engaged in a social exchange. Thus the boundary dividing the public and private domains becomes blurred.

Barbara Herman (1993, vii) complements this interpretation of the social character of Kantian ethics by arguing that "Kant's ethics has been the captive of his critics" (by which she means, by and large, rights-based deontologists), and rather than a deontological ethics of duties and obligations, Kant's project is better regarded as "a correct analysis of "the

Good" understood as the ultimate determining ground of all action" (p. 210). Shifting from a rule-based ethics, centered on duty, to a value-based morality focused on defining the Good, Herman is moving against the historical tide of traditional Kantian scholarship, but she and Korsgaard are seeking to rescue Kant from the atomistic individualists who would claim an individualist-based autonomy as the motive force of morality. In contradistinction, Herman and Korsgaard argue that autonomy is better regarded as in the employ of finding the common good. Accordingly, each person exercises moral choices within the commonality of public reason. Autonomy then becomes the challenge of exercising the rationally based individual choice within the context of communal rationality. The importance of this approach will become apparent when we consider moral theories that contrast with those based on a nineteenth-century ideal of individualistic autonomy.

In sum, autonomy, according to Kant, resides in the person's rational ability to independently perceive and act on an a priori moral dictate in the particular setting of contingent and individual moral choice. Self-governance has thereby been elevated further. Indeed, Kant "held that we are self-governing because we are autonomous" (Schneewind 1998, 6). The moral is both understood and followed by our own free choice and through this self-imposition humans are provided with the motive to obey, or as Jerry Schneewind (1992, 327) puts it, "Practical [moral] reason generates its own unique motive."

In other words, each of us is not only responsible for acting ethically, we are ultimately responsible for formulating those actions rationally. And if action and legislation are generated by individual interpretation of a universal moral ideal, how does a society of free people sustain a just community? The Kantian three-part answer: (1) everyone is endowed with the ability to interpret moral truth, and like the laws of nature comprehended by "pure reason," a unified moral order is analogously revealed by "practical reason"; (2) our human character dictates that we follow this perceived "ought" as best we might because we are *rational*; and (3) a social ethic evolves from an appreciation that our rational choices are consistent with those of our group from which a "public" rationality emerges.

The Self and Its Passions: Hume

The Kantians are fighting a pitched battle against the skeptics. For instance, Bernard Williams (1985) represents those who see little hope for Kant's formulation, because it resides on a prevailing uniform rationality, which he believes no longer appears correct in our pluralistic era. In this view, the Kantian idea of autonomy and its operation arose within the culturally homogeneous social and intellectual milieu of the European Enlightenment. That milieu is gone forever, and the concept, accordingly, has metamorphosed over the past two centuries. Obviously, our rational faculty is central to Kant's understanding of human freedom, moral choice, and ethical action, but the centrality of reason was already contested by David Hume, and it was to this challenge that Kant originally responded. Hume maintained a commonsense view of moral behavior: it is impossible for reason alone to account for ethical motivation, because passion and desire are each elements in the complex calculus of morality, and emotion is neither rational nor irrational (Lindley 1986, 26ff.). There can be no categorical rational imperative, for people determine their actions not solely by a rationality that might "fix" upon such a universal directive (nor even a communal rationality), but also by their individual goals motivated and governed by nonrational "passions." From this perspective, one choice cannot necessarily be classified as more "rational" than another.

Hume's essential insight was that not everyone has to reason in the same way, and consequently individuals might arrive at divergent choices, each of which may be reasonable. Indeed, it is a truism that people hardly reason impartially, nor are they immune from idiosyncratic inclinations or feelings. But Hume went further. In *A Treatise of Human Nature*, he wrote: "In order to shew the fallacy of all this philosophy [the superiority of reason over passion], I shall endeavour to prove *first*, that reason alone can never be a motive to any action of the will; and *secondly*, that it can never oppose passion in the direction of the will" (Hume [1739] 1978, 413). Hume reconfigured the relative roles of reason and emotion, proposing that reason was only a tool for deliberation and hardly could suffice as the source of moral choice and motivation. He maintained that preferences or desires cannot be motivated by reason alone, and that reason can only help direct our choice: "A belief, desire, feeling, or action may be rationally required, rationally permitted, or rationally proscribed, [so that] unless they derive from false beliefs, they are all rationally permissible" (Lindley 1986, 30). From this perspective, goals are determined by a complex array of psychological and cultural factors, of which rational order may play only a small part. In what has become a famous hyperbole, Hume asserted, "Tis not contrary to reason to prefer the destruction of the whole world to the scratching of my finger" (Hume [1739] 1978, 416). No wonder Kant was outraged!

The essential disagreement between Kant and Hume is over the putative role of reason in moral decision making. For Kant, reason is the sole arbiter of self-governance. Hume was skeptical of reason's hegemony, because he believed that the sentiments fix the agent's ultimate ends and reason is left to determine the best way of achieving those goals. So where does this leave autonomy in Hume's moral philosophy? Autonomy per se is not a category in Hume's writings, but its place may easily be located as we unpack his notions of liberty and freedom.

For Kant, freedom was the critical factor in moral action, otherwise how might we be held accountable? In seeking moral action freed of determinism, he found that freedom in the exercise of reason (Allison 1990). Accordingly, if one reasons freely, moral choice is concomitantly free. As noted, Hume was skeptical both of reason's freedom from self-interested emotional influences he called the sentiments or passions, and of reason's power. Hume devised a more subtle attack on a rationality-based morality by arguing that determinism was compatible with liberty and any confusion was the result of a linguistic snarl. *Liberty* and *necessity* are often paired as opposites, but the true opposite of *liberty* is *compulsion*, and necessity's opposite is *chance* or *randomness* (Lindley 1986). Actions, including human actions, may be explained as "necessary" in the sense they do not occur at random. And *liberty* should be understood as any act performed without compulsion—that is, against individual choice. A prisoner may be forced to act in a certain way; whether I get up and leave my house or not is freely chosen according to my will (Hume [1748] 1975, 95). Autonomy then corresponds to

Hume's understanding of liberty, namely that "to be autonomous is simply to act on those of your rationally permissible desires, which most take your fancy—to do as you choose" (Lindley 1986, 33).

Criticism of Hume's position generally dwells on the unsure footing of "proper deliberation" that determines whether the suppositions underlying reason's exercise are true or false. To act with false suppositions destroys the entire enterprise, and thus how to ensure that reason's grounding is firm has remained a crucial sticking point (Brandt 1979; Parfit 1984). How is all relevant information assured access, and perhaps more to the point, how do preferences necessarily follow ideal rational deliberations? The entire rational inquiry is set by a host of underlying suppositions and forces—cultural, historical, and personal—so that "ideal deliberation" cannot attain neutrality and complete closure. In short, rationality is context-dependent and value-ridden, which is not to say that we do not act rationally, but at the same time, acting morally requires more than just rationality. The Humean position only asserts that moral action derives from a deeper sense of obligation or choice than that dictated by reason alone. For instance, a beggar approaches me for money. I may have reasons for or against responding to him, but the decision is not solely decided by some neutral rationality. I may be in a rush; I may be repulsed; I may have no small change; I may be financially strapped myself. But given these rational strictures, I give anyway, perhaps too much for reasons that have little to do with rational choice as framed by some neutral rational construction about charity, philanthropy, social justice, or the like. As a Humean, I give because I feel compassion or sympathy, and by giving I feel better about myself. These emotions are not rational in the ordinary sense of the word, but they are rational in the context of choice Hume defines as a composite of emotion and rationality. And more to the point for our concerns, the choice is "free." Some would give; most would not.

Simply, from Hume's point of view, rationality and autonomy are not coextensive; pure rationality is a conceit and furthermore, it cannot ensure moral responsibility; finally, actions cannot be reduced to rational choice considering the complex array of social, existential, and personal factors that come into play in any decision. Hume offered a minimalist conception of autonomy. To be autonomous is simply to do as one chooses, provided one is not acting irrationally—that is, by using faulty reason. The crucial caveat is that the agent must be able to stand back from desires and beliefs in order to scrutinize them skeptically and allow for deliberation about the value of those ordering sentiments. In that process, conflicting desires and the actions resulting from differences with others must be resolvable. Hume offered no perspective on this central problem of ethics.

The Humean position has been extended by at least four prominent postmodern critiques of selfhood: psychoanalytic theory, Foucault's theories of power and agency, feminist theories of gender differences and otherness, and, finally, various poststructural philosophical schools ranging from Derrida-inspired deconstructions to post-Wittgensteinian analytics. What holds these various perspectives on the "critique of the subject" together is the recognition that the ideal self is hardly self-transparent, psychically unified (or rational), or able to achieve self-mastery (Mackenzie and Stoljar 2000). Autonomy becomes highly problematic when the moral agent is depicted as conflict-driven, often self-deluded, fundamentally opaque to themselves, and driven by archaic drives and desires that they are unaware of and consequently unable to control. These forces may be intrapsychic (Freud) or social (Mead)—that is, persons constituted within and by regimes, discourses, and power of which they have little knowledge or control (Rose 1990, 1998)—or by historically specified cultural ideals that masquerade as universal norms (Butler 1990). In any case, in these views, self-will, self-determining free choice, is a delusion of unrecognized configurations of psychic, political, or historical forces. In short, current fashion dresses Hume in the garb of a debunked rational deliberation—a garment that reveals the Emperor's nakedness!

In an age marked by an explosion of information (often contradictory), sensitivity to other cultural views (sowing a moral relativism), and a well-earned skepticism of our own rationalities, I believe Hume's skeptical position has generally prevailed. In regarding moral distinctions as arising from our subjectivity, inner drives, and the emotions, which are subsequently given rationales to gain authority, he set the groundwork for our post-Freudian self-consciousness of the fallibility of rationality and the determinism embedded in the deep structures of our psyches.

Most would regard Kant's principle of free will as a philosophical construction whose demands for human conduct cannot be fulfilled, and by warning us to act with "reason independently of inclination" (Kant [1785] 1996, 66 [4:413]), his "view of *theoretical* man is hopelessly estranged from *real* man" (Katz 1984, 109). Reason and unreason must be taken into account, because human beings are subject to the influence of both. Reason as the mediator of moral action simply places too high a premium on rationality, which increasingly appears, outside the natural sciences, as itself culturally and historically contingent. In Foucauldian terms, ethics becomes an exercise in power, and morality, as an execution of rationality, simply has left the playing field to others.

Kantian ethics still has much appeal, and we would be derelict to cede the playing fields too easily to the followers of Hume and Foucault. We recognize that the "truth" lies somewhere that still allows for reason. Indeed, Reason still makes its claims and for those eager to save a Kantian perspective, I review Onora O'Neill's vivid interpretation of "principled autonomy" in the next section, and then in the following one, I consider John Stuart Mill's attempt to synthesize the Humean and Kantian positions.

Principled Autonomy

The rescue of Kantian ethics resides in its social consciousness, as mentioned in the writings of Rawls, Korsgaard, and Herman. Their "social interpretation," as opposed to libertarian ones (e.g., Nozick 1974), rests on an important distinction: Kant never refers to an *autonomous self* or an *autonomous person* or an *autonomous individual*, but rather to the *autonomy of reason*, the *autonomy of ethics*, the *autonomy of principles*, and the *autonomy of willing* (O'Neill 2002, 83). (Autonomous individualism, associated with a liberated self, freed from political, religious, and social bonds, is a distinctly post-Kantian modification attached during the romantic era (Tauber 2001).) Properly, Kantian autonomy is "principled autonomy," not "individual autonomy" (O'Neill 2002). Persons choose their moral actions according to how principles of action could be chosen by all—that is, moral principles are those that might be universalized, or fit to be universal laws. Hence, so-called principled autonomy is not something one *has*, nor is it equated with personal independence or self-expression. Rather, it is the self-legislated moral behavior prescribed by principles that could be laws for all. In other words, "For Kant autonomy is *not relational, not graduated, not a form of self-expression*; it is a matter of acting on certain principles, and specifically on principles of obligation" (O'Neill 2002, 83–84). Accordingly, autonomy only makes sense as duties or obligations are met, of which respect for the rights of others is paramount.

Allen Wood (1999, 156) points to two potentially fatal flaws in Kant's formulation. Given the centrality of the autonomy of the will as the ground of moral obligation, he suggests that (1) if one's own will is the author of an individual's obligations, it seems as if individual discretion is allowed in determining the content and binding of those duties (thereby contradicting their obligatory character), and (2) if Kantians counter that it is the rationality of these laws that makes them binding, the source of obligation is only transferred from an individual's will to the canons of rationality. If the second objection is correct, Kant is rightly accused of retreating from grounding morality in principled autonomy, and substitutes some previously given conception of the good or of reason. Onora O'Neill (2002, 90–91) addresses these criticisms by showing how Kant regarded principled autonomy itself as the fundamental principle of reason: "The power to judge autonomously—that is, freely (according to principles of thought in general)—is called reason" (Kant [1798] 1996, 255 [7:27]). Moral agency is thus grounded in our ability to discern moral principles—to judge and choose, to act and execute according to what might reasonably be applied to others. In short, principled autonomy is a formulation of the basic requirements of all reasoning. Thus, according to O'Neill, moral will is primary, not reason, and moreover, this will is the foundation of reason itself! Interestingly, on this reading, reason's function is delimited quite clearly: (1) the antecedent standards of reason are unknown and unknowable, and (2) reason is like a currency—ideas must be exchanged, justifications must be accepted, options and choices must be understood, and actions must be explained. And most important,

Reason must subject itself to critique in all its undertakings, and cannot restrict the freedom of critique through any prohibition without damaging itself and drawing upon itself a disadvantageous suspicion. Now there may be nothing so important because of its utility, nothing so holy, that it may be exempted from the searching review and inspection, which knows no respect for persons. The very existence of reason depends upon this freedom, which has no dictatorial authority, but whose claim is never anything more than in the agreement of free citizens, each of whom must be able to express his reservations, indeed even his veto, without holding back. (Kant [1781, 1787] 1998, 643 [A738/B766])

In this famous quote, Kant encapsulates the Enlightenment project: reason is both the medium of morals and action, but it has no final dictatorial authority and is thus always subject to criticism. In what Adam Seligman (2000) calls "modernity's wager," Kant presents the gambit to liberate the modern individual from external social expectations and religious norms by supplementing them with the rational self as its own moral authority. But we cannot appeal to some final rational authority, or even rationality itself, to discover the foundations of morality:

Reasoning . . . is simply a matter of striving for principled autonomy in the spheres of thinking and of action. Autonomy in thinking is no more—but also no less—than the attempt to conduct thinking (speaking, writing) on principles on which all others whom we address could also conduct their thinking. . . . Autonomy in action is no more—but also no less—than the attempt to act on principles on which all others could act. Wood's dilemma is avoided because Kantian autonomy is neither derived from an antecedently given but unjustified account of reason (hence unreasoned), nor lacking in structure (hence willful and arbitrary); principled autonomy itself supplies basic structures of reasoning. (O'Neill 2002, 94)

In this scheme, (1) reason becomes the vehicle of moral discourse; (2) moral agents, discover and act according to principled autonomy; (3) the will that might discover a universalized moral imperative has no prior antecedent or given moral code; and (4) the exchange of reasons generated by autonomous individuals creates a community's rationality that may be freely understood and then chosen. So in this view, Kant dispensed with all sovereignty, including reason's own claims, established self-governance as the basic characteristic of ways of thinking and willing, and in so doing, created a moral "space" in which external authority was replaced with individual responsibility and communal normative standards. He thereby set the foundations for later conceptions of the self and its moral structure.

Mill and Contemporary Utilitarianism

I wish to follow one more line of criticism that seeks to place autonomy at an appropriate resting place between the original Kantian and Humean positions. John Stuart Mill's *On Liberty* ([1859] 1972) and *Utilitarianism* ([1861] 1972) offer a reconstruction that has had a vast impact on our own understanding. Mill's inquiry is framed by Hume's position: To what extent is moral reason in the employ of hidden motives and thus fixed by ultimate ends? Despite Hume's valid claims, Mill still asserted that theoretical rationality is intrinsically desirable, apart from any instrumental value it may have, not only serving as the means toward achieving the most harmonious social interactions, but also constitutive to the flourishing of individual growth and development (Lindley 1986, 49). Accordingly, the quest for truth is a good in itself and essential for autonomy, because individual fulfillment or avoidance of harm—more broadly, the control of one's life—depends on minimizing or eliminating the influence of false beliefs or incomplete information.

The crucial turn following Hume is that not only does autonomy require that people optimally (rationally) pursue their nonrational goals as best they can, they actually should not be deluded about the nature of their goals and the consequences of their actions. Mill is espousing the liberal credo of free choice informed by knowledge, because irrational beliefs compromise free and thus informed choice, which is essential to decision making by autonomous agents. Mill thus situates himself between Kant and Hume by critically acknowledging the role of hidden motives and emotional needs—that is, the extrarational influences on our choices—but at the same time by elevating reason he claimed that humans may, through deliberation, arrive at ethical choices, which modify base inclinations.

Mill is credited with being the first to attempt an account of individual autonomy within a naturalistic account of action. *On Liberty* asserts that character and individuality require that persons "own" or identify with certain desires, by making them their own in the sense of both acknowledging them and assuming responsibility for acting on them. To choose, then, is not arbitrary but rests on some sense of inner selfhood and moral identity, and so emotion and desires are molded into character. Mill thus admits the passions, but sees their control as the critical element of moral agents.

By championing the role of reason, Mill asserts autonomy as the result of reason, which permits human self-determination and self-discovery of capacities and limits. One might challenge whether such "higher" pursuits are superior to "lower" ones, but Mill argued that reflexive thought and deliberate choice allow human beings to realize their full potential by the ongoing revision of their goals and options (Gray 1983, 85). Reason, instrumentally directed at attaining human flourishing, confers the capacity to make a distinctly human, that is, freely chosen, world (a widely held romantic idea (Tauber 2001)). Of course, one may dispute that self-determination is an ultimate value, or that deliberation might stem the flood of determinative influences on our lives. Be that as it may, Mill's understanding of autonomy or individual liberty, which contains a hefty dose of autonomous choice and which is based on judicious reason, offers a foundation for later philosophers, and indeed, has launched several influential contemporary models of autonomy.

But this balanced position still leaves considerable scope for reason to govern moral choices. We might still ask, If we discard the notion of a universal moral imperative, what takes its place? What, indeed, grounds our own morality and that of society? A constellation of individuals without such an orienting structure may be doomed to chaos as they argue their own rational choices, and there are some, to be sure, who believe that we actually live with various forms of moral anarchy. The optimists think we are only philosophically confused, for we do, in fact, have stable political institutions supported by a common law. The crisis, if one exists, does not seem to be in self-governance per se—we continue to tax ourselves quite ably to build bridges and educate our children. Rather, the issue is whether such a pragmatic attitude suffices for a moral code in the absence of some comprehensive philosophical understanding.

Pragmatists from John Dewey (Dewey [1888] 1997; Diggins 1994) to Richard Rorty (1999) have trusted the common sense of reasonable persons, who in free exchange derive the best (right) course based on reasoned judgment and informed opinion. This attitude may be traced back directly to Mill ([1859] 1972, 88):

Why is it, then, that there is on the whole a preponderance among mankind of rational opinions and rational conduct? If there really is this preponderance—which there must be unless human affairs are, and have always been, in an almost desperate state—it is owing to a quality of the human mind, the source of everything respectable in man either as an intellectual or as a moral being, namely, that his errors are corrigible. He is capable of rectifying his mistakes, by discussion and experience. . . . Wrong opinions and practices gradually yield to fact and argument. . . . The steady habit of correcting and completing his own opinion by collating it with those of others, so far from causing doubt and hesitation in carrying it into practice, is the only stable foundation for a just reliance on it.

But dissenters abound. From Nietzsche ([1887] 1967) to Williams (1985), philosophers have despaired at establishing a rational basis for ethics and mistrusted the pragmatic strategies offered by Mill and his followers, who trust that in the process of orderly discussion and debate a reason-based decision emerges. Skepticism rightly abounds from such attitudes, but it seems to me that we have increasingly become moral pragmatists, in Rorty's (1999) understanding of the term, with regard to how we determine moral action, both personally and in the public arena. I particularly like Tristram Engelhardt's (1996, 79) formulation: "Ever more individuals live more of an aesthetic than a moral life. . . . They are more than tolerant. They are ecumenical cosmopolitans who have framed a morality of shifting content and unburdensome obligations."

Now, *autonomy* often means political independence: individuals acting in self-assembly and self-governance under the principle of permission, "justified in terms of the morality of mutual respect" (Engelhardt 1996, 119). Thus persons remain "the source of general secular moral authority" (p. 119). But this is certainly a dilute potion, as forthrightly acknowledged by Engelhardt himself, when he notes that he has "rebaptized 'the principle of autonomy' with the name 'principle of permission' to indicate better that what is at stake is not some value possessed by autonomy or liberty, but the recognition that secular moral authority is derived from the permission of those involved in a common undertaking" (p. xi). In other words, the moral focus has shifted from the individual making independent choices to the individual consenting to be part of collective decision making.

Part of this contemporary formulation is dictated by the nature of our complex culture, where we must delegate decisions too technical for non-experts to comprehend. General citizens do not expect to become fully conversant with the complexities of those choices—contending matters of fact, the context of those facts, the diverse social and political implications of choices, the history of the problem, and so on. Decision making becomes a technical endeavor, informed by experts and delegated to offer options in a most general sense. This leaves our personal ethics much closer to Rousseau's social contract than to Kant's ideas by subordinating our individual choice to others, who we deem better informed. Indeed, the Kantian elaboration of autonomy has been recast as a form of contractualism, whose deontological flavor has been retained as "respect for individuals."

Contractualism accommodates a moral pragmatism composed of various strands. A virtue component heavily invests morality; a reflexive equilibrium adjudicates competing demands for justice; and given the moral and political complexities of vying interests and the danger of a power-dominated system of justice, a rights-based individualism has staked out the limits of communal interests. These are potentially disparate orientations, and I regard each element as part of a mosaic of values and strategies that are assembled in various ways to accommodate differing social challenges. Our pragmatic approach is ultimately a contingent product in a galaxy of options, each of which might be assembled into a different order depending on the particular social or political context. But an overriding precept is dominant: because we have competing moral coordinates, our ethics are largely directed at accommodating diversity. We seek to protect the insularity of those living in disparate lifestyles, as Mill advised in *On Liberty*.[11] Only through tolerance does our diversity support coherence. And that diversity is reflected in the moral strategies adopted to achieve our utilitarian goals.

This is, simply, a pragmatic accommodation to the moral heterogeneity of our society. We steadfastly hold on to the fundamental notion of autonomy as a basic value, but it has mutated into a principle that enables individuals to find their place in communal decision making and action. We obviously remain persons, but our individuality has been largely subordinated to the collective in ways hardly imaginable to Emerson and Thoreau. We adjust our ethical compass to operate in competing force fields, each of which claims legitimacy. Our moral plight, then, is to find an acceptable balance of differing interests in order to preserve the fragile equilibrium of free association. After all, permission is granted only as long as persons of different moral persuasions believe that their greater interest remains within the larger group.

We practice a form of self-governance to be sure, but Rawls, Herman, Korsgaard, and others have interpreted *autonomy* from a communal perspective and thus configured personal individuality with an eye toward a more self-conscious social orientation.[12] I believe this general attitude is a response to the need to find common ground for a common morality. And that common ground is not to be found by constituting society as a conglomerate of disconnected atomistic selves pursuing self-defined, self-centered needs, but rather by a collective embrasure of individuals into a collective venture of mutual interest. To achieve that kind of integration, successful configuration of interpersonal relationships is crucial, and to that end we require an understanding of persons as achieving their identity in relations. Once that is accomplished, we will have established a groundwork for medicine's ethics.

Another Self, Another Autonomy

Despite the philosophical caveats attached to *autonomy*, the lingering sense of personal independence remains. And well it should, because our sense of selfhood firmly rests on our rights to freedom of choice coupled to the image of the free-ranging cowboy or frontier pioneer. Images of the American hero are always based on his or her self-determined will and struggle against control. One facet of our national character celebrates, if not demands, personal self-reliance and sovereignty to enact standards of individual moral and political independence determined not from some universal moral imperative, but rather from the individuality of our personhood. Such authority requires that each citizen independently determine for himself or herself the parameters of knowledge and judgment for independent inquiry, assessment, and action. In short, "Trust thyself" and understand that "Whoso would be a man must be a nonconformist" (Emerson [1841] 1979, 29). While the Enlightenment stressed the promise of objective knowledge and universal rationality, our own postromantic understanding is centered on the sanctity of individual judgment that must arise from the confidence of personal knowing. For an agent to assume such autonomy, reliance is placed within the individual to know the world and rely on his or her own faculties. This includes a newly found voice of self-expression, one that Charles Taylor (1989, 368–390) calls the "expressivist turn." This new self-confidence, so eloquently expressed by Emerson, for instance, bestowed on the knowing agent a newfound freedom of imagination and feeling. Instead of reliance on rationalism, tradition, and formal harmony, the romantics affirm the deeper insight of the inner voices of personal knowledge and expressive nature. Truth is to be found within us, through our feelings, as well as by our rationality. Truth is personal; belief is radically individual; morality is self-responsible.

This is one stream of romantic thought, but there was a second conception of selfhood, one that appears to oppose it, or at least complements it with a radically different conception. I am referring to the notion of the subject as emerging only as a product of his encounter with another. In this latter construction, selfhood is determined by relationship, and individuality is subordinated to a metaphysical understanding of the dialectical character of the world. How they are reconciled takes us well beyond our narrative, but a partial answer might consider "individuality" as best expressed in the political domain, while "person-in-relation" better defines the metaphysics of the self. The psychological ego then becomes a tensioned combination of each understanding. While we may not be satisfied with the apparent contradictions of this formulation, romanticism is beset with such antinomies. Indeed, as Isaiah Berlin (1999, 14 ff.) shrewdly noted, following a long line of despairing critics, contradictions abound in any characterization of romanticism, since the variety of aesthetic and philosophical visions that have held the attention of the romantics seems boundless. The exuberance of possibilities, and the ability to hold contradictory sentiments and opinions, is typical of the literatures and discourse of the period. As Emerson ([1841] 1979, 33) so simply stated, "A foolish consistency is the hobgoblin of little minds."

In acknowledging that the romantics extended the notion of individuality—the unique expression of personal values, the privilege of personal knowledge, the power of individual authority over his or her person—this sense of identity was challenged, not so much in terms of the values it celebrated, but at a deeper level. We have already witnessed that even as Emerson celebrated self-reliance and the promise of self-fulfillment, hidden within the deeper recesses of the American Hero was reliance on the other, on God in his case. And with Emerson, ironically, perhaps, considering how he is typically regarded, two philosophical streams at last converge: in the 1840s, we finally witness the collapse of the atomistic, circumscribed ego. Søren Kierkegaard, writing five years after Emerson published "Experience," describes a reflexive, dialogical self-consciousness built on Hegel's insight that the "self" *is* a product of self-reflection.[13] Persons engaged in the world are normally unaware of themselves as entities of action or thought. Unless musing about the source of our own thoughts or behavior, the issue of personhood never arises. But the source of our reflection on our thoughts, perceptions, and feelings is irretrievable, remaining as a continual generator of new experience that must in turn be contemplated. Because the self-conscious review process is fundamentally oriented as a retrospective act of analysis, it can never be the primary act itself. The reflection itself is a thought about the thought, which initiates a recursive spiral that has no end (Tauber 2001, 198ff.). In short, introspection is perpetually incomplete in its attempt to capture primary experience and the "self" remains a post facto postulate of our self-consciousness (as Hume and Kant observed earlier). In sum, the self is best regarded as an activity (or "a relation of a relation") connected in time, which organizes, creates, and judges experience, both external and internal. And more to the point, the self is not *known*. Only construed, it can be neither "captured" nor "defined," and in this sense, "the subject" does not exist.

This depiction of self-consciousness arises directly from Hegel's dialectical formulations and, more specifically, from the Hegelian construct of selfhood. Hegel applied his dialectical schema to metaphysical ideas ranging from history to rationality to personal identity and thereby inaugurated a radical transformation in Western thought, including the understanding of the self. The basic dialectical synthesis describes the transition of A's engagement with B, where both are changed and a new product, C, is created. Thus no entity, event, idea, or being could be understood without recognizing that each was a product of an evolutionary encounter with others of similar, or dissimilar, kinds. In Hegel's famous Master-Slave schema (found in the fourth chapter of *The Phenomenology of Spirit*), self-consciousness itself initiates the process of discovering the "self." In the meeting of two primordial persons, the recognition of another consciousness dawns on the naive consciousness of each. Hitherto the world was encountered without cognizance of individual identity, but on recognition, a struggle ensues. One prevails and becomes the Master; the other succumbs and is the Slave. Ironically, the Master is dependent on the Slave for his sustenance, and thus the Slave is ultimately free to work for himself (and the other) and to struggle against the other. The dialectic thus continues, and in Nietzsche's rendition of this archetypal relationship, the weak must overcome the rulers in their never-ending will to power. Putting aside further details, the crucial point is that for Hegel and all those who followed him, the self scrutinizes not only the other, but itself and thereby recognizes, and constitutes, personal identity. In this dialectical formulation, the other not only confronts the self, but it turns consciousness to scrutinize itself and thereby become self-conscious. In this process, the other does not act as a "mirror," but rather in acknowledgment and response, becomes constitutive of identity.

Thus the self is transformed from an *entity* into a *process*, ever-changing and forever synthesizing itself into new conformations in response to every new other. Accordingly, there can be no unchanging self, no core identity, no final definition of personhood. The introduction of the conception of the self in Hegelian terms initiated a fierce philosophical debate among nineteenth-century philosophers (most notably Schopenhauer, Kierkegaard, Nietzsche, and James (Tauber 1994)), each of whom responded to their Hegelian Master, who had set the terms of discussion: the self was in flux and radically elusive.

In the twentieth century, the ensuing discussion was dominated by the phenomenologists,[14] but here I wish to dwell on an interesting comment about the moral implications of deconstructing the self as an entity. The self cannot be construed as an object, for as Charles Taylor argues, the conception of the self as an *object* (or entity) must fulfill certain criteria: it must have objective status, standing independent of any description or interpretation.[15] Most importantly, an object can and must be understood without reference to its surroundings or contingent circumstances (Taylor 1989, 34–35). The core self conception cannot fulfill these criteria, and when the second aspect of identity (the relational basis) is included, the question moves from *What* is the self? to *Who* am I? Indeed, this is the basic issue of the Hegelian interpretation of the birth of self-consciousness. The first question, Will I be a Master or a Slave?, arises directly from the immediacy of self-consciousness. The *who* inquiry demands a social answer, totally dependent on human categories of personal and social action.

In this context, the self, then, is perceived as a moral description or category that fulfills criteria of human identification, and thus is fundamentally social in character: no ready definition of the self outside of larger groups and relationships is plausible. (For instance, selves as citizens have certain rights and obligations as defined by law; soldiers as selves are defined by their military roles and duties; patients are defined by their respective pathologies and reports of illness.) So when we speak of "the self," we must differentiate between that self-conscious sense of being (which ties together all of the various identities enacted) from the roles themselves (which form out of the contingency of social functions fashioned in a particular time and place). *How* those roles are fulfilled remains individualistic, and in this sense, open.

While social identity confers certain obligations and behaviors, individual choice opens a spectrum of ways such roles are enacted. A balanced tension then emerges as identity is formed and expressed between these two poles of personhood. Of these two senses of selfhood—the personal, individualistic and the social, relational—I will now focus on the latter depiction. I find ample justification inasmuch as the self, conceived in its atomistic sense, reduces identity to a simplistic formulation and thereby fails to provide the framework for the task at hand. The moral philosophy I seek directly emerges from the other orientation.

At last I return to defining autonomy, and I do so not from the vantage point of atomistic selves, each protected and insulated from others, but rather viewed as constituted by the relations in which all persons must partake. And from this grounding, autonomy must reflect a relational ethics. From this point of view, in the meeting of an individual with other persons, moral choices are defined by the nature of those relationships.

And here a crucial turn is made: embedded in relationship are reciprocal duties, obligations, and expectations of a general kind. In other words, to look at autonomy as simply the vector of interest originating in an individual's desire or action is to ignore the social context in which those individual choices or behaviors are made. To achieve choice, the very act of choosing must be respected. This then becomes the domain of the respondent who acknowledges a complex of responsibilities as constitutive of any social relationship. I am making no further claim than stressing that human rights are grounded in obligations (O'Neill 2002, 78–89). Accordingly, rights and obligations are mutually determining, and thus where there are no obligations there are no rights. From this perspective, the social relationship is the ontological grounding of autonomy, which now has "obligation" attached as firmly as "rights" to its definition. In other words, individuals exist by virtue of their relationships with others and thus reciprocal rights, as well as duties, arise from that social encounter. In short, once a social concept of the self eclipses atomistic formulations, individualistic notions of autonomy are radically challenged.

Notwithstanding the oversimplification I have presented, autonomy, at least in the common imagination, builds on the notion of a self that resides independent of other relations, and the various meanings attached to *autonomy* reflect this sense of personhood as atomistic, selfdetermined, and self-supporting. And indeed, there are those who have been reluctant to abandon the notion of a core self as the basis of an autonomy-based medical ethics (e.g., Pellegrino 1979b; Meyers 1989), but I follow those who would attempt to salvage autonomy by refashioning our concept of personhood with an eye toward its relational character.

I begin by noting that individuals have multiple identities conferred by different social roles. To be a mother, wife, waitress, juror, consumer, driver, congregant, singer, army reservist, and so on, means that different kinds of responsibilities, opportunities, obligations, rules, and fulfillment are associated with each role, and correspondingly the moral agency associated with each identity differs. To assume that a single autonomous identity supervenes and orders the others is not only simplistic, but falsifies the character of selfhood. This aspect of social identity is closely associated with a constellation of ideas that might be grouped as the "conceit of independence." Instead of ignoring the complexity of social identities, this view regards them as somehow removable personae, masks of identity that cover a deeper true self. In this interpretation, the "autonomy obsession" of contemporary American culture offers a biased picture of human nature, because instead of presenting a more realistic relational depiction of persons, it substitutes a symbolic representation under the label of individualism (Code 1991). Indeed, individualism, the bedrock foundation for various understandings of autonomy, claims that agents are causally isolated from other agents—that is, an agent's sense of herself is independent of family and community relationships in which she participates. Consequently, an agent's essential properties are intrinsic and are not comprised, even in part, by the social relations in which she might participate.

But feminist critiques have focused on how "independent selves" are in fact highly integrated into myriad relationships and locked into determined behaviors as a result of these social commitments. Thus a radically independent, autonomous person is at best an idealized portrait of a fictional character, part of an elaborate ideological cartoon of Western culture. Accordingly, the notion of self-sufficient independence promotes only one of several depictions of persons, a picture that celebrates self-reliance over relationship. This understanding of persons has profound moral implications, because the idealized autonomous person forfeits trust, friendship, loyalty, caring, and responsibility as secondary attributes to those primary values of self-direction, self-determination, and self-realization. This is not to say that these other interpersonal values might not be honored, but their subordinate standing to an atomistic quintessence carries ethical import. Another way of looking at this point is that values, social practices, relationships, and communities that are based on principles of cooperation and interdependence, threaten or at least compromise atomistic autonomy.

From these considerations, Carol Gilligan and other feminist philosophers initiated a rigorous debate over the diverse ethics of "care" and "justice" as the ideal types of two contending ethics.[16] The ethic of justice begins with an assumption of human separateness; freedom is fundamental. In contrast, the ethic of care begins with an assumption of human connectedness, and its goal is to correct detachment, for in this view relationships are fundamental and must be protected. Consequently, fundamental relationships are defined in answer to opposing agendas, inasmuch as the ethic of justice has some form of equality as a priority, whereas the ethic of care gives prominence to the maintenance of relationships, sometimes equal, sometimes not. The net result of these divergent views is a "conflicting value of autonomy."

So while individualistic autonomy is naturally situated in an ethic of justice, the ethic of care is founded on obligation and connectedness. In the latter formulation, autonomy shifts from an expression of radical self-governance in a world organized and determined by the individual, to one in which individual actions are decided and constituted within a universe of complex social interests and demands. Thus, two understandings of autonomy emerge: an atomistic variety that asserts that one should be free to define oneself as long as one does not "interfere with the autonomy of others" (Clement 1996), and another more social, relational conception that regards atomistic autonomy as dangerous because it is maximized through isolation from others and is consequently disruptive to the cooperative venture of communal interactions. In short, from differing conceptions of selfhood divergent visions of autonomy arise, and the task is to reconcile them if possible.

These contentious visions are often seen as alternatives to one another, but arguments for their intimate complementarity are compelling (Clement 1996), and, indeed, as discussed above, certain neo-Kantians have arrived at the same moral resting place, but from a reinterpretation of the Kantian construction. Both perspectives converge on the following rationale: the potential conflict between justice and beneficence, between autonomy and care, is reconciled by understanding autonomy as a primordial product of social relationships. Rawls and his various followers arrive at this position by acknowledging the social *responsibility* of rational moral agents. Feminists and phenomenologists place the *response* to the other as fundamental. *Responsibility* and *response* derive from the same Latin root, *respondere*—to promise in return, to reply, to answer. From each philosophical perspective, responses to the call, demands, and obligations of human relationships are the means to individual fulfillment and achievement. Instead of assuming the primacy of individualism, they claim that isolated persons are not only incomplete individuals, but their isolation beleaguers them with burdens that actually impede their self-actualization. Accordingly, autonomy is "not merely an internal, or psychological characteristic, but also an external, or social" one (Clement 1996, 22). This insight highlights a fundamental social fact: no one is fully autonomous, because everyone relies on a vast social network to provide goods and services, and each of us enjoys (or regrets) complex and numerous interpersonal relationships. Thus an "autonomous individual" is not some Robinson Crusoe stranded alone on an island, but rather a person who *exercises* autonomous choices. Thus we distinguish "autonomous persons" from "autonomous acts." The latter is a characteristic or property of persons, and the former is a nebulous ideal that has no bona fide standing in the real world of social relations. So part of the murky philosophy enveloping "autonomy" is cleared by recognizing that none of the criteria defining autonomy precludes interdependence.

Conclusion

But a deep tension between "autonomy" and "relationship" is not easily overcome. At one level this is perhaps surprising, considering how myriad testimonies to "love" have surely made commitment to another a central theme of our culture. Given the romanticism of our era, and the emphasis of happiness as eros-fulfilled, one must wonder at the confusion holding seemingly contradictory cultural ideals together—love, relationship, commitment, on the one hand, and autonomy, independence, self-centered self-fulfillment, on the other hand. In the typical scenario, love is reserved for intimates (family and lovers), and the circle of intimacy is carefully guarded, notwithstanding the fundamental Judeo-Christian precept to love one's neighbor! The point is so obvious that it requires no further clarification, and the social critic can only marvel at our ability to follow, simultaneously, different trains of emotional needs and social ideals. Despite our conflict, we must still place ourselves along a continuum of self-identification. I choose, almost at random, a physician's own musings on the issue:

As I've gotten older, I understand how conditioned I am to see the world in terms of "either/or" or "I" or "you"—the adversarial world-view that makes lawyers rich and science seem triumphant. From time to time I've been offered glimpses of what now seems a more authentic world, the world of "and" (which includes and affirms "either/or") and the world of "we" (which includes and affirms "I" and "you"). This is the world in which . . . I cannot see you or me with clarity unless I can see the connection between us. . . . I've come to see healthy growth not so much as the growth of a self, but as the growth of a self-in-connection. Mutuality is a more authentic description of humans and nature than dichotomy. (Shem 2002)

Generally I favor this position, and believe, perhaps naively and idealistically, that it must serve as a guide toward finding a place for autonomy that minimizes its competitive opposition to a relational ethic.

To seek such a resolution, we need to define the basic requirements of autonomy within a relational construct: (1) decision making must be one's own and free of coercion; (2) in order to fulfill the first requirement, one must critically reflect on one's choices to ensure that they are solely self-motivated (per the Frankfurt-Dworkin model discussed in the next chapter); and (3) one must assume responsibility for one's choices. *None of these measures precludes interdependence.* Given the reality that few choices in fact fulfill all of these requirements, autonomy must be placed in a social context where supporting relationships enable individuals to achieve various degrees of autonomy and thereby act as freely as possible according to the criteria just presented.

By emphasizing the ultimate relational character of autonomy, justice and care may be seen as complementary to each other and thus mutually interdependent (Clement 1996, 109).[17] Unable to prioritize one principle over the other, we should recognize that they are indispensable to one another. This is an important corrective, for until the emergence of the care-justice debate, the ethic of justice dominated moral philosophy and imposed a definition of autonomy that arose from limited notions of selfhood. If the self is defined in terms of some splendid epistemological isolation, then that identity must construe autonomy as supporting that epistemological conceit, an individualistic construction that oversimplifies and thus distorts identity. The consequence? A particular atomistic account of autonomy displaces the complex ethical choices characteristically determined by the social milieu, where identities derive from several sources and options exhibit corresponding complexity. In sum, the focus on the ethic of justice reflects an excessively individualistic conception of autonomy, which ignores the social conditions necessary for self-determination. Moral knowledge is then seen exclusively as an individual achievement, a product of rational reflection independent of its social locus (K. Baier 1995; A. C. Baier 1997).

Relational autonomy offers a corrective to a severely atomistic orientation by emphasizing moral knowledge as the product of the interdependence of persons and their mutual negotiation of options and choices. In the end, moral knowledge depends not only on individualistic rationality, but on socially determined factors as well. This theme will be further developed later in the book, but the key point I wish to establish may be clearly stated now: substituting a relational understanding of selfhood for a narrowly atomistic notion fundamentally shifts the definition of autonomy from the exercise of moral choice by a fully independent agent to one who is embedded in relationships, which of themselves, confer identity. "Relational autonomy" then becomes a more complete, and honest, depiction of the doctor-patient relationship, because it more accurately describes the agency of each party. Once autonomy is configured as achieved in cooperation, the defensive and distorted moral posture of the patient may be replaced with a more appropriate understanding, which allows for a better fulfillment of the healing encounter: the recovery of independence and a sense of self-authority.

Although my view is clear, I am uncomfortable with doctrinaire pronouncements, even my own. So let me point to a path that should appeal to even the most stalwart libertarian: autonomy has no single definition or standing, and consequently it must find its place in the flux of social demands and claims that balance the needs of individuals and their society in a complex, dynamic relationship. Thus neither atomistic autonomy nor the ethics of responsibility can claim hegemony, for they are mutually interdependent, and a complete account of the moral axes in patient care requires that they be integrated. It seems clear that *both* ethics capture something real and important about morality, and that insisting on ranking these principles trivializes the contributions of the principle deemed less basic. It also seems to presuppose that one of the two ethics, in its standard form, is *correct*, ruling out the likelihood that their interaction weaves the moral fabric by which we live (Clement 1996).

Allowing for my own bias and for this dualistic, balanced approach, how might such a synthesis be configured? On the one hand, I believe that only by recognizing a social view of morality, where the individual is seen as functioning within relationships, might we appreciate the insufficiency of atomistic autonomy to serve as the governing principle for health care. On the other hand, autonomy must be recognized for what it is in our culture, a prime value of authenticity and self-fulfillment. Perhaps paradoxically, I suggest that we use a relational ethic to achieve an individualistic ideal.

In the clinical setting, perhaps more than in any other, patients are not self-sufficient, and an expansive definition of autonomy is required to preserve their sense of self-governance and their ability to assume the responsibility of making choices even under dire circumstances. An *ethics of responsibility* is based on a relational morality, where response to need guides its actions. Indeed, an ethics of responsibility serves as a powerful moral paradigm of how support for those choices is oriented to preserve self-determination, promote authenticity, and protect autonomy. This is a "process ethics," in which moral choices are made by ongoing, open negotiation. Such a dialogical process requires self-reflection, and the physician is best situated to guide that exchange. (This moral "negotiation" is based on a professional commitment to responsibility and trustworthiness, matters further discussed in chapter 5.) Characteristically, this process is articulated by informed consent. So, we are now poised to move from the abstract realm to the bedside and ask, What does *informed* mean, and how is it attained? If the primary goal is, in fact, to allow individuals the full freedom of choice, an ethics committed to meeting patients' needs and supporting their aspirations requires a corresponding conception of autonomy that is consonant with these goals. I next turn to exploring such a formulaton.

4

Balancing Rights and Responsibilities

The chief task of a theory of autonomy . . . is to reclaim the distinction between real and apparent desires.

—Meyers 1989, 26

Despite the dominance of autonomy as a political and judicial ideal in American civil life, the application of autonomy-based ethics to ill persons has been criticized as a conceit (e.g., Schneider 1998). Given the apparent disparity between the technical expertise of doctor and patient, the basis of cooperative decision making was seen as too often creating an obstacle to full patient participation in deciding clinical options. While autonomy remains an aspiration in the clinical setting, a fair appraisal shows that its attainment requires accepting "varying degrees" of autonomy or, better, "respect" for individual choice, as a substitute for full patient participation in decision making.

I believe this critique is essentially correct and highlights the difficulty of applying certain moral definitions in differing contexts. Standards in one setting may not be appropriate to another. So in medicine, the question of autonomy assumes a particular cast: What is autonomy, and if it is not "full," is it adequate? Posing the question in these terms recognizes that the principles of civil autonomy apply with significant restrictions to persons who cannot exercise their full freedom of choice. Because of this ambiguity lawyers and ethicists are left scrambling to find appropriate caveats, provisos, and adjustments to a moral principle that relies on assumptions of competency and knowledge that simply may not apply to patients as they might pertain to other social identities.

Despite the confusion, we should acknowledge that autonomy is a plastic concept exhibiting different "degrees of freedom," for in the highly technical arena of contemporary medicine, the power relationship between physician and patient is profoundly unequal. Patients, simply out of deference to superior knowledge and technical expertise, agree to delegate varying degrees of their freedom and entrust their care to others. It is precisely at this point that current medical ethics fails to make the appropriate adjustment of modifying a restrictive definition of autonomy and complementing it with expanded physician responsibility.

I am dissatisfied with how informed consent has become a stopgap measure to protect against abuses of trust, and therefore I seek, instead of a moral space filler, an understanding of autonomy that accommodates itself to a broader conception of an ethics of responsibility. The foundations for that understanding were set forth in the preceding chapter, and its rationale will be explored in the next, so now we may pointedly ask, How might we reconfigure patient autonomy at the bedside and in the clinic to achieve a balance between patient rights and physician responsibilities? How do we transform defensive medicine into a model of health care in which autonomy is more fairly aligned with beneficence? How might autonomy more effectively serve the telos of care? What is the structure of a medical ethics that reasserts the relational principles in alignment with the claims of patient autonomy, both theoretically and practically? And finally, What is the end point? Instead of assuming an ethics of suspicion that places patients and doctors in opposing courts, we should promote an ethical medicine in which the clinical encounter again enacts an ancient covenant (discussed in chapter 5).

The difficulties we face in establishing such a balance of moral principles arise from several sources: (1) the economics of care that has made health care a commodity; (2) the technical and scientific reductionism so characteristic of contemporary clinical medicine (chapter 1); (3) the rise of defensive medicine resulting from malpractice claims (chapter 2); and (4) an overtaxed version of atomistic autonomy (chapter 3). With this background, we are now prepared to seek a strategy that strengthens individual choice compromised by what currently passes for patient protection. To that end, I proceed, not so much to "solve" the crisis, but rather to offer a philosophical orientation toward an ethical medicine that must, if effective, help to offset the other forces at play in dehumanizing health care.

Salvaging Patient Autonomy

Today, most commentators would agree that *autonomy* has no single, coherent meaning, except in the most general sense of drawing on two understandings of freedom (Berlin 1969): one is negative, the freedom from oppression or interference by another, and the second is positive, the freedom to participate in the process by which one's life is controlled. At least four closely related meanings link *autonomy* with different references or capacities: (1) the capacity to govern oneself, (2) the actual condition of self-government, (3) an ideal of virtue derived from that conception, and (4) the "sovereign authority" to govern oneself (Feinberg 1986). While a vast literature has attempted to sort out the relationships of these various aspects of autonomy, we can cut to the chase by identifying the core idea that holds each of these aspects together, namely, a psychological ability, and the self-assurance, to be self-governing. This aspect I will call the "psychological" or "political" meaning. It is to be distinguished from the meanings used in the "moral" domain, which consists in the acceptance of responsibility for one's choice.

We begin with motivations. One need not be a Freudian to appreciate that individual motives and self-understanding are subject to seemingly endless reflection. Whether we accept the "unconscious" as a section of the mind or not, cognitive scientists have confirmed that we are subject to myriad unconscious factors and experiences that make decision making less apparent (and thus less self-aware and rational) than we might otherwise hope (Wilson 2002). But just because we are subject to certain hidden or disguised forces of our culture or personal experience does not mean that we are products of a capricious determinism. Indeed, a theory of autonomy seeks to understand that choices have varying degrees of self-understanding, that the freedom exercised in comprehending those choices involves deliberate selections, and that in the end, to whatever degree we exercise independence in making a choice, the final arbiter must always be a moral one, namely, assuming responsibility for that action. The search for justifications may be endless, but the process rests when responsibility is accepted.

Choices and acts are judged autonomous when the process of exploring the reasons for our selections is completed. We enter an intricate maze to sort out immediate desires from deeper commitments. By what criteria can we decide? How are they adjudicated? Isn't the recursive spiral of analysis endless? Where is the Archimedean point for judgment? Sophisticated answers have been offered, and they fall into three general categories:

1. *Insight into the socialization process.* Autonomy is putatively achieved by autobiographical understanding, which is designed to liberate oneself from stultifying aspects of socialization (Young 1980; Richards 1980). Basically a Freudian argument, advocates of such self-knowledge theories must still contend with unconscious factors in a never-ending attempt to seek cause. While psychoanalysis may yield a new tranquility and harmony, any final resting place is unlikely to be found for true motivation.

2. *Testing the phenomenal self for coherence.* Acknowledging the power of social influences to mold individual choices, a critical examination of those underlying social beliefs will yield an array of options (Benn 1976). The moral character of an individual is thus expressed by the choices exercised, which in turn are molded by a critical faculty that determines moral action. Accordingly, autonomy resides in the integrity and coherence of this behavior and is the expression of those choices. But coherence, in and of itself, hardly confers autonomy. Putting aside the issue of what constitutes coherence, how does a series of choices manifest autonomy? Certain actions may be consistent but not freely chosen, or more dramatically, an insane individual may be consistent in his beliefs, but he is hardly acting autonomously. Self-examination alone is insufficient to account for autonomy.

3. *Stratifying desires and identifying dominant ones.* This third approach, probably the most influential, argues that the self-awareness conferred by the first two approaches is necessary but insufficient to account for autonomy, and instead seeks a correction by adding a procedural account.[1] This "procedural" theory uses a structural approach—

a hierarchical organization of various desires, emotions, traits, values, objectives, and the like—to describe how autonomy is exercised. Influentially promoted by Harry Frankfurt (1971) and expanded by Gerald Dworkin (1988), this understanding of autonomy is based on how potentially conflicting forces must be aligned and coordinated by higher-order desires to achieve morally autonomous actions. The so-called lower-order desires have as their object immediate or primary actions of the agent: a desire to *do* X (e.g., eat a sundae, steal a lemon); higher-order desires, Y, have as their object these lower-order desires, so that the formula becomes a higher-order desire or choice, Y, acts on the desire to do (or not do) X (Christman 1989, 6–8). In other words, humans are endowed with the capacity to reflect on their wants and beliefs, and ultimately these yearnings must be stratified, so that some impulses will be acted on immediately, some deferred, and some ignored (Lindley 1986, 64–66). I may want a candy bar, but I more powerfully want to lose weight in order to be healthier, in order to live a longer and more productive life, because I have aspirations that require longevity, and on and on. I monitor my craving, and choose to deny my hunger for the chocolate. There is perhaps no end to how many higher-order desires might be invoked, and one need not identify them all to act. The point is not the number, but rather recognizing the hierarchy of desires and the ability to act on the highest ones.[2]

Illustrations may be useful: being incarcerated in prison, regimented in the military, or following religious orders each refracts "autonomy" in different ways. How might we account for such ordinary circumstances (not to speak of the hidden Freudian or Foucauldian ones!)? Imprisonment offers no confusion, but what about the autonomy of soldiers or priests? Dworkin (1988) maintains that we must seek another level of inquiry to judge autonomy in such settings. Accordingly, a soldier following an order to clean latrines is, in fact, acting autonomously, because his initial decision to join the army was voluntary. (Of course, if he was drafted, this assignment takes on a very different cast!) He understood that once inducted in the military, orders must be followed and personal choices of many kinds would be severely compromised. But the decision to enlist was (at least in this example) a purely voluntary one, based on rational expectations. So while we might observe that onerous duty may not have been freely chosen, the overall context of the soldier's behavior is autonomous. The essential feature is the assumption of responsibility for the choice exercised, perhaps not in the particular instantiation (washing latrines), but in choosing the life of a soldier.

This example highlights how autonomous persons need not always be fully autonomous in their actions, and in fact, social roles proscribe certain behaviors, different degrees of regimentation, and loss of personal choice, but these regimens in and of themselves are not necessarily restrictions on personal autonomy as understood as a regression to some fundamental choice. Simply put, we forgo the freedom to do what we want because of a larger social, ultimately moral context in which we function. Autonomy is determined at this higher level. If we choose to be teamsters, teachers, judges, artists, salesclerks, or whatever, each role assigns a set of determinants: show up at work on time; fulfill assigned duties efficiently and correctly; comport oneself appropriately; and so on. Some jobs are more restrictive than others, but that is not the determining parameter, for the autonomy of individuals is established at an existential level of choice, for example, how to conduct oneself in a chosen job; how to enact religious and political beliefs; how to establish and maintain interpersonal relations; how to achieve self-fulfillment; and, most importantly, accepting responsibility for those determining choices. How such autonomy is then *exercised* becomes a different kind of problem.

By making the higher-lower desire distinction, "autonomy" is rescued from the panoply of disguised and unknown forces that mold our wishes and inspire our desires. Freed of ceaseless analysis, the Frankfurt-Dworkin model readily admits that persons are subject to social and psychological influences that defy a full accounting, and in that admission it follows a pragmatic strategy. By understanding that autonomous acts are context-dependent, "free choice" assumes varying expressions, answers heterogeneous demands, and is judged by relativistic standards.

The model melds the central elements of its philosophical heritage: on the one hand it salvages rational choice as crucial to autonomy (Kant), while at the same time it acknowledges the emotional influences on making such choices (Hume). By seeking a balance between them (not so different from Mill's strategy), the Frankfurt-Dworkin model high-lights how choices are determined by our ability to regulate primary desires with rational controls, which serve to regulate responses to lusts, hungers, aspirations, and so on. The rational, self-reflective aspect of a higher-order desire becomes the moral faculty writ large and confers what Frankfurt calls "freedom of the will." Without this contemplative higher-order faculty of deliberation, where all of an agent's motivational forces take their final form, humans would simply act on their strongest immediate impulses:

The weakness of this construction resides in the choice of covering values, which may become ever-wider as the agent seeks to account for viable options. While the danger of a never-ending regress looms, a viable escape from this spiral of justification is found in a coherence theory of values, where a choice is justified by how well its underlying value coheres with other values. However, one must still face the choice of which values to start with, as well as all of the choices among competing values that cohere equally well with the initial set once adopted. Thus it seems that choosing one course of action over another must end in either a brute choice or a brute fact about what value is to be optimized. (Richman 2004, 123)

This dilemma is of general concern, but in medicine, *health* is an over-riding value for a person (Richman 2004), and thus the regress essentially stops, at least in the clinical setting, with the value of restoring or maintaining health. Of course, how we define health is itself an issue (see especially Canguilhem [1966] 1989), but assuming a needs-wants, person-centered, goal-oriented ideal, the regress of values usually comes to a tidy end (see chapter 1). To the extent that a patient has the ability to fulfill her higher-order desires—that is, health (and is cognizant of those choices as rational and reasonably coherent)—she is autonomous. Accordingly, freedom of the will is a necessary condition of autonomy, and, true to Kant and Mill, rationality and judgment remain its lynch-pins. While we might acknowledge the limits of such deliberation, the moral faculty remains grounded on some semblance of rational control. It makes no absolute claims of what constitutes the rational, but the model asserts an operative ideal, which in the clinical setting seems quite appropriate when structured on the value of health.

While I am sympathetic to the Frankfurt-Dworkin approach, I would go one step beyond it, especially in the medical setting, with another standard, where a grounding in agency is unnecessary. While rationality is preferred, in the end, given all of the uncertainties plaguing choice, freedom of will, and the identity of moral agency, perhaps self-responsibility suffices. Indeed, I feel more closely aligned with those who get directly to the root of the matter: "Autonomy requires only that we are morally responsible, or capable of self-revision. It does not matter that our desires may arise from sources within or external to ourselves that we do not control, nor does it matter that we did not invent the values that guide our lives. What matters is that we are capable of revising ourselves in light of critical reflection" (Mackenzie and Stoljar 2000, 29).

This discussion profits from distinguishing between *being* autonomous and *exercising* autonomous choices (between asserting selfhood and more simply recognizing choice and responsibility). Broadly construed, autonomous acts possesses certain intellectual and practical characteristics that reflect self-governance, principally, that one has chosen among various options of action without being coerced into picking one or another. But being free of coercion does not necessarily ensure free choice, since various predicaments restrict personal options. While the self-reflective component is emphasized, the final common denominator for exercising autonomy is to assume responsibility for one's choices and actions.

No set standard for exercising autonomy is possible or even desirable considering the myriad kinds of choices that must be made in ordinary life, and instead of some Golden Rule, a sense of choice is retrieved as sufficient, because the underlying responsibility that accompanies such choice grounds the moral decision. In short, in this view, two dimensions are at work at once in the exercise of autonomy: a psychological one (we must *feel* that we have choice), and a moral one (we assume *responsibility* for the choice selected).

I am deliberately choosing a "fence" philosophy (one that has openings as opposed to a solid wall), for while I wish to contain the idea of autonomy, at the same time I wish to entertain a certain flexibility to either expand or contract this principle for particular applications or interpretations appropriate to medicine's myriad needs. In short, by containing the basic idea within circumscribed boundaries, we map a moral space for autonomy to function in the special domain of medicine. Our operative conception of autonomy entails (1) a distinction between being autonomous and exercising autonomy; (2) a recognition that autonomy may be exercised by relinquishing certain choices and maintaining other, more basic ones; and (3) in the special case of medicine, an admission that autonomy is only one of several moral principles governing medical care and it must be accommodated within that constellation of competing principles. Perhaps the better goal is protecting patient dignity, which may be understood as encompassing autonomy. But I will put aside that suggestion for the moment and rest with these three basic tenets that allow autonomy to assume its rightful, yet measured place in medical ethics. With this background, I can now proceed to my primary concern, namely, to describe the moral posture physicians might assume given the demands of patient autonomy.

Autonomy in the Clinic

Few decisions even approach an ideal of autonomy in a strict sense, but in admitting that most instances of moral decision making are made with incomplete knowledge, a method of accommodating that restriction must suffice. The Frankfurt-Dworkin procedural model provides an approach, by allowing patients to make autonomous choices by entrusting themselves to physicians—that is, their fundamental autonomy is honored in delegating technical decisions to caregivers. After informed consent, under ordinary circumstances, patients adopt a role in which decisions are made for them with the understanding that such decisions are made in their best interest. They have, in short, accepted responsibility for delegating responsibility. The question then is not whether they have choice, but whether patient choices are fully, or adequately, understood. Informed consent is based on the presupposition that "full" disclosure of information will provide patients with enough knowledge for them to confidently entrust their care to others. Almost universally, patients are incapable of assessing *all* clinical information, or even possessing the judgment so determined by prior experience that might enable them to make *all* choices relevant to their care. This is simply due to the radically differing technical competence between doctor and patient.

Again, patients may exercise their autonomy by opting for technical deferral to others. In other words, "autonomy" in the clinical setting according to this understanding provides the latitude of moral choice that permits an unequal relationship between a highly trained professional and an unsophisticated patient to be brought within the boundaries of a flexible understanding of personal autonomy.

Two general approaches to this end have been formulated (Emanuel and Emanuel 1992). In the so-called interpretative model, the physician is regarded as helping to select medical interventions that realize the patient's overall values. Acting as an advisor, the doctor offers information, helps to clarify values, and suggests ways of implementing the patient's global goals. Doubts as to the efficacy of this approach concern the inability of many (perhaps most) physicians to remain neutral with such demands, their poor communication skills, and perhaps most importantly, their tendency to slip into a paternalistic role. Alternatively, the "deliberative model," presents the physician with a more limited role "to help the patient determine the best health-related values that can be realized in the clinical situation" (Emanuel and Emanuel 1992, 2222). Remaining confined to the professional arena, the doctor assumes a more neutral posture and thus, according to this last model, patient choice is less guided and allowed a freer rein. I concur with others (e.g., Brody 1992; Richman 2004) that notwithstanding the problems inherent in the interpretative role for doctors, it remains the most viable for two principal reasons: (1) patients are seldom able to process the highly technical information required to make informed decisions (the epistemic dimension), and (2) a physician cannot offer informed, deliberative advice without understanding the context of a person's needs and values (the moral dimension).

In a sense, we are witnessing a stalemate in regard to defining physician advocacy, and our dilemma has been resolved to a certain extent in the law, specifically in the requirements of informed consent. Informed consent, as an exercise of autonomy, embeds the *patient's* responsibility for making the delegated choices. In other words, physician responsibility is to fulfill the professional obligations so contracted, but the underlying and directing mandate remains the patient's. And when violated, civil injury may be claimed.

Although informed consent is based on respect for autonomy, the law has evolved to protect related rights and duties derived from this principle. Informed consent arose from the common law of torts—that is, from cases of civil injury resulting from intentional or negligent actions inflicted by another (Faden and Beauchamp 1986, 23ff.). So, while the right of privacy and protection from battery are complementary legal elements, the law concerning negligence has been the dominant theory of liability informing the doctrine of medical consent. Negligence is the tort of unintended harmful action or omission. In the clinical setting, medical negligence, as applied to informed consent, "assumes that there is a professional duty of due care to provide patients an appropriate disclosure of information before obtaining authorization for treatment. Lack of informed consent is treated as professional negligence in essentially the same respect as is careless performance of a surgical procedure" (Faden and Beauchamp 1986, 29). The disclosure requirements (professional-practice standard, reasonable-person standard, the subjective standard) are debated and since the courts have not applied precise criteria, the appropriate standards exhibit heterogeneity in practice. Be that as it may, informed consent has largely become both (1) a routine part of the administrative process of health care (legal formulations are well established that direct patients to sign consents and waivers), and (2) a second dimension of consent that occurs at the interstices of doctor-patient relations that follow no proscribed rules or regulations.

Important distinctions must be made between general policy rules and requirements that comprise consent in the institutional context, which may have little direct relevance to individual patients, and a second sense of informed consent in which autonomous authorization is made with the attendant criterion of authentic responsibility assumed by the patient for the delegation of decision making. The latter constellation of concerns is referred to as "autonomous authorization," and the former, "effective consent" (Faden and Beauchamp 1986, 274–287). Faden and Beauchamp elaborate on the distinction as follows. In autonomous authorization, consensus or congruence between physician and patient is not required, for the patient authorizes independently: "It is a matter of indifference where or how the proposal being authorized originates" (p. 279). The patient's intentions and understanding remain the lynchpin of the consent process and the responsibility for choice remains firmly within the domain of the patient. "Effective consent" is not necessarily concerned primarily with autonomy, but rather addresses the institution's legal obligations. Effective authorization obtained through defined rules and regulations is the focus of malpractice law, but this is not my primary interest. Here, I am concerned with autonomous authorization, where certain moral issues are prominently at stake:

1. *Are the intentions of the patient protected?* Intention resides at several levels. For example, an intention may be purely mental and have no consequence in action, or an intention to accomplish one goal may involve associated sequels that are anticipated, or not. Degrees of intention vary from deliberate acceptance to willing acquiescence. The two are not equivalent, and more to the point, they may not be distinguished under certain circumstances.

2. *Does the patient understand the choice being made?* Obviously, "to understand" invokes various kinds of comprehension: the practical competence to know how to do something; propositional knowledge that reduces understanding to an analysis of knowledge; or comprehension of another's point of view or statement, without necessarily concurring with that assertion or belief (Faden and Beauchamp 1986, 249ff.). Given variable interpretations, analytical skills, background supporting concepts, ability to think probabilistically, and a myriad universe of other factors, "understanding" has a problematic status in the realm of informed consent.

3. *Are decisions made free of coercion and thus autonomous?* Distinctions between "influenced," "persuaded," and "controlled" draw out the nuances of voluntary choice. At one end of the spectrum, patients require instruction, which embeds certain subjective points of view, values, and assumptions. Manipulation lurks in the background of the education process, and the aspiration for an objective accounting of risks and benefits, foreseeable consequences, and the implications of one strategy versus another leaves the freedom of choice as an abstract ideal in typical scenarios.

Experienced clinicians recognize that all of these elements—freedom of choice, competence, understanding, intentions—are highly problematic for typical patients, and while respect for patient autonomy is an abiding value, its instantiation remains a beguiling problem.

In an age that celebrates autonomy, the abdication of *any* choice is often regarded as anathema. But given the limits of autonomy in the clinical setting, the moral logic of balancing other principles against its demands, and the simple pragmatics of caring for the ill, it is foolish not to admit that physicians assume authority—sometimes greater, sometimes less—in the execution of their professional skills on behalf of their patients. This task is normally accepted without any moral compunction. Indeed, doctors are trained to exercise authority in the forms of expertise and technical skills. Agonizing moral reflection as to the appropriateness of such authority for most medical decisions is not only impractical, it is counterproductive. With this understanding of physician responsibility, the moral challenge is to help the patient identify the *pertinent* personal and ethical issues that should be factored into medical decision making. The doctor as patient-advocate assumes a dual role: on the one hand she asserts her command of a complex process of disease and situates it within a larger social context in which it must be managed, and on the other hand, she guides her patient with respect for the maintenance of personal choice and, optimally, the fully restored sense of autonomous agency. The physician thus enacts the traditional role of care provider, but now on a larger moral axis: fully asserting physician responsibility (beneficence) requires that patient dignity (autonomy) be respected. The site of action configured on these coordinates must precisely define the parameters of care and harmoniously assemble the components of such care to promote the global health of the patient. The problem to which I now turn concerns balancing the exercise of patient rights against other moral principles.

The Debate

The paradigm of patient autonomy holds a strong place in the law and ethics of medicine. Indeed, "The notion of rights in medicine . . . has . . . become part of the culture of medicine itself" (Zussman 1992, 85), making the empowered patient a different agent from the one enrolled in the traditional doctor-patient relationship. A dominant lobby of ethicists and lawyers assert a strong form of patient autonomy: in their respective roles, the doctor is the provider of knowledge and facts regarding treatment, while the patient selects treatment that reflects personal values. But this interpretation begs the question of how far this new autonomy should extend. In other words, what choices should patients make?

To counterbalance the more assertive position, critics such as Carl Schneider have argued that the notion of patient autonomy is vague and has been too readily adopted as an extrapolation from civil life to the clinic. He observes that the continuum of patient participation is long and elaborate, even though "the overwhelming weight of bioethical opinion endorses not just the autonomy principle, but a potent version of it" (Schneider 1998, 9). He counters that a more refined interpretation of patient autonomy is required to address the different needs of patients, many of whom might fall victim to the false assumption that more assertive forms of autonomy better capture their self-interest (pp. 35–46).

The fundamental precept from which I have launched my own critique resides squarely in the acceptance, congruent with the imperative of patient autonomy, of the physician's abiding care of his charge. What does this mean? Most simply, patient autonomy does not mitigate physician responsibility. Although medical decisions must be made in light of the patient's values, health-care providers heavily influence how those choices are presented and thereby set the context in which they are understood. And we know from exhaustive psychological studies that the manner and context in which choices are offered largely determine a person's response.

Choices float in a river of various currents, of which the psychological is too often neglected. Aside from the issues about unconscious desires and motives, a more immediate element is simply the nature of the information presented to patients from which they must make decisions. Information can never be neutral. Medical facts are attached to personal values, and, indeed, how information is given, the frame or context of presentation, will have an enormous influence on how the facts transmitted are understood and acted on (Tversky and Kahneman 1981; Kahneman and Tversky 1984, 2000). When choice is framed in terms of gain, people are risk-averse, and when choice is presented in terms of loss, risk taking is increased. This so-called framing factor may be so powerful that patients may make choices that fail to satisfy their own values, and experienced doctors understand that how options are presented largely determines patient selection (McNeil et al. 1982).

As discussed in chapter 1, objectivity remains an ideal and the conceit of neutrality belies the vested interests and biases of the professional, whose own values and experience must influence their opinions and advice. Indeed, because judgment is at the crux of decision making, in what situations do we want professional advice that is restricted to naked facts—that is, devoid of guides and interpretations? To serve as a clear-inghouse of opinion, studies, data, and all those elements that go into clinical judgment, patients seek a mediator and counselor. Indeed, to serve as a resource is one of the doctor's fundamental functions! This raises the specter of physician values (or less kindly, bias), and perhaps the best one might expect is that physicians reflect on how their own values might be effectively integrated with those of a patient, with which they may clash. Julian Savulescu observes that physicians must acquire a sensitivity to these issues as well as new skills to understand the place of value judgments. Reiterating the discussion in chapter 1, facts and values are inseparable:

It is relatively easy to be a fact-provider (though how to present facts itself presents a problem). It is easy to turn decision-making over to patients and say: "There are the facts—you decide." It is difficult to find all the relevant facts, to form evaluative judgments, and critically examine them. It is even more difficult to engage a patient in rational argument and convince him that you are right. If doctors are to avoid the shortcomings of being mere fact-providers, if they are to function properly as moral agents, if they are to promote patient autonomy, they must learn these new skills. They must learn these skills for another reason: ... Gone are the days when they did not have to provide a justification for the position they were advocating. And that justification goes beyond the fiction of a "purely medical" justification. (Savulescu 2000, 79)

The responsibility that physicians and nurses accept in helping a patient understand his illness and the options to deal with it is rarely a straightforward matter. To derive a course of action most consistent with the particular needs of that patient is a self-reflexive exercise that must weigh both the health-care provider's medical judgment and the patient's preferences. As discussed below, paternalism is not being invoked when direction is asserted. A negotiation must occur, and if conflict arises, patient wishes must override other opinion. But, and this is the critical caveat, physician responsibility remains whatever degrees of patient autonomy are exercised. Indeed, the entire debate over patient autonomy results from the tension arising from the medical point of view versus the patient's. The latter always trumps the former in the United States, but the moral calculus of care does not change, only its legal implementation.

My position may be stated too starkly, but I wish to stake out a larger ethical space for physician beneficence, which I hope may be accomplished by reconfiguring autonomy's own standing in the clinic. The argument has already been presented effectively by Schneider, who describes two models of autonomy: first, optional autonomy, where patients may, but are not required to, make decisions about their treatment, and second, mandatory autonomy, where patients must exercise their autonomy regardless of their desire to do so. Indeed, an autonomist like Haavi Morreim argues that people should not burden others with their life decisions, and, what sounds suspiciously like a prescription, she opines that "it is this capacity to be an agent, to bear responsibility for decisions and actions that are truly one's own, that renders a person worthy of moral respect, dignity, as beyond merely considerate treatment" (Morreim 1995, 134). This view may be called "mandatory autonomy," which is based on a rationale that patients must make their own decisions to confirm their self-dignity, and secondarily curb the potential abuse of power by doctors. This attitude assumes that doctors have, and exert, domineering power over the patient, and that the dependent and weak require assistance against what can only be construed as an adversary. Of course, patients are free to select and dismiss their physicians, and given the legal protections of informed consent and malpractice, patients have potent recourse to professional abuse, which effectively offsets physician authority. But more to the point, Morreim is exhorting all to exercise a version of autonomy that makes demands on the ill that few are capable, or even wish, to respond to.

Another tack taken by the strong position is the so-called prophylaxis argument, which asserts that patients benefit medically from participating actively in their own care, because of the salutary effect of being in control. This attitude may hold for some patients, but there is no evidence that it is widely applicable, or that more than some unidentified small group requires this sense of self-governance. Some certainly do, but most probably do not (Schneider 1998, 151). But the strong autonomists will insist that most people suffer from false-consciousness, another speculative and uneven belief that "if people . . . just saw their interests more acutely, they would want different things" (p. 151). Accordingly, education of an unsuspecting consumer will result in a more assertive patient. The counterposition simply avers that most people are satisfied with the ordinary clinical dialogue, and that the overwhelming majority of patients do, in fact, satisfactorily understand their own situations, their own interests, and their own minds (p. 153).

Facts would, of course, help settle this dispute, and the majority of studies that have examined this problem have concluded that most patients are pleased to have their doctors inform them of their clinical options, but when it comes to making a final decision as to what to do, the typical patient delegates that decision to their physician (pp. 92–99). Most physicians would concur with Schneider's measured assessment: Because patients fall on a continuum of decision making, no prescription suffices. We require a process by which the complex spectrum of patient behavior might be accommodated, and in this process, a moral structure must be in place to satisfy the extremes at both ends.[3]

That process must acknowledge an existential fact: the medical scenario makes autonomous persons inescapably dependent. In situations where individuals simply do not possess the experience to exercise informed decisions, "The strong view of independence imposes an obligation which cannot be met but is culturally so basic that it can be neither escaped nor forgiven. . . . Indeed, dependence is a feature of life at any time" (pp. 173–174). Here, "relational autonomy" makes its claims. As discussed in chapter 3, when autonomy is configured in the web of social relationships, choices become negotiated in light of those relationships and not artificially situated in an enclave of individual isolation. In short, decision making may be regarded as cooperative or selective.

Uncertainty abounds at every step of medical treatment. In addition, communication between doctor and patient is not only impaired by the barriers posed by medical jargon, the knowledge base of bioscience, and the fear and anxiety that may overwhelm a sick patient. Sickness itself may rob the patient of his rational faculties and may also blur the distinct beliefs and values that are so necessary to the exercise of autonomy. In addition to these formidable obstacles, the bureaucratic nature of modern medicine as well as various forces that dehumanize the patient converge to make the free exchange of ideas and options often difficult, if not impossible. The sick devote enormous energies to their illness, recovery, and countless other new issues.[4] Most physicians would agree with Schneider (1998, 74–75) as to why patients might not crave the decisional authority the autonomy paradigm envisions for them: "Those decisions are so complex, so foreign, so tumultuous, so recalcitrant, so confounding, so demanding that patients might reasonably hope to escape them. . . . Delegating medical decisions is not the only reasonable strategy for patients, nor always the wisest. . . . But . . . many patients delegate medical decisions because they believe someone else will make them better than they can."

How is autonomy to be exercised if a patient becomes "preoccupied" and unable to take part in making medical decisions? Though such persons run the risks associated with paternalism, they generally exercise their autonomy by distinguishing (per the Frankfurt-Dworkin model) higher and lower decision making and so avoid the burden of executing lower choices they feel incapable of making. Patients delegate such decisions, because they reasonably believe that physicians are more capable of assessing technical choices for them. Anxious and frightened, "Patients clearly make medical decisions in ways that are less than optimal and quite different from the ways lawyers and bioethicists assume" (p. 99). In sum, "Many patients seem to have declined to seize the power of decision bioethics has proffered [because they] believe themselves poorly situated to understand and analyze medical problems, [and] too ill to face serious decisions" (p. 108).

Schneider adopts what I believe is a commonsense approach to these matters, but a deeper philosophical agenda awaits us. Key to the exercise of autonomy is moral competence. According to Tristram Engelhardt (1996, 139), people demonstrate such competence by (1) being able to conceive of rules of action for themselves, (2) exercising rationality, (3) exhibiting moral sensibility, and (4) thinking of themselves as free. By these criteria, Engelhardt appropriately discounts the autonomy of fetuses, infants, or retarded adults. But I would go further. The ill are not fully autonomous either, if one understands that to act rationally and freely (criteria 2 and 4), one requires the intellectual competence and emotional wherewithal to make informed decisions. Patients frequently (if not usually) lack full competence in two ways. The first is simple ignorance. Medically unsophisticated, or at least untrained, patients cannot be expected to fully understand and integrate the vast body of technical and scientific information required to make informed clinical decisions. Although motivated patients can be rapidly familiarized with the knowledge base, nevertheless, health-care providers attain their professional standing precisely because they possess a greater fund of knowledge and experience, and more to the point, a frame of reference that allows for more objective decision making. On account of that expertise, patients authorize them to make decisions. This delegation of authority is the basis of beneficence.

The second issue pertains to a more primordial level of experience, namely the dependence of the ill on doctors and nurses. Frightened and in psychological, if not also physical distress, the patient is fundamentally dis-eased. To think rationally and dispassionately about life-and-death choices is all too often beyond normal human ability. Indeed, fear about sickness or death is the appropriate response when we ourselves are the subject of calamity.

A third factor, while not a general concern, is cognitive impairment. Patients with fever, insufficient brain oxygenation, and short-term drug effects (e.g., from sedatives) are quite easily recognized as exhibiting compromised competence. But less obvious are the long-term cognitive impairments resulting from chemotherapy for cancer, which produce more subtle alterations in rational functions. Beyond experiencing decreased physical capacity, including exhaustion, these patients often exhibit defective abilities to organize, multitask, and maintain routines, as well as to perform memory tasks, including word finding (Cull, Hay, and Love 1996; Bender, Kramer, and Miaskowski 2002; LaTour 2002). These so-called chemo-brain effects (unrelated to anxiety, depression, or fatigue) appear related to the dose and duration of chemotherapy, and perhaps even more disturbing, the cognitive defects may be long lasting

(Wieneke and Dienst 1995; Schagen et al. 1999). One is hard pressed to attribute full competence to such patients, yet their choices are not typically scrutinized in the context of subtle thought disturbances.

Any experienced physician recognizes the diversity in patients' expression of autonomy. The need for information is highly variable, with some seeking a comprehensive explanation, some wanting or expecting little information, and some exhibiting different degrees of discussion at different times in the course of their illness. Many patients only seek reassurance or basic information. In their effort to understand the general parameters of their welfare and prospects for health and happiness, information alone often serves to satisfy these needs. Thus, patients may legitimately seek information without wanting to make the relevant medical decisions, and they may shun control for fear that they might misuse it, or because it is cumbersome.

Medical decision making is a dramatic example of the variable nature of voluntary choices writ large.[5] From this perspective, it is clear that ongoing negotiation needs to accompany the presentation of patient options and that voluntary choices may or may not be desirable. The key point, then, naturally follows: the exercise of autonomy, like the related notion of voluntariness, is best regarded as a variable moral exercise (O'Neill 2002, 37).

Because medical decisions exhibit a colossal variety, it is pointless to make sweeping generalities as to whether patients should or should not make particular choices. Different contexts, different personalities, different clinical scenarios all demand individualized assessments to determine the appropriate degree of patient autonomy. When all of these considerations are weighed, it seems obvious that autonomy is a question of degree and that its exercise should be determined by myriad factors, which may be reduced to the simple determination of whether the patient is comfortable delegating authority. By the Frankfurt-Dworkin model, the total relinquishment of medical decision making to a physician may still be an exercise of autonomy, and from a practical standpoint, this seems a viable formulation in most settings. To insist on a more extreme enactment of autonomy seems simply misplaced.[6]

To illustrate the continuum on which patient autonomy and physician responsibility are enacted, I will sketch two cases drawn almost arbitrarily from my personal experience. Each illustrates how autonomy is an interpretative project, and in that hermeneutic, various approaches are not only possible, but inevitable. (Names have been changed, but otherwise the accounts have not been fictionalized.)

Case 1

"Mama's Jehovah Witness. So am I."
"I know."
"Then you also know she can't have no transfusion."
"I know. But I want to give her a blood substitute.
Something new. It's made from blood, but it isn't
blood"
"So, what are you asking?"
"Mrs. Jones, do you understand that without a
transfusion the risk of you dying is very high?
You are in the Coronary Care Unit, because your heart
isn't getting enough blood."
"I know."
"Do you want a transfusion?"
"She don't want no transfusion!"
"Mrs. Jones, do you want a transfusion?"
"Is it blood?"
"No."
"Then I want it."
"Does that mean you'll take the transfusion?"
"Yes. The new stuff."
"Mama, the Elders don't allow that."
"We'll worry about the Elders later."

Comment:
This dialogue clearly illustrates disparities of power, inasmuch as the doctor's voice of authority overwhelms the daughter's protestations. Indeed, a power brokerage has been established between the doctor and Mrs. Jones, and the daughter was displaced while her mother negotiated with the physician. The doctor suspected that the Church Elders were

unlikely to view the chemically modified blood substitute as sufficiently different from the natural substance to warrant its use. But in his moral calculus this was subordinated to what he perceived as his patient's deeper wish to live, albeit in sin for which she might seek absolution. One might argue that the doctor manipulated the patient, and thus violated her autonomous choice by offering her biased information. But the rebuttal holds that in this instance, the deeper motives of the patient are in question. According to the Frankfurt-Dworkin formulation, the choice for life trumped that of religious rectitude. Using a liberal interventionist strategy, the doctor assumed responsibility for a morally ambiguous exchange by rationalizing that the desire to live was dominant, and in offering a rationale for the blood substitute (a moral trespass in its assertions according to Jehovah's Witness doctrine), he was effectively enacting the patient's truest desires. Alternatively, a negative assessment might easily be formulated and the doctor vilified for inappropriately imposing his values.

Case 2

November 13, 2002
Herod le Grand, M.D.
Julia Heidegger, M.D., Ph.D.
Buster Display, M.D.
Re: Tumor Board consultation on November 9th, 2002
Dear Drs. Grand, Heidegger, and Display:
I am writing to let you know how extremely disappointed I am in my experience with your consultation at the Tumor Board on November 9th, 2002. Your Tumor Board has an outstanding reputation and, thus, my expectations were high. I hoped to hear an innovative and creative approach to treating my obviously serious diagnosis of stage 4 non–small cell lung cancer. As you recall, I am 40 years old, have no risk factors, am tolerating chemotherapy extremely well, and am otherwise in excellent health. My recent CT scans and a recent PET scan showed that my tumors have stabilized and are shrinking in response to chemotherapy.

I was shocked to receive a death sentence from you during our consultation. Your casual delivery of it was unbelievably cold and insensi-

tive. I have spoken to quite a few oncologists over the past few months since I was diagnosed in December of last year. No other doctor has ever spoken to me in the way that you did and given me no room for hope. I know that there are lots of new treatments in development that may, in the next few years, be able to extend my life. I did not need to hear the words from you, Dr. Grand, that it is the cells that have spread outside my lung "that are going to kill you." Nor did I appreciate your telling me, not just once but twice, that this cancer will "take your life." Dr. Heidegger delivered statistics to me about the number of years I may live, from one to three years. She did mention something about the possibility that it might be able to be treated as a chronic illness in the future, but then Dr. Display was quick to jump in, repeating for the second time that the cancer certainly "will take your life."

The three of us, myself, my husband and a close friend, left the consultation speechless. While I am well aware of the dismal statistics regarding survival rates with lung cancer, I also know that there are exceptions to statistics and everyone is a case of one. More importantly, I can't stress enough how much more helpful it would have been to me for both of you (another doctor in the room whose name I do not remember said very little) to find a more humane way to speak to patients. When you are talking to another human being about their life (especially someone who still has young children), it would be more appropriate to be more tactful and sensitive in delivering devastating information.

You left me in a horrible state of shock and severe depression. I will try to find a way to put it behind me because I believe that having a positive outlook and cautious optimism is key to trying to heal and live my life, however long it may be. No one should ever play God and tell people how long they have to live. No one can predict the future in such a certain way as you chose to.

Dr. Grand, please think twice before you make statements like I've already quoted, including your statement that it would be a good idea to get a brain MRI because lung cancer cells "like to go up into the brain."

My husband is a psychiatrist and my friend who was at the consultation and I are both clinical psychologists. We are well trained in the value

of how, what, and when you say difficult things to people so they can hear it in a way that is helpful and hopefully productive. I suggest that doctors at your medical center, if they don't already, receive training in bedside manner to learn more humane ways than we experienced to talk to people with life-threatening illnesses.
Sincerely,
Jessica Strong, Ph.D.
cc: Chief of Staff
Chair, Board of Directors

Comment:
This case is reminiscent of one I described in *Confessions of a Medicine Man* (Tauber 1999a, 119–20), where a woman was brutally informed of a diagnosis of terminal cancer. What went wrong there, and here? The members of the Tumor Board informed Jessica Strong of their best medical judgment concerning treatment of her lung cancer, and in this sense honored their commitment to her autonomy, namely, the right of the patient to be fully informed of her condition. In this regard, they undoubtedly believed that they were fulfilling their professional responsibility of full disclosure and the need for transparency. Unfortunately, this approach was not appreciated by the patient, husband, and friend, and, indeed, from the perspective of the care of the patient, the consultative opinion was woefully insufficient . . . not because it was *wrong*, but because it was incomplete in presenting the full horizon of possible outcomes and insensitive because it dismissed the empathetic dimension entirely. The Strongs felt, and there is no reason to question their responses, that the stark conclusions drawn and the way the information was transmitted were hardly appropriate to this particular patient. In a word, she felt assaulted, and in this sense her autonomy was violated. Interestingly, the professionals' error in judgment arose because the physicians did not know the patient beyond her medical record, and this gaping hole in the doctor-patient relationship highlights how care of the patient must extend to a minimal appreciation of those dynamics that will enhance trust and lead to the best therapeutic outcome. Hope was a vital ingredient for Jessica Strong, and she was unceremoniously robbed of it. At the very least, a more judicious balance of opinion might have been offered without distorting the clinical reality. In short, the

mistake, and I believe one was committed, resided in the board's inability to relate to Mrs. Strong as a person, as opposed to an individual with a disease.

Despite the consensus that doctors and patients should share in the decision-making process, we see in these two illustrative examples, the difficulty of correctly predicting the patient's own understanding of autonomy and the hidden impediments in reaching mutual understanding. And more, we see how patient autonomy may easily by compromised by even well-meaning physicians, whose power is exercised in subtle and not-so-subtle ways (Brody 1992; Levi 1999). In this regard, it is perhaps surprising that little comment has been made about conflict over control, about situations in which patients assume an apparently ill-informed control of the treatment process. If one appreciates the dominant moral and legal standing of autonomy (e.g., "no competent patient in the United States has ever been forced to undergo medical treatment for his or her own good. No matter how tragic, autonomy should always win if its only competitor is the paternalistic form of beneficence" [Veatch 1996, 42]), then conflict resolution deserves serious examination. Dan Brock and Steven Wartman (1993, 80) have suggested a taxonomy of the different sources and forms of what appears to be irrational patient decision making in order to give practitioners tools for distinguishing between a patient's apparent irrational choices, which the physician may wish to change, and merely unusual choices that should be respected. The general attitude advocated here is what Ronald Dworkin (1993, 224) calls "the integrity view of autonomy":

The integrity view of autonomy does not assume that competent people have consistent values or always make consistent choices, or that they always lead structured, reflective lives. It recognizes that people often make choices that reflect weakness, indecision, caprice, or plain irrationality—that some people otherwise fanatical about their health continue to smoke, for example. Any plausible integrity-based theory of autonomy must distinguish between the general point or value of autonomy and its consequences for a particular person on a particular occasion. Autonomy encourages and protects people's general capacity to lead their lives out of a distinctive sense of their own character, a sense of what is important to and for them. . . . If we accept this integrity-based view . . . our judgment about whether incapacitated patients have a right to autonomy will turn on the degree of their general capacity to lead a life in that sense.

Accordingly, in finding a balance between professional authority and patient preference, physicians are obligated to negotiate choices based on their own best judgment but, in the end, yield to their patient's final selection. This must be a deliberate process of sorting out rationally held beliefs that may be in conflict from irrational choices:

Being autonomous may not require that one's choices and actions are rational. But it does require that one's beliefs which ground those choices are rational. If this is right, what passes for respecting autonomy sometimes consists of little more than providing information, and stops short of assessing whether this information is rationally processed. Some of what purports to be medical deference to a patient's values is not this at all: rather, it is acquiescence to irrationality. Some of what passes for respecting patient autonomy may turn out to be less respect than abandonment. (Savulescu and Momeyer 2000)

Irrational choices may be made by patients due to ignorance, abandoning rational deliberation, or simply making mistakes. The antidote is for physicians to sort out the crucial difference between belief and choice. Whenever competent patients appear to be making irrational choices about treatment that are contrary to their own well-being, physicians must determine if such choices are made because of conflicting belief systems (then little can/should be done to persuade patients to shift their values). But if the choice is based on irrational choices, the physician is obligated to assume an educative posture in an attempt to persuade the patient that other choices are better and still conform to his individual values.

Rationality is framed by circumstances and driven by underlying emotions and social forces, so patients and their surrogates still do, at times, exhibit what appears to their doctors as irrational choices. These include (1) a bias that gives disproportionate weight to securing benefits and avoiding harm in the present and near future as opposed to the more distant future; (2) a denial reaction in which an "it won't happen to me" irrationality allows patients to feel invulnerable to certain harms; (3) an escape defense where fear of pain or the medical experience elicits irrational decision making. Even though Brock and Wartman allow that patients' choices should be respected, this does not mean that a selection must "be simply accepted" when it is irrational. But their prescription is weak indeed (p. 91), and in the end these authors conclude, as most would in the present climate of rights protections and assertions, that even a truly irrational choice is not a sufficient indication of a patient's incompetence that would allow the physician to override that choice.[7] Coercion, intimidation, and co-optation are exchanged for counseling and cajoling, because "sometimes, the best that physicians can do is present the choice in alternative ways in the hope of minimizing framing effects" (p. 88–89). And sometimes, despite the best-placed efforts, "wrong" decisions are made. Of course, "wrong" is being defined by the medical authority, by no means a final arbiter in any case.

In short, the doctor must navigate the treacherous shoals of what she believes are choices likely to maximize the patient's well-being, at the same time recognizing the ultimate right of patients to make decisions when they are able. A rational choice rests on the coherence of values and beliefs, based on a patient's own deep commitments, aims, and priorities, and "an irrational choice is one that satisfies those aims and values less completely than another available choice" (Brock and Wartman 1993, 83). This standard subordinates physician values to the patient's right to self-determination, and at the same time offers parameters to guide the doctor in counseling her charge.

Expanding the Fiduciary Function

Is there a protected site for patient autonomy, and what are its limits? Much discussion has ensued as the balance of physician authority and patient autonomy has shifted over the past thirty years. Indeed, various formulations and prescriptions have been offered to address these questions (e.g., Childress 1982). But the practices that are proposed for securing or respecting autonomy in the medical context have been too often reduced to informed consent, and the "much-discussed triumph of autonomy is mostly a triumph of informed consent requirements" (O'Neill 2002, 38). In other words, a procedure, informed consent, has been substituted for what is, in fact, an extremely complex moral action. "Sign on the dotted line" captures typical practice, and perhaps more importantly, too often distinguishes informed consent from patient autonomy.

So the question remains, given the concerns summarized above about the exercise of informed consent, at what point does a particular patient lose the ability to make free and rational choices? Tom Beauchamp and James Childress (1994, 101), in their pragmatic approach, offer a wise intermediate opinion: "Merely because our actions are never *fully* informed, voluntary, or autonomous, it does not follow that our actions are never *adequately* informed, free, or autonomous." "Adequate" is a freely floating designation, one that may be adjusted to any given clinical setting. It is a practical accommodation to a problem that does not readily lend itself to a prescribed formula of abstract principles.

My concerns about patient autonomy, especially as exemplified by "informed consent, " are hardly radical. Indeed, most medical ethicists have reduced the role of autonomy by introducing other ethical principles that must be factored into the moral setting (e.g., beneficence, justice, nonmaleficence) and thereby acknowledge the limits of an autonomy-based morality for medicine, and they have also weakened the concept of autonomy itself within the medical scenario. As an example, allow me to again cite Beauchamp and Childress, who pursue both strategies. First, they offer a loose definition of autonomy—intentionality, understanding, and freedom from controlling influences—to render consequential decisions as "substantially" autonomous if these criteria are met (1989, 69; 1994, 123; 2001, 60). Driven by context, as opposed to some inclusive general principle, they allow a flexible approach to informed consent, where the various elements (disclosure, understanding, voluntariness, competence, and consent) need not always be fulfilled to satisfy "autonomous authorization" (1989, 79ff.; 1994, 133ff.; 2001, 69ff. [this edition is substantially revised]). Sensitive to the varying degrees of competence of the ill, they measure autonomous authorization by a set of capability criteria, which may be applied with varying degrees of stringency to determine whether an individual is capable of making an informed decision. Conflict then arises as to how strict such rules should be and how judiciously they might be applied in any given setting (see note 7).

This approach then opens the door to the role of beneficence in decision making, and we immediately recognize that autonomy cannot be divorced from the responsibility health-care professionals assume in the care of the patient. In fact, this is the entry for other moral principles that must operate in the clinical setting, the second mode by which autonomy's dominance has been effectively challenged:

Making respect for autonomy a trump moral principle rather than one moral principle in a system of principles, places an inappropriately high premium on autonomy.

Although respecting autonomy is more important than biomedical ethics had appreciated until the last two decades [1970s and 1980s], it is not the only principle and should not be overvalued when it conflicts with other values. (Beauchamp and Childress 1989, 112; 1994, 181; 2001, 104)

Increasingly, this pragmatic, multivariant approach has gained influence, but Beauchamp and Childress lament, perhaps with some resignation, "So influential is this autonomy model at the present time that it has become difficult to find clear commitments to the traditional beneficence model in contemporary biomedical ethics" (1989, 210; 1994, 272, but omitted in 2001!). Yet their approach seems appropriate to me. Instead of pitting one principle against the other, they seek an appropriate balance of competing ethical interests, whereby beneficence might incorporate patient autonomy, a position I follow, albeit in a different way:

No premier and overriding authority exists in either the patient or the physician, and no preeminent principle in biomedical ethics—not even the admonition to act in the patient's best interest. This position is consistent with our earlier claim that beneficence provides the primary goal and rationale of medicine and health care, whereas respect for autonomy (and nonmaleficence and justice) sets moral limits on the professional's actions in pursuit of this goal. (Beauchamp and Childress 1994, 273; similar wording 2001, 177)

Despite their eloquent espousal of a plurality of moral principles, their measured and ecumenical strategy finds little acceptance among factious contenders who seek to define contemporary medical ethics along other, more doctrinaire lines.

Perhaps further analysis will help. The conundrum about patient autonomy resides squarely in the very character of informed consent. Informed consent is a *propositional attitude* (O'Neill 2002), which for philosophers means it is "opaque" (Quine 1963)—one might see no further than the specific descriptions it contains. So, in the medical context, the "vision" of the patient must necessarily be, for all the reasons enumerated above, myopic with respect to understanding consequences, risks, and other options. Competency encompasses many degrees of freedom, and none should be assumed. In the end, we are left with a pragmatic approach, one that must be resilient to differing patient needs and clinical demands. This position is a realistic appraisal of typical moral choices in the hospital or clinic, and serves as a pragmatic working model for decision making. But I am left contemplating what "*adequately* informed, free or autonomous" (Beauchamp and Childress 1989, 101) means.

One response invokes an expanded notion of physician responsibility, both legal and para- or extralegal. Within legal confines, physicians perform fiduciary-like roles and generally regard themselves as adhering to a fiduciary ethics. But American law regards such functions only in narrow contexts (Rodwin 1995). "Fiduciary" is now largely a metaphor, and no longer, at least legally, possesses much relevance to the doctor-patient relationship. While one might presuppose that physicians act on their client's behalf, fiduciary principles have only been applied for specific purposes. Physicians cannot abandon their patients, they must keep clinical information confidential, and they must disclose to patients any financial interest in clinical research (Rodwin 1995). That physician fiduciary authority is so limited seems counterintuitive to our basic notions of health care (one might reasonably assume a wider legal basis for physician responsibility), but aside from professional competence and these specific fiduciary responsibilities, the law makes little demand on beneficence as a governing moral principle in medical practice. This is hardly the ethic endorsed by an entire pre-1970s generation of physicians, clearly articulated by the Harvard surgeon, Francis D. Moore (1959 vii): "The fundamental act of medical care is the assumption of responsibility . . . complete responsibility for the welfare of the patient."

That adage now too often seems quaint, at best, and paternalistic. Nevertheless, if one embraces a weakened traditional model for the doctor-patient relationship, a broadened fiduciary role of the doctor is assumed and current American law seems anomalous. After all, the oldest tradition in medicine makes physician responsibility to the patient sacrosanct, and, indeed, empowers the physician to act on behalf of the patient. And while some have argued that this relationship remains at the core of medicine (e.g., Pellegrino and Thomasma 1988; Tauber 1999; Pellegrino and Harvey 2001), others regard this classic formulation as naive and "woefully inadequate and inappropriate" to present realities (Wildes 2001). In this view, medical care is a commodity: patients are clients or consumers, who should be able to freely choose their health-care options, and if they did so, the quality of care and price effectiveness would improve (Herzlinger 1999, 2003). (Accordingly, if health-care customers had better consumer information and choice, competition among providers would follow other capitalist markets to the benefit of patients.) In this scenario, physician responsibility then resides solely in providing specific professional services, and no more. The critics are legally correct, and responsibility has been diffused as the corporate dominance of contemporary medical care has taken hold.

But physicians have dual responsibilities in the managed-care setting—to the employer and to the patient—and while the doctor's legal persona demands allegiance to the company, the deeper moral commitment to the care of the ill creates an ethical tension (see Jacobson and Cahill 2000 for comprehensive references). And most saliently for this discussion, medicine as a commodity draws on a model based on consumer-patient autonomy. In the contract model of care, the autonomous free choice of the parties binds and defines their relationship, and thus autonomy makes its easy transition into the medical culture in no small measure because of its ready extrapolation from a commercial construct and the politicojudicial principles governing it. Perceived in the master narratives of medical ethics, which are often developed from case law, the underlying preoccupation with conflict resolution reveals the basic *legal* structure of the contemporary doctor-patient relationship. But this is not necessarily an accurate description or formula of medicine's *moral* praxis. This is a crucial distinction and a dilemma not easily resolved. Despite autonomy's ambiguous standing in medicine's moral universe—the complex dynamic governing its balance within that ethical canon, which includes beneficence, justice, and nonmaleficence—it remains the trump card because of its legal standing. Indeed, because of the primacy of the principle of patient autonomy, fiduciary options are severely restricted. And because beneficence has not been given broad sanction by the law, conflict between commonsense ideas of professional responsibility and patient autonomy often arises. In short, the legal and moral universes do not necessarily coincide, and therein is the rub. The casualty is trust, and to this issue I now turn.

5

In Search of a Moral Glue

It is a characteristic of human life that we naturally trust one another. . . . This may indeed seem strange, but it is part of what it means to be human. Human life could hardly exist if it were otherwise.
—Løgstrup 1971, 8

One has to be struck by the deep inconsistencies in our notions of moral agency in medical ethics. We espouse the ideals of autonomy, and yet we must admit the limits of autonomy in the clinic and hospital. Patients settle for varying degrees of choice, believing, from a practical standpoint, that the options exercised are sufficient to maintain a sense of freedom. And medical ethicists justify this compromised version of autonomy, more often than not, by employing such qualifying terms as "sufficiently informed" or "adequately understood," implicitly acknowledging the limits of patient understanding and freedom. Informed consent then becomes a prescribed process, much like following a dance routine. This is not "bad" in any ordinary sense. After all, virtually every study that has examined patients' efforts to learn about their disease and therapy shows that they shy away from decision making, to the undoubted consternation of those who insist that they protect themselves (Schneider 1998).

Patients, like individuals in other social roles, allow themselves to fit into a structure in which they trust that their basic rights will be protected. By and large, they are concerned far less with their political or legal autonomy than with getting better. They prioritize their various definitions of selfhood, and autonomous individuality—at least in this setting—is almost always subordinated to other identifications. Indeed, being a patient alters the fundamental sense of personhood. Patients want to facilitate the process of healing, and to do so they usually readily admit their dependent status. In short, autonomy in the medical context is an *aspiration* of the curing process—a goal, not a starting position.

To direct our efforts, we need a better understanding of the nature of trust between patients and their caregivers. Trust and trustworthiness are basic to each element of our discussion of patient autonomy—legal, political, psychological, and sociological. But as the doctor-patient relationship has changed in recent decades, former modes of implicit trust have been exchanged for patient rights and defensive medicine. This chapter examines this issue with a lens that sharpens my argument against a particular kind of autonomy, and at the same time widens the scope of our inquiry to include the vast social and economic forces that have weakened the doctor-patient relationship.

As already discussed, advocacy of patient rights is a response to a loss of trust as contemporary medicine has been caught up in a general social crisis, where each of our basic institutions—government, education, medicine—has been forced to adjust since the turbulent 1960s to a new balance of power and expectations between power brokers (in this case, health-care practitioners) and their constituency (i.e., patients). Autonomy-based medical ethics originated when disgruntled patients and their advocates reacted against what they regarded as physician arrogance, and drew on legal precedent to demand informed consent in medical practice. The pendulum swung forcefully and unwaveringly toward patient autonomy and away from the older tradition of physician paternalism. In the words of Ruth Faden and Tom Beauchamp (1986, 94–95), "This [language of rights] emphasis is a new kid on the block in medical ethics. Its tone and connotation carry a message, usually reserved for law, that has never before been a part of physicians' thinking about patients. When turned in the direction of medical decision-making, it literally invites the replacement of the beneficence model with the autonomy model." This assertion of a new doctor-patient relationship was based on a shift in the basic contract of care, as a result of a breakdown in older patterns of trust. As discussed in chapter 2, informed consent was used by the courts and the legislatures to ensure and expand patients' rights to have access to information, to participate in decisions, and to determine whether procedures should be performed. In short, as Paul Root Wolpe (1998, 48) wryly observes, "Informed consent is the modern clinical ritual of trust." He might have added that medical ethics reflects the erosion of that trust. And such a profound realignment has not only had consequences for local doctor-patient interaction, but has necessitated broad changes in the terms and conditions of medical practice more generally.

The irony, the one prompting this book, is that these efforts to safeguard patient autonomy and offer protections against possible abuse have failed to reestablish trust. After exhaustively reviewing the relevant surveys and studies, Onora O'Neill (2002, 11) correctly observes that public trust in medicine "has faltered *despite* successes, *despite* increased efforts to respect persons and their rights, *despite* stronger regulation to protect." She then asks the obvious question: Why?

The short answer: contracts (exemplified by informed consent) cannot substitute for beneficence and the trust accompanying it. This claim will require some exploration (provided below), so here let me simply observe that the contract "solution" falls directly out of the commodification of contemporary medical practice. Patients have become consumers and doctors have assumed the complex identity of "provider." The purchase of care, the contractual agreement framing that commercial arrangement, and the resulting defensive autonomy adopted by the client are all products of a basic shift in the doctor-patient relationship from one dominated by a sense of personal commitment to a more distant and circumspect delivery of service. Doctors have always sought economic gain, but in earlier periods the business end of their practice was usually subordinated to their interpersonal relationship with their patients, rather than reflecting the consumerist mentality that dominates health care today. In short, medicine's ethics arise directly from the system in which they operate—to facilitate, coordinate, and order its inner workings. Bioethics has only a limited ability to realign the identities and the behaviors arising from, and in response to, that system. This is a simple admission that the social and economic forces have coalesced to present Americans with a new alignment of patient and doctor. To better understand the "logic" of these relations and the ethics that regulate them, I now explore the matter of trust.

The Problem of Trust

Consider an interesting paradox, which for now at least is presented as a proposition: an augmented requirement for trust is intimately related to (alternatively, reflects or parallels) the ascendancy of autonomy. As we assume greater degrees of social atomism and move between multifarious social roles (based on the autonomy of individual choice), trust becomes increasingly important, because more traditional ways of defining interpersonal relations are in transition. If one *knows* the prescribed actions that accompany a particular role, the expectation that the role will be fulfilled is enhanced. When the actors are not known to each other and/or the roles are less well defined, trust must replace the expectation. In other words, in this era of fluid interpersonal relations, trust has become *more* important as a "regulator" of behaviors. And ironically, as the need for trust rises, so do the requirements of trustworthiness. If discordance appears, mistrust grows. With the commodification of health care, we witness a potential conflict, because the *traditional* role of caregiver is less well defined. By this reckoning, patients easily fall prey to misgivings, inasmuch as the traditional expectations are often not met. Countermeasures to reassure patients may not be effective, and consequently the intimacy of the doctor-patient relationship is stressed and often broken. In this new context, mistrust takes hold and defensive postures are assumed. This is the fertile ground in which "autonomy" arose as a key principle of bioethics.

For me, the interesting problem is not so much how to guarantee patient rights, as worthy as that might be, but rather how to configure "autonomy" in the medical setting so that it no longer represents the defensive position of a threatened person, but instead becomes integrated into an apparatus of care in which trust is enhanced. In what might appear as a paradoxical alignment, I believe that autonomy is best served by reconfiguring notions of individuality and self-determination in a more intimate patient-physician dyad. If trust was enhanced, the *requirements* of autonomy would be lessened. Accordingly, we enhance patient autonomy by fortifying an ethics of responsibility that presumes an ongoing negotiation of choices and decisions between patient and physician. This in turn posits a high degree of physician responsibility, which is then perceived as trustworthiness.

While I am focusing in large measure on characterizing trust, trustworthiness is the moral issue at stake. Interestingly, as I will review below, defining trust dominates the philosophical and sociological literatures, but the moral question is truly framed by how well trust is established by the actions of the one seeking the trust of another. The calculus thus depends on how well the physician fulfills the ethics of responsibility, from which *trustworthiness* is derived. Trust then is a psychological response to the success of that ethic, and mistrust is, in turn, the failure of that moral demand.

I proceed by beginning to unravel the intricate web of social, psychological, and moral strands comprising "trust," and in doing so, I draw on a rich literature as the question of trust/mistrust has emerged as a topical issue.[1] In medicine, specifically, the unsteady standing of trust has received increased attention as commentators have focused on both the macrosocial factors and microinterpersonal elements that seem to have adversely affected the doctor-patient relationship (Annison and Wilford 1998; McKinlay and Marceau 2002). The health-care dyad, traditionally characterized by trust on the part of the patient, seems too often plagued by doubt.

Two dimensions of mistrust spring to mind. The first concerns confidence in professional ability and judgment; it stems from the increasing evidence of physician error (Institute of Medicine, 1999; Berwick 2003), and, perhaps even more important, patients' increasingly sophisticated knowledge of the controversies and uncertainties that plague the science of medicine. (I am referring to the debates that arise over the efficacy of new advances in diagnostics and therapies.) Doctors are increasingly facing an informed consumer, who often presents a skepticism toward medical authority. Such suspicion may be well placed and appropriate, but it is not my concern.

The second dimension of mistrust involves moral interpretations of trust. Sown by cynicism and cultivated in a climate of social wariness, patient autonomy assumes its defensive character in a climate of unsteady relationships. Putting aside the degree of patient confidence in their physician's technical ability and the prestige of medical science, a deeper, and perhaps more menacing question looms concerning the ethics of responsibility. In the corporate setting of an HMO, in the emergency ward of a municipal hospital, and even in a private doctor's office, patients increasingly wonder, "Will my doctor do what is best for me?" This question is not directed toward pondering professional competence, but rather concerns the personal commitment of the caregiver who increasingly must account for her divided loyalties.

As discussed in chapter 2, in this era of managed care, the doctor-patient relationship is now an "encounter" and the doctor has become a "provider," while the patient has become a "client." This corporate vocabulary reflects a different moral tone than that traditionally governing medical practice. Prior to World War II, a close coincidence of interest between physicians and patients was generally regarded as emblematic of their relationship. Today, the "trust question" is the disparity between this older norm and what is now too often only a nostalgic (perhaps romnnticized) memory of a more intimate relationship. Putting aside the accuracy of this idealized past, the yearning for a more personalized relationship between doctor and patient seems widespread. After all, physicians in the corporate environment do have conflicts of interest, which may give rise to patient mistrust. Patients are aware of these competing agendas (Emanuel and Dubler 1995; Mechanic 1996; Mechanic and Schlesinger 1996; Kao et al. 1998a, 1998b; Shortell et al. 1998; Buchanan 2000; Jacobson and Cahill 2000), and physicians have been known to compensate for their corporate affiliations—sometimes by lying to extract benefits for their patients (Freeman et al. 1999; Wynia et al. 2000) and sometimes by not offering potentially useful services because of perceived coverage restrictions (Wynia et al. 2003).

To be fair, the ethics of managed care are complex and hardly reducible to a "them-us" formula: the broad economic requirement of limiting health-care costs has powerful utilitarian motives, and within the political context these are hardly disputable. The debate rages as to how the resources are best used. In that discussion, the costs of administration and the reaping of profits cut into the health-care dollar with huge moral implications. But patients know, and worry, that the ethics of providing good returns on investment are strikingly different from the morals governing health care (Illingworth 2000). Perhaps the most interesting formal response to the challenge of split allegiance has been made in the Charter on Medical Professionalism (Blank et al. 2003), a broadly adopted code of ethics. Beyond outlining the specific responsibilities to advance the well-being and dignity of their patients, the charter urges physicians to improve patient quality of care, access, and more equitable distribution of resources as part of their moral code. This code of ethics clearly places the physician's loyalties squarely with the patient (see chapter 2, note 15).

While an argument might be made, on the contract model of care (discussed below), that autonomous subscribers make their own choices that do not rely on older forms of trust (Morreim 1995; Mariner 1995; Goold 1998), this is patently false. Employees typically have little or no choice as to which health plans are offered them (Davis et al. 1995). How can autonomy be invoked when patients perceive that they are victims of economic forces that restrict the health care they or their loved ones have access to? A defensive posture is a natural response (Bodenheimer 1996; Blendon et al. 1998).

But the managed-care setting presents only the most obvious example of the shifting relationships between patients and their caregivers. I maintain that a more general ambiguity has replaced the traditional trust characterizing the patient-doctor dyad, and the sources of this misalignment are deeply embedded in contemporary society. Physician accountability is one way of reassessing this vanishing ideal, and a myriad array of studies, regulations, legislation, and reactive risk-management measures now mark a profession that until quite recently conducted its business with little concern for maintaining its own professional standards of behavior (Shortell et al. 1998). The shadowed presence of others at the bedside to protect the patient is a symptom of deep mistrust between health-care providers and their patients. As Francis Fukuyama (1995, 27) observed, "People who do not trust one another will end up cooperating only under a system of formal rules and regulations, which have to be negotiated, agreed to, litigated, and enforced, sometimes by coercive means." While an invigorated standard of patient autonomy signifies one aspect of the changed social and economic climate in which medicine exists, neither informed consent nor regulations can substitute for primary trust.

Clearly, trust is highly correlated with patient satisfaction (Anderson and Dedrick 1990), and while many theories thrive as to why trust has been eroded, few measures and little data can accurately ascertain the general impression of trust's decline in the clinic (Pearson and Raeke 2000).[2] To quantify this problem is difficult, inasmuch as the categories of assessment are not standardized (Hall et al. 2001). The kinds of questions that must be addressed include how thoroughly clinical problems are evaluated, how well health-care providers understand and empathize with a patients' individual experience, and how effectively they communicate and successfully build a relationship with their patient that is both honest and respectful (Thom and Campbell 1997). These interpersonal parameters then must be meshed with, and also kept distinct from, the perceptions of providing appropriate and effective therapy. Despite patients' continued high levels of trust in their primary physicians (Blendon and Benson 2001), the data do point toward patient mistrust as a growing problem. Sorting out the mistrust directed at the individual physician versus the system at large is vexing, but by and large, current studies suggest that patients have a higher degree of trust in their physician than in the system in which they are enmeshed (Hall et al. 2002). The strength of the interpersonal commitment is strained by the powerful economic forces in which clinical practice is embedded, and several emerging trends suggest that interpersonal trust will be increasingly undermined in coming years due to a perceived competition of interests.

While interpersonal trust has until now provided considerable insulation against serious conflict (Hall et al. 2002), the warning signs are apparent. With a particular eye toward the doctor-patient relationship, I want to outline the complex character of trust and thereby highlight how integral it is to any discussion of autonomy. Indeed, I believe that the dilemma underlying this entire discussion of the doctor-patient relationship is the problematic status of trust in contemporary American culture. These comments are directed not so much at offering either a psychological analysis or a philosophical anatomy of trust, as at illustrating how trust serves as the moral glue of society. I seek to show that the particular issues we have been concerned with here cannot be understood independently of the greater social and historical contexts in which autonomy resides. Our review of the erosion of trust in contemporary American society will offer a better understanding of why the autonomy question in medicine has become so difficult to resolve. And from this broad perspective, I hope to better situate patient autonomy in medicine's social and moral universes.

Eroded Trust

The search for reliable bases for social solidarity, cooperation, and consensus has arisen from recent challenges to the most basic sources of the social: reconfigurations of traditional values around family, work, and personal lifestyle, the appearance of new patterns of normality determined by a changing social, political, and economic life, and the redrawing of national identities due to globalization and an increasingly pluralistic culture. Thus, the questions of how social trust is established and how it might be strengthened have become increasingly insistent (Misztal 1996, 4).

Since the 1960s, Americans have redefined the relationships of citizens to their basic institutions—educational, governmental, medical, military, corporate—because of what can only be characterized as a crisis in trust (Wolfe 1991). The general consensus that trust has become increasingly precarious in America is supported by numerous empirical studies that show variation in levels of cooperation in different political and social environments (e.g., Fukuyama 1995; Putnam 2000). The specifically American historical roots of this issue may be traced to the 1830s, when Alexis de Tocqueville first coined *individualism* to describe the ethos of antebellum Americans. Perhaps he was particularly prescient in recognizing the political and social ramifications of this identity, when he observed that in democratic societies, a high degree of voluntary participation in civic associations took the place of aristocratic forms of centralized government. He saw that individualism actually weakened social activity and that countermeasures were required to achieve collective goals: societies that stressed equality became most reliant on voluntary associations to achieve common aims (Tocqueville [1840] 2000, 490).

He offered an ironic explanation: In democracies, "All citizens are independent and weak; they can do almost nothing for themselves, and none of them can oblige those like themselves to lend them their cooperation. They therefore all fall into impotence if they do not learn to aid each other freely" (p. 490). Tocqueville saw the economic segmentation of the workforce as negating independence, so that at the heart of individualism resided a paradoxical denial of personal emancipation. Democracies, precisely because governmental authority was diffuse, required an active citizenry to achieve their own social objectives, both within government and without. He drew an important political, and moral, lesson from this observation: "In democratic countries the science of association is the mother science; the progress of all the others depends on the progress of that one. Among the laws that rule human societies there is one that seems more precise and clearer than all the others. In order that men remain civilized or become so, the art of associating must be developed and perfected among them in the same ratio as equality of conditions increases" (p. 492).

Robert Putnam has used Tocqueville's measure, now called *social capital*,[3] as a sensitive indicator of social cohesion. Studying membership in a variety of social associations (ranging from bowling leagues to civic and religious voluntary groups), he has shown that Americans, in generations born since World War II, have become increasingly disconnected from each other. As a result, fundamental social institutions—for example, church groups and PTAs—have suffered collapse as a result of new social patterns emphasizing atomistic behaviors at the expense of collective communal ones. Echoing Tocqueville, Putnam (2000, 134) observes that "the touchstone of social capital is the principle of generalized reciprocity"—the general understanding that my helping you now is done with the expectation that you will help me later. Confidence in reciprocity is based on deeply ingrained patterns of trust, and empirical evidence shows that those engaged in community life are both more trusting and more trustworthy than those who isolate themselves (Putnam 2000).

Putnam maintains that social trust is a measure of cooperation between individuals and is distinct from trust in institutions or political authorities. (Luhmann (1979) calls these relationships *trust* and *confidence*, respectively.) Various surveys have measured both, and while correlations may exist, for my purposes, the measure of the former is most important in establishing a context for the doctor-patient relationship. The data are consistent: since the mid-1960s, Americans have increasingly been suspicious of each other and doubted the honesty of others (Putnam 2000, 139ff.).[4] Using an array of measures, the empirical evidence only verifies what most of us already intuit: relying on trust alone in American society is increasingly regarded as naive, if not dangerous. Instead, legal recourse, regulations, imposed strictures, and policing agencies have substituted for what used to be settled by trusting another to fulfill the expected task: "For better or worse, we rely increasingly—we are forced to rely increasingly—on formal institutions, and above all on the law, to accomplish what we used to accomplish through informal networks reinforced by generalized reciprocity—that is, through social capital" (Putnam 2000, 147). And so medical ethics and malpractice law appeared in tandem with a general decline in social trust, whose replacement with regulations and legal mandates saw the substitution of patient autonomy for older forms of trust. From this wider social standpoint, the suspicion of physician authority (and accompanying responsibility) simply reflected the major shifts occurring in society at large.

Though medicine as an institution is still trusted more than education, television, major companies, and Congress, confidence in medicine's leaders has fallen precipitously (Blendon, Hyams, and Benson 1993). Though poll data from the period before 1970 is limited, a 1949 Gallup survey asked American adults to look at a list of six "well-known professions" and identify those they trusted most. Doctors of medicine topped the list. By 2001 they had fallen to fourth, placing behind nurses, pharmacists, and veterinarians. Interestingly, as a group, health-care providers remain at the top of the list, and doctors remain high on the list of professions, despite their diminished status relative to other health-care providers.[5] Yet, the "quality of communication and trust" continues to deteriorate (Murphy et al. 2001, 126), which most commentators regard both as a reflection of general trends in American society, and due to particular problems in health-care delivery. The impersonal system of managed care is generally identified as the most influential of these local factors. Doctors are no longer perceived as solely governed by their interest in the patient's health and welfare, and the public now seems skeptical regarding physicians' motives. Due to the nature of managed care, economic incentives place "the interests of patients and doctors in direct conflict" (Mechanic 1996, 178). The perception of care as part of a "medical marketplace" is troubling—but hardly to all critics (e.g., Herzlinger 1999, 2003)—and many patients feel that they must now be "on guard" (Mechanic 1996, 177).

Given the centrality of trust in assessing contemporary American social changes, there has been renewed interest in defining the problem on the part of various academic disciplines, which have endeavored to offer a sociological analysis of how trust operates and of what it represents morally. These discourses are, of course, complementary, and while I will make no attempt to comprehensively review them, I believe by teasing out their major themes we will have a clearer picture of how to place autonomy and responsibility on the axis that connects them.

Defining Trust

What is trust? A prominent approach is to regard trust as a means of negotiating risk and acknowledging the unpredictability of the future. Trust refers to the endangerment arising from the "discretionary power of the other" (Baier 1994b) or the "fundamental inscrutability of the other" (Seligman 1997, 69). To account for such an assessment, trust is seen as coping with one type of risk by trading it for another type of uncertainty (Sztompka 1999, 32), which in turn is based on an "individual's theory as to how another person will perform on some future occasion" (Good 1988, 33). Each of these refractions of the idea involves two ingredients: uncertainty (of risk) and dependence (on another), each of which is largely determined by the roles the actors play.

In his influential book *Trust and Power* (1979), Niklas Luhmann argued that contrary to the notion of trust as characteristic of traditional societies, the growing complexity, uncertainty, and associated risk of postindustrial societies made trust a crucial component of effective inter-relationships in Western cultures as well, if not more so. Adam Seligman (1997) built on this line of argument and went further in arguing that trust is a specifically modern phenomenon linked by the division of labor, the pluralization of roles, and the nebulous character of role expectations in a highly specialized society, where self-reliance as traditionally understood has become a vanishing ideal. The consequence is that risk becomes a factor that must be self-consciously weighed as one increasingly relies on others. Accordingly, trust is not only a means of negotiating risk, it implies risk, and precisely because one cannot necessarily expect a return or reciprocal action, trust can only be offered and accepted (p. 63). This dependence on others led Seligman to opine that trust acts as what I will call a "solvent" in which various roles are enacted.[6] And, indeed, the ability of human agents to assume their individuality depends on the ability to move from one role to another, which in turn is conditional on the solvency provided by trust: "It is not the space between roles per se which leads to individualism or to trusting as a form of social relations. . . . Rather, the emergence of individualism . . . rests on the ability to move between roles and role expectations, and trust emerges precisely from such movement or rather from its very potential" (Seligman 1997, 59).

Individuals now have an aggregation of roles, enabling them to mediate and blur their identification and movement between roles by a self-reflexive, private process, as opposed to some normative group-held injunctions (Seligman 1997, 129). (This is a fancy way of saying that a person can be a corporate executive during the day and a disc jockey in the evening as he or she effortlessly switches group affiliations.) This fluidity of assumed roles, each carrying its own moral vectors, demands a matrix by which negotiation occurs. Trust holds respective identities in juxtaposition to one another in the public domain. Since the roles of others are similarly fluid, each party must assume a predicted behavior, and because of the complexity of roles and the latitude in which they are enacted, assumptions must prevail. The assumption that expectations will be met is trust; the suspicion that failure looms is mistrust; determination of their respective likelihood is risk assessment.

Trust encompasses various types of relationships—personal, categorical, group, institutional, commercial, technical, systemic—and in describing them, various methodological and theoretical approaches have been employed.[7] For instance, Mark Hall (forthcoming) notes that descriptive, normative, and prescriptive discussions of trust are often intermingled. He offers a framework based on three different attitudes toward medical trust: predicated, supportive, and skeptical. The predicated stance, exemplified by informed consent, takes trust as a factual premise that imposes obligation. This form is discussed below in connection with the so-called contract model of care, which is firmly grounded in commercial law. A supportive stance describes the unstated, assumed sense of responsibility a patient entrusts his physician. This form of trust is described below with respect to the covenant model of care and is based on physician beneficence. Finally, the skeptical orientation begins with the understanding that trust cannot be sustained or even justified. Instead, distrust is institutionalized, as exemplified by the regulation of managed care.

Such descriptive formulations are complemented by various philosophical perspectives. For example, rational-choice theory examines whether it is rational to trust and if so, under what conditions (e.g., Gauthier 1986; Williams 1988; Hollis 1998). These arguments, often involving game theory, hinge on the definition of rationality, and thus acquire complex philosophical constructions about the nature of rationality—that is, its social (e.g., Baier 1997) and moral (e.g., Baier 1995) character. Others emphasize the emotional character of trust, correctly observing that as often as not, one does not trust based on careful deliberation and assessment of evidence, but rather on implicit assumptions that reflect unconscious emotions and experience (e.g., Govier 1993; Lagerspetz 1998; Lahno 2001). And there are those who have attempted to balance the claims of each school (e.g., Jones 1996). Closely related to the cognitive/affective debate is the question of whether altruism is natural—that is, whether human trust and generosity have an evolutionary history (Sober and Wilson 1999). Apparently, advocates of the biological basis of altruism believe that efforts to enhance what apparently is inborn and not simply acquired in culture, assume renewed legitimacy if they can demonstrate the natural status of cooperative social behaviors.

Irrespective of these various conceptualizations, I note, like others before me (Williams 1988; Hardin 2002), that the philosophical literature is preoccupied with "trust" when, in fact, the issue is "trustworthiness." Trustworthiness is the true locus of moral concern, for it requires fulfilling a commitment of one to another. Responsibility, indeed, an *ethics of responsibility*, is the moral foundation of the trust/mistrust phenomenon, which itself is a psychological or social product of the moral engagement: trust follows as the acceptance of that ethical action. Once trustworthiness is established, trust follows within the variables of how the "dependent" psychologically assesses that presentation, both as a variable of personality and within the larger context of previous experience. Bernard Williams (1988) succinctly outlined the so-called macro- and microlevels of enactment and pointed out that the motivation for generating trust required self-interest, since he was skeptical of the social or religious power of some benign commitment to ensure trustworthy behavior. Russell Hardin (2002) built on this argument and defined "encapsulated interest" as the vehicle for promoting trustworthiness and thereby trust. This essentially sociological account subordinates the moral challenge of fulfilling obligations and duties by translating the deontological question into the domain of assessing motivations and self-interest. Rather than relying on benign goodwill and moral rectitude, these authors are more confident in the practice of balancing power and interests.

I demur. I still hold that morality goes beyond power relationships and cannot be guided solely by utilitarian ends. Yes, we follow a pragmatic course to answer the demands of divergent beliefs and pluralistic traditions, but in the moral intimacy of the doctor-patient encounter, I am reaching for a more personalized moral commitment. I have had occasion to discuss this issue in detail in chapter 3, where the Hume-Nietzsche line of argument was contrasted with the tradition beginning with Kant and extended by neo-Kantians (e.g., Rawls, O'Neill, Herman, and Kosgaard), as well as feminist ethicists from a different perspective. Both groups seek to ground a social ethic in a deeper metaphysics of identity. But the challenges remain: How do these relation-based formulations help us better address the moral encounter of doctor and patient as one in which patient trust is engendered?

To respond requires that we consider one more philosophical matter: the ethical nature of the doctor-patient relationship. Indeed, why is *relation* the lynchpin of the entire question? This issue runs as a constant stream beneath, and sometimes rises to the surface of, our various discussions in one form or another. I venture that an answer requires different strategies, so here I take one more approach, one firmly planted in the everyday life of the clinic and in the ordinary behaviors of its moral agents.

A Groundwork for an Ethics of Responsibility

The ethics of everyday life, the morality of the ordinary, is the "place" in which medical ethics is enacted. The routine interaction between doctor and patient, not the dramatic life-and-death decision making that dominates the thinking of bioethicists, defines the "space" of relationship, where the quiet, ongoing administration of care is most characteristically enacted. The case studies filling ethics textbooks do not typically address the moral dynamics of the everyday care of patients. Extraordinary decisions are not routine. An ethics of the ordinary is also required.[8]

A conduit to the "ordinary" is opened by recognizing the fundamental social character of clinical practice. As Martin Heidegger configured human coexistence as *Mitsein*—our being together with one another in the world—the ethical follows an "ordinary" course (Olafson 1998). Eschewing the theoretical and abstract for a moment, let us dwell on the social dimension in which the moral grounds behavior. Instead of erecting theories to structure or formulate medical ethics, let us simply observe the moral as it emerges in the everyday exchange of health-care providers. There we will find the moral in the interstices of effective social interaction, and more germane to our current inquiry, the source of trusting relationships. To the extent that philosophy captures and understands those behaviors, it becomes a philosophy of the ordinary—an analysis that offers insight about the parameters of an ethics of responsibility in the everyday life of the clinic. If that philosophy rings true, it should enhance physician self-awareness of what it is to be ethical.

How might one describe "the ordinary" life of the hospital and what does it tell us? Sometimes, the intimate is unrecognized. Indeed, to appreciate the mundane, I, as a physician, must dissociate and peer at myself as an anthropologist might observe a village scene. Donning that disguise, what do I see? As I walk through the halls of the hospital, discussing cases with the residents and fellows, stopping to talk with colleagues, negotiating with nurses, laboratory personnel, and administrative types of all varieties, and, of course, conferring with patients and their families, the vast clinical spectrum of biomedicine with its various diagnostics and therapies assumes aspects of an intricate drama involving chesslike characters played on a multidimensional board. The board in this schema is the health-care complex, which structures care; the pieces move about to "capture" or eliminate patient-based problems; and as I observe all of this movement, it begins to appear that we are enacting a "game."

Games in a general sense need not be won or lost, but more generally engage actors in activities governed by rules. Generically, *game* covers the spectrum of chess, word play, puzzles, building sand castles, roleplaying, and so on (Wittgenstein 1958). And games need not be entertainment. Designating a social activity as a game confers a certain way of thinking about the relationships of the actors, the rules by which they function, and the organization of their activity. Game theorists apply different kinds of logical analysis to discern choices and behaviors; sociologists seek structures by which to codify functions; policymakers and the military employ games to predict outcomes. In short, games have assumed a standing well beyond fun and frolic. For me, *game* is a way of describing the "ordinary," and so to follow our present tack, let us consider medicine as a game, one composed and regulated by its own peculiar rules, interactions, and assertions of diverse wills working within a multidimensional system of competing interests.

As I watch myself and those around me, I have pondered, If this were a game, what are the rules? Who are the players? What are the objectives?

The pieces of the game (e.g., the diagnostics and therapies) moved about the playing board are only artifacts of the game, and these have different meanings for the players employing them. For instance, the physician regards the chest MRI ordered for his patient quite differently than would the hospital accountant or the insurance comptroller. For the former, the test represents data for evaluating disease and more broadly caring for the ill person. For the accountant, the MRI is a cost item, and its significance hinges on whether it is reimbursable. The game then is played at several epistemological, economic, and social levels simultaneously, and its complexity arises not only from the interactions at any single level, but also from the intersections between those levels.

Dispensing with any further descriptive characterization, the game, at any level or composite of different levels, essentially remains a value-based schema of behaviors. These values, of course, vary, depending on the roles played by the agents. The physician is concerned with an ethics organized around the care of the patient (and even at this single level, autonomy, beneficence, and justice vie for dominance), while the financial agent is responsible to a different constituency with a different set of values altogether. Indeed, the two are playing by different rules, albeit related to each other. Simply because the game appears as a win-loss scenario, the patient ponders who will prevail. Here, mistrust develops, because one's health care is not typically regarded as a purchase. Something is profoundly amiss when a person must *protect* himself to attain a service so basic to his life. So, as doubt emerges, the social alchemy of defense works a peculiar chemistry to "protect" the patient.

Patient mistrust arises from this general concern as to whether his best interests will be protected. In the metaphor used here, the patient is unable to understand, and thus play, the game. And no wonder; clinical medicine is not even a single game, but rather an ensemble of games, always intricate, often mysterious and even hidden. Various agents play by different rules and yet they still must interact with others aspiring toward different goals, some competing and others in line. Consider how health-care professionals—doctors, nurses, allied health workers, and administrators—follow one set of related rules, while corporate engineers, government administrators, and industry profiteers follow others. And even when one focuses on the health-care professional—that is, doctors and nurses—their professional logistics do not always coordinate with each other! Each group of actors must interact and their successful negotiations depend on subtle clues that hinge on the fluidity of the relationships.

Given their competing interests, traditions, rules, and aspirations, what ties these various players together? One obvious answer is the patient, but other contenders beckon. After all, beyond the patient, physicians answer to their professional ambitions, economic needs, and social roles. While the ethics of care largely orders the doctor's behavior, those ethics compete with others. Accordingly, the ethics governing patient care is a subset of a much larger moral universe, where the ethics of ordinary clinical life encompasses different domains with interlocking, yet distinct sets of interests. The call of the patient is dominant, but not entirely. Here, we must probe to find the wellspring of trust.

If physicians are playing diverse roles with differing rules and goals, no wonder moral confusion might reign. Trust emerges when the patient recognizes that the doctor is focused on his care and the other contending matters competing for attention are subordinated. This message, enacted by explicit actions and more subtle messages, aligns the doctor with the patient to form a couplet that then moves confidently on the game board. When the patient recognizes this bond and the promise it signifies, trust emerges. On the ethics game board, physician trustworthiness is the basic rule. Win, lose, or draw, the doctor plays well only when he fully joins the patient in the quest for restored health or any of its conjugates (e.g., palliation, chronic adjustment, rehabilitation, and so on).

This "process" ethics, dynamic and dialectical, requires a moral compass. Physicians are constantly making value judgments ranging from interpretations of data, to choosing a clinical strategy, to forming relationships with patients and hospital personnel. In a broad sense these choices are ordered by ethics—the ethics of care, of professional integrity, of personal belief. And underlying each of these ethical structures is an "ethics of responsibility." By this I mean that physician identity, irrespective of all the other contending personas, is formed in response to the physician's obligation to the patient. Most would designate this constellation of values as the "ethics of care," but an "ethics of responsibility" better addresses the moral intimacy of the doctor-patient relationship. It calls on the primordial recognition of the other, or in other words, an ethics of responsibility is metaphysically situated as a response to an other (Tauber 1999a).

The ethics of responsibility orients all other contenders, including self-definition. By this I refer to the Hegelian construction of identity as arising from the self-consciousness of self-recognition in the encounter with another (see chapter 3). In enacting the ethics of responsibility, the physician is not only defining her personhood, she is also authenticating it (Tauber 1999a). Many might find these ethical metaphysics distasteful, and I well recognize that my position may be dismissed for any number of reasons, so I offer a critical caveat: the self-image of the doctor is determinative of her ethical persona, and while I am espousing a deep commitment to the patient, other attitudes beckon.

Here I must admit to an obvious bias. Undoubtedly, doctors may assume a more distanced stance and still fulfill their professional responsibilities. Indeed, as discussed in detail in the next section, a "contractual" relationship, as opposed to one determined by a "covenant," may be more appropriate, even realistic, in responding to the demands of contemporary health care. Below, I elaborate on that argument, but suffice it to note that my entire presentation is based on a presupposition: physicians, in donning their professional mantle, accept an abiding responsibility for the care of their patients. We can argue about how comprehensive this responsibility is, but the ethical dimensions are certainly wide and demanding. In the clinical scenario, an ethics of responsibility defines its values in relation not only to the biomedical treatment of disease, but also to the broad social and psychological experience of a patient's illness. Consequently, physician actions follow from judgments and options governed by an array of considerations, in turn determined by the patient's best interests at various levels. The "game" is exceedingly complex and the patient requires a trustworthy guide. In short, trust is derived from ordinary doctor-patient interactions, and the kind of trust is defined by that relationship. To that matter I now turn.

Contracts, Covenants, and Clients

The analysis of trust relies on a characterization of personhood and the nature of relationships, which in turn determine the character of moral commitments. This platform then sets the stage on which the ordinary ethics of health care are practiced. The *perception* of risk translates into varying degrees of trust. Trust, in itself, is subject to many variables outside the doctror-patient dyad—for example, personal history, psychological propensities, cultural context, and "treaties" of interpersonal relationships. This is the domain I now wish to explore more fully, and to do so I again return to formulations of selfhood, where trust assumes two different characterizations. If persons live in a social world of conflict, one in which the moral commitments of autonomous individuals to each other are based on independence and self-interest, trust is negotiated. But if persons are characterized as connected and responsible for each other, then trust assumes a different character. Instead of regarding trust as the means of negotiating risk, in this latter formulation, trust is constitutive to the relationship itself, and in this sense is ontologically part of it. In both formulations, trust is the basis by which persons interact successfully, but in the former it is, in a sense, a product of an ongoing negotiation, while in the latter, it is assumed as part of the identity of the parties.

In my view, medicine is, or perhaps only ideally is, the exemplar of this latter kind of trust. Many contest that opinion, so to draw the lines more clearly, I now contrast two models of the doctor-patient relationship, one based on a legal understanding (emphasizing the encapsulated interest formulation) and the other on a voluntary pledge (residing squarely in a deontological construction). The two domains certainly overlap, but they are distinct, and as I draw out their ethical portraits, it will become clear how differently personhood might be understood when placed into one construction or the other, and what role trust plays in each. The moral implications are apparent.

More than thirty years ago, Robert Veatch (1972 and further developed in 1983a) and William May (1972) debated the character of the doctor-patient relationship. Each described what they took to be the most appropriate model characterizing the moral structure of care, and in so doing revealed the difficulties of reducing such a complex interaction to its ethical essentials. Veatch began by rejecting three candidate models: the engineering, priestly, and collegial models. The engineering model suggested that the basic relationship between doctor and patient was valueless, because the physician was regarded as a scientist or technician; the priestly model captured the paternalistic dominance of the physician; and the collegial model depicted doctor and patient as colleagues pursuing mutual goals. Instead of these, Veatch proposed that a contract model was most appropriate, where physician and patient negotiated a sharing of ethical authority and responsibility, and each would fulfill those stipulations. Aside from its strengths in clearly defining that specific obligations and duties were incumbent on both parties, Veatch recognized the sociological fact that by the 1970s most health care in the United States was administered in anonymous institutions and that the doctor-patient relationship was hardly intimate or premised on the friend/physician model (Veatch 1983b, 196).

The contract model is characterized by mutual agreement between equals. Informed consent is integral to this relationship, and a specific enunciation of rights, duties, conditions, and qualifications both limits the contract and establishes the basis for legal enforcement of terms on both parties. The contract thus offers each party some protection and recourse under the law to make the other accountable. By dispensing with a nebulous sense of charity or beneficence to account for physician responsibility, the contract model defines the dignity of the patient within a specific array of legal parameters that are both definable and enforceable (Veatch 1972; 1983a,b). Contractual relationships "intend to laicize authority, legalize relationships, activate self-interest, and encourage collaboration" (May 1983, 118). And most importantly, autonomy is honored and preserved.

May argued that the contract model was not only too restrictive as a moral description of the doctor-patient relationship, but it was distorting as well. Because of its legalistic bent, contracts highlight a formal, business relationship, and, indeed, "Promises [contracts] have no natural obligation, and are mere artificial contrivances for the convenience and advantage of society" (Hume [1739], 1978, 525). Instead, May (1983, 116ff) presented the covenant model, and argued it was at odds with the contract model at a deep moral level. The most obvious shortcoming of the contract approach to the doctor-patient relationship is that it eliminates, or at least minimizes, beneficence, and "tends to reduce professional obligation to self-interested minimalism, *quid pro quo*" (p. 118). But a more fundamental problem is also evident: no contract can exhaustively predict or cover the needs of patients, and the kinds of services rendered by physicians in terms of empathy or compassion can never be specified. In other words, "Covenants cut deeper into personal identity" (p. 119) by enjoining human resources that defy description and prescription. Contracts determine only what is required, not necessarily what is just, while a covenant "obliges the more powerful to accept some responsibility for the more vulnerable and powerless of the two parties" (p. 124).

Since contracts are made between equals, their playing field is equalized by the law; relationships based on trust in its looser meaning are typically between parties that are unequal in power and authority (Baier 1994b). The contract is a device designed for traders, businesspeople, and capitalists, not for children, spouses, or patients. Building from Hume's *Treatise* ([1739], 1978, 521ff.), Annette Baier (1994b, 106ff.) clearly illustrates how promises (contracts) are artifices inasmuch as they enable us to accept an invitation to trust, whereas in general we cannot trust at will. Prescriptions are simply too cumbersome, too rigid, too limited to allow for the free exercise of social interaction. In short, the contract model is hardly enough to describe the paradigm of trust between doctor and patient, considering its limited applicability, but it is enough to govern managed care (Jacobson 2002). After all, managed-care organizations are bona fide businesses and thus have been held accountable through contract law rather than tort law (which, incidentally, generally results in more limited monetary damages than does tort law). HMOs have not been regarded as exceptional to other industries, and the courts have consequently allowed them great latitude in pursuing cost-containment controls. The advocacy role of the physician for her patient has thus become more self-conscious, and, as already noted, conflicted for physicians aware of divided loyalties and responsibilities.

But medicine is obviously more than a business with self-interests protected by contract, for beneficence remains as a guiding ethos for the clinical encounter. Here the covenantal character of medicine is prominently displayed. We normally think of such responsibility as exclusively serving the patient's interests, namely, physicians act in accordance with the ends of medicine to relieve suffering and effect cures, and this is broadly regarded as a good. But the rub is whether the values of the physician coincide with those of the patient and whether the solutions offered reflect the best options for a particular case. Autonomy in this model is of a different character than that in the contract model, where the independence of the patient must be guaranteed in order to allow a free association with the physician to take place. In the setting of the covenant model, patient autonomy is used to trump physician values in determining clinical choices when a conflict arises. So, in a simple way we think of physician responsibility in terms of service to the patient, but the inequality of that relationship, essentially a bestowal of physician largesse on her patient, is balanced by a counterprinciple of patient independence and free choice. Indeed, beneficence is limited by patient autonomy in the covenant model, whereas in the contract model, individual autonomy is assumed and presupposed as part of the relationship. So we might say that autonomy is "outside" the covenant model and "inside" the contractual. Autonomy thus assumes a characteristic role that depends on the nature of the relationship between the parties. And, perhaps more to the point, trust assumes a different meaning in each model.

A hierarchy of trust is determined by the social context in which interpersonal relationships are played out. On one end of the spectrum are contracts, which are designed to limit ambiguity about expectations. As John Locke observed, contracts are written promises that define not so much *whom* one trusts, but *what* is entrusted (Baier 1994b, 101). Precisely because they are part of a legal system, contracts are designed to clearly define services and limit liabilities, so, if necessary, adjudication may occur within specified legal channels and with defined rules.

Trust in more intimate settings places relationships within implicit expectations, and because they remain largely unarticulated, they encompass actions that are not, indeed, cannot be specified. The trust between parent and child, teacher and student, doctor and patient must allow for seemingly infinite possibilities of interactions. They remain "liquid" and "open." Here we find a key difference between contracts and covenants. Because contracts elicit promises that reflect no human kindness (Hume [1739], 1978, 521), they show the limits of trust, not its full character. For Hume, the caustic critic, contracts were designed to protect the contractual parties from each other and thus to stabilize what he regarded as expected selfish behavior (pp. 519–521). In clarifying fragile or uncertain relationships, "the beauty of promise and contract is its explicitness." (Baier 1994b, 117). Conversely, trust is implicit and must adapt to myriad social challenges. Reflecting the deepest moral obligation to humanely answer another, medicine becomes an exemplar of trust. When trust fails or is denied, the doctor-patient relationship loses it moral bearings and uses instead a contract for a business venture governed by certain specifications. This hardly suffices to describe the trust that must ground the healing act.

Tom Beauchamp and Laurence McCullough (1984, 22–51) observe that the beneficence and autonomy principles of health care are at odds simply because of the different perspective each adopts. Beneficence is organized around clinical medicine's point of view, that is, what physicians might deem best for a patient, while the principle of autonomy is organized around protecting the independent values and beliefs of the patient. Thus an implicit bias is at play in the physician covenant inasmuch as the determination of value, of what is most appropriate, does not necessarily coincide with that of the patient, and as the rise of a rights-based culture has affected medicine, bioethics has been burdened with attempts to reconcile this basic difference.

One major approach tries to salvage the contract model on the basis of a Rawlsian notion of justice (e.g., Veatch 1981), and with the benefits of an ethics based on the sociological reality that patients and doctors increasingly meet as strangers (Veatch 1983b). But to admit a sociological reality—medicine is undeniably a business with self-interests prominently displayed in a market economy, where financial forces commit physicians to contractual relationships with their clients—begs the question and challenge of medicine's moral mandate. Indeed, while the current health-care lexicon often supplements *patient* with the descriptive terms like *client, customer, consumer,* and *covered lives,* this vocabulary only embarrasses us to admit how profoundly the ancient covenant model has been displaced by market models (Wildes 2001).[9] But the ethics of responsibility remain paramount despite the too often opposing demands of a commercial medical economy. To understand that claim, a philosophical characterization of trust is required.

Trust, a Moral Category

Sociology merges into ethics when the social scientist constructs his frame of reference on a moral foundation: "Viable society is perceived not only as a coalition of interests, but as a moral community" (Sztompka 1999, 4). Morality of course refers to how persons relate to each other, and *moral community* refers to the ethical habits and reciprocal moral obligations of community members (Fukuyama 1995, 7). Moral communities have three components, all closely aligned. The first is trust, the expectancy that others will behave in an expected virtuous manner; the second is loyalty, the obligation to refrain from breaching trust; and the third is solidarity (or perhaps identification with another), the sense of caring for the interests of others (Sztompka 1999, 5). But most important, from the perspective adopted in this book, is how a moral community configures and determines personal identity, or in other words, where the individual finds his place within the larger moral space of the group. The coordinates of that "space" define one's obligations "to trust, to be loyal, and to show solidarity to others. In other words it is the indication of the 'us' to which 'I' feel that I belong" (Sztompka 1999, 5).[10]

To address this ethical dimension, we come full circle, returning to the Scottish Enlightenment, when modern medical ethics had its first stirring (chapter 2). Francis Hutcheson, Adam Smith, and their colleagues championed individuality in the context of communal interests, and their program of developing the moral sentiments sought a balance between the needs of satisfying the growing sense of choice and the responsibility of autonomous agents against the wider needs and demands of the larger group (Seligman 1997, 107ff.). The atmosphere in which the doctor-patient relation was scrutinized reflected a general concern with an understanding of "civil society" that would promote a moral agenda of reciprocity, mutuality, and cooperation. This tradition joined an older public philosophy of "civic virtue"—originating with ancient Greek and Roman political philosophy and carried into the eighteenth century by Rousseau on the Continent and by the neo-Harringtonians in England. Their political philosophy subordinated individual interests to the collective good, and in the form of republicanism, citizenship itself was defined in terms of allegiance to, and identification with, the state. Thus civic virtue was less a private attribute than one defined in, and by, the communal context. But by the end of the eighteenth century, this public-based morality was increasingly eclipsed by one grounded in the private personal domain, and this move not only heralded a shift in the very conception of the state, but moved the focus of morality from one centered in the public domain into the private realm. And thus modern liberal individualism was born.

Understanding the philosophical foundations of "civil society" shows how self-consciously it described an ethical program (Seligman 1992). The major emphasis on individual agency grew from Protestant self-responsibility and personal conscience (detailed in chapter 3). Indeed, defining public morality in the face of a new individualized morality depended on an entire philosophical construction that posited an inner moral sense. The Scottish Enlightenment devoted itself to this project, whose basic tenets included the declaration of "moral sentiments" independent of reason and arising as a function of individual moral psychology. This ethics moved from an external authority to an inner morality, one based on the assumption that humans possessed an innate benevolence, a fundamental constituent of the human character. As Adam Ferguson wrote in *An Essay on the History of Civil Society* ([1767] 1782):

Mankind, we are told, are devoted to interest . . . but it does not follow that they are, by their natural dispositions, averse to society and mutual affection . . . human felicity does not consist in the indulgences of animal appetite, but in those benevolent heart; not in fortune or interest but in contempt of this very object, in the courage and freedom which arose from this contempt, joined to a resolute choice of conduct, directed to the good of mankind, or to the good of that particular society to which the party belongs. (pp. 57–58; quoted by Seligman 1997, p. 110)

Although radical individualism may have been born in these sentiments, its full flowering awaited later developments. What interests me in this history is the core idea of personal morality private (dominantly so), but still addressing social concerns and interests. In the mid-eighteenth century, Ferguson, Smith, and their fellow travelers assumed an "interactive self," one whose existence is fundamentally social, not atomistic. The self in their formulation was thus linked to the social whole by responding to an internalized social or communal "other" (Seligman 1997, 111).[11]

This ever-present sense of the individual situated firmly within his social context accounts for the natural sympathy and moral affections on which the Enlightenment moral community is predicated. So while "civil society" and "civic virtue" placed the realm of virtue in different domains (private and public, respectively), most strikingly different between what became modern liberalism and an older republican tradition is the conception of selfhood. Under the domain of "civic virtue," the self is constituted by its identification with a greater collective whole (Durkheim's "conscious collective" (Seligman 1997, 115); in a "civil society," the self is reflexive and thereby divided in seeking its proper action in response to inner needs as contested by public demands. In the *Theory of Moral Sentiments* ([1790] 1982), Adam Smith posited an internalized "impartial spectator," who allows moral choice to remain private and individualized (see note 11), but that internal judge probes the community to orient its options. Thus, this impartial adjudicator is the moral embodiment of a Januslike faculty, one that simultaneously peers both at the private and public moral domains to find the balance between personal aggrandizement and communal duties.

Smith configured a complex moral agent. Although ethical choices are private, the reflexive individual answers to a divided moral agenda, one prescribed by personal wants and the other by obligations to the community. In seeking the judgment of an impartial spectator, virtue ostensibly shifted from a public morality to an inner one. But I believe this internalization oversimplifies the duality of Enlightenment morality, which is truly an amalgam of the private and public. The tenet that conscience was private and that choice was personal must be balanced with the deeper idea that there was, in fact, a universal morality, one exercised in the public domain and accessible to all rational persons, which, while leaving moral agency to the individual, placed moral authority above him (see the discussion of Kant and neo-Kantians in chapter 3).

By the end of the twentieth century, the moral logic established 200 years earlier had borne fruit. Individualism made morality increasingly a question of personal choice. Indeed, in a pluralistic society characterized by a plethora of social, political, and religious groups from which to choose identification, personal morality became the key precept for autonomous agents. But the historical origins of autonomy assumed a reflexive self that contemplated the moral choices offered by personal desire or need and those of the collective. Without a guiding public morality, the requirement for a social glue, trust, grew.

As postindustrial society has imposed new identities and new relationships, trust must substitute for a public ethos to which all may subscribe. Indeed, trust is increasingly regarded as a valued and scarce resource in maintaining the dignity and independence of individuals, for what must transpire with the erosion of a public morality is either more rigid legal strictures to guide behaviors or the more elemental solution of trusted reciprocity between strangers.

The orientation adopted in this book reflects one prominent response to this challenge: recognizing the group character of identity, emphasizing the relational basis of personhood, placing rights within a broader moral context of reciprocal duties and obligations, and identifying the domination of community-based identification of individuals playing multiple social roles, all point to trust as the common stage on which all of these moral and social dramas are best enacted. The law certainly holds us together, but it is cumbersome if not antithetical to fluid social interaction. Most would concur that when the law must be invoked, normal trust has been replaced by a procedure of mechanistic design. Law appears when trust fails.

The Politics of Trust

The shrinking "public space" of contemporary Americans is reflected by many parameters, one of which is growing mistrust. There are many ways of describing this state of affairs, but the sociological tradition that begins with Durkheim's *Suicide* ([1897] 1951) is a compelling account of the anomie imposed by mass society. This tradition typically laments the social isolation characterizing such a society. And, indeed, new values replace the old. Autonomy becomes a cherished value as more traditional communal identifications recede. Ironically, the "problem" of anomie has, in certain contexts, been converted into a virtue. Asserting autonomy, at least in the form of individualism, is now an ideal, and the fact that it is a response to this crisis, converts the predicament into an opportunity. Autonomy makes no effort to reform the problem, because it leaves the quandary unresolved. We are left with the restrictions of communal space and the dilemmas of navigating it successfully, but we do so with a sense of self-sufficiency and concomitant self-satisfaction. We trade communal identity for a private one; we pursue private gains at the expense of public ones; we seek self-aggrandizement at the cost of social benefit. The antidote, at least as I have argued for the setting of the doctor-patient relationship, is a relational ethic.

The relevance of rebuilding the level of trust in society seems self-evident. We have become more interdependent as society has become increasingly factionalized and allowed a flourishing of subcultures and lifestyles. The diversity and specialization of modern life have spawned a hitherto unimagined diversity of roles, where each of us, under the umbrella of autonomous choice, ironically has become more dependent on trusting others to do what we cannot do for ourselves. The greater the number of roles, the greater the likelihood for role conflict; the greater the complexity of roles, the greater the need to negotiate role expectations; the more the negotiation, the more need for trust, because the boundaries, and even the content, of roles and expectations become more fluid, less determined, less specified by codes. Here, in the interstices of roles, trust serves as the moral "glue" binding us together in coherent groups.

As we each become more immersed in the individually created world of our own making, all the other persons on whom we are dependent must reliably fulfill our expectations. Is our mistrust in fact due to the disparity between expectations and results, or is there at the heart of our disquiet, the implicit acknowledgment that we are, in fact, hardly autonomous of others, only at best believing or hoping that our choices reflect autonomy? If so, we are then left with a tension between the ideal independence that free choice offers and the uncertainty that low levels of trust bequeath. I have maintained that if individualism is to thrive, we must recognize a beguiling paradox: autonomy in its atomistic posture must recede as a cherished value. Relational autonomy must take its place.

Bolstering trust becomes an effort within a political and ethical orientation that regards the strengthening of interrelationships as crucial for contemporary society. So by advocating a program of enhancing social cohesion and strengthening the trust that holds members of a diverse society together, I am proposing to reconfigure autonomy and its underpinnings, and I agree with Barbara Misztal (1996, 7) that this is an ambitious political project:

The re-invention of civil society, the renewal of the importance of personal bonds and the adaptation of the post-modern and post-industrial schemes as features of Western development relate to sociological attempts to find a balance between the competing nature of the different values. . . . Trust cannot be seen any more as an automatic by-product of macro-social or macro-economic processes, but rather it needs to be perceived as an active political accomplishment.[12]

That strengthening the claims of trust might now be construed as a political goal is interesting in its own right. Misztal suggests, and a large critical coterie would agree, that if the communal character of American life is threatened, we need to try to identify what is missing and then attempt to remedy that ill. In this sense, medicine is part of a grand social challenge.

Doctors and their patients are caught in a social and moral confusion, which I see as reflecting the precarious role of trust in contemporary society. If trust is the ultimate basis of the doctor-patient relationship, no wonder, considering what is occurring in the wider culture, that the clinical dyad is under stress. I have surveyed the legal response to the challenge and found it wanting. Contracts serve as poor substitutes for a more fluid interaction. Once mistrust is established, the law only can adjudicate the dispute.

So what is a remedy? Two domains of the trust issue need to be demarcated—one situated in the macro-overview and the other in the micro-interpersonal environment. In the first, the general cultural moment has realigned values of individuality and with that shift a change in patterns of interpersonal relations has placed new challenges on how Americans interact. Medicine is simply one of those arenas that is undergoing a change in more traditional relationships as a result of this cultural movement. This immense issue, its causes and possible resolutions, I cannot address. What I can do, albeit only in summary fashion, is to address the microarena of the clinic. Specifically, in what ways might local medical practice address the ascendancy of mistrust? (The assumption, of course, is that a more intimate doctor-patient relationship is worth pursuing.)

As already discussed, trust and mistrust are the resulting attitudes generated from a sense of *trustworthiness* (Hardin 2002), and this places the onus on the medical profession. Relevant questions then include the following: in what ways have health-care providers distanced themselves from their patients? How has the professionalization of young doctors supported the dehumanization of their patients? In what ways can the moral milieu of clinical practice be fortified to offset the corporate character of health-care delivery and the dehumanizing technology of modern diagnostics and therapies? These are crucial questions with no ready answers, but to ask them is to ponder to what extent doctors might better instill a sense of trust in themselves.

Consistent with the argument of this book, I believe certain changes in how physicians regard their patients should be considered. Specifically, what might physicians do to better personalize their interactions with their patients and treat their needs more comprehensively? How might they fortify the moral intimacy of the doctor-patient dyad? The next chapter points to several areas in which reforms and reconciliations might be attempted to address these concerns. So now we move from analysis to programs of action, from theory to praxis, from the predicament to possible solutions.

6

Reforms and Reconciliations

Medical ethics are divorced from everyday clinical practice.
—Walton 1998, 175

Now we consider practical responses to the foregoing critique. While each is designed to protect the dignity of patients, the topics presented are only several of dozens of possible approaches to reforming clinical care. But at least for my purposes, each points toward a more humane medicine and should be plainly visible as complementary to the discussion of earlier chapters. The translation of a theoretical orientation can take many forms, and these are offered in that spirit. I do not consider them radical, but their appeal has thus far seemed too limited and thus they deserve another airing, now with a more thorough philosophical underpinning.

The first is an alternative view of medicine's dominant biomedical clinical model, which focuses on the science of disease. Here I will again revisit the rationale for a more comprehensive psychosocial consideration of the patient. Proponents of a more humane medicine appeared, perhaps not surprisingly, at about the time medical ethics was born, and their goal was similar, namely, to protect the dignity of the patient. In addition to informed consent and all that it implied, these medical reformers sought to shift the emphasis of the clinical approach from a *diseased patient* to an *ill person*. The adoption of this alternative model to the dominant disease approach has had some success in achieving its goals, but the power of reductive science and the allure of powerful technologies continue to undermine this so-called patient-centered medicine. A plea for a reorientation is again offered.

To achieve the kind of moral sensitivity I espouse, a major commitment to promoting a morally sensitive approach to patients is required. My approach here is twofold, one long-range, the other immediate. I outline a proposal (first formulated with Richard Cooper (Cooper and Tauber, forthcoming)) for a dramatic shift in the guiding parameters of medical school education, with an appeal to move the curriculum into a paradigm that accepts the integration of fact and value, science and ethics, disease and illness. The patching that is now being done and the further reforms being discussed at all levels of education review are, in my view, inadequate without a firm commitment to changing the current paradigm. That is my quixotic ideal, and although it is briefly sketched here, I focus on more pragmatic, immediate concerns.

Appropriately, then, I fix my gaze on the role of current medical ethics training. My general perspective is that the basics of medical ethics should be taught to entering medical students, like any other preclinical subject, but more emphasis on moral reasoning must occur at the bedside and in the clinic. By experience and by example, students are too often allowed to overlook or simply ignore ethical issues. They learn to make decisions based on a clinical perspective that focuses on objective accounts of disease rather than on a moral perspective that scrutinizes the ill person. This professional socialization, which includes the acquisition of "detached concern," is thought necessary for effective professional performance. In other words, the student is conditioned to employ the objective perspective, giving only secondary consideration to the ethical aspects of their practice. This issue, closely related to the first, is reviewed to highlight how true respect for the patient requires a deliberate effort to expand the focus of interest beyond the science of disease to include multiple dimensions of the ill. In short, medical ethics should be integral to practice, not just an appendage to risk management. This must be taught in the clinic and become part of the professionalization of doctors.

To this end, the last section of this chapter discusses a mechanism that is immediately accessible to make the patient's personal world more available to the doctor. To do so, a deliberate identification of the moral issues must be accomplished. Irrespective of individual physician sensitivity, an entrance must be provided into a domain that has hitherto remained obscured by vapors of good intentions. To construct such a portal, I propose that a portion of the medical record be designated to specifically address the moral concerns of caring for a patient. The gathering of such information must become integral to the clinical assessment. By demanding attention to the ethical dimension of patient care, the health-care provider is mandated to take seriously this dimension of care. Rather than wait for major curricular reform, we can place bioethics squarely in the center of care by a relatively simple effort.

Diagnosing Disease, Treating Illness: A Conceptual Framework for Comprehensive Care

Effective physicians must fulfill two complementary moral imperatives: they must respect patient autonomy and assist in identifying those concerns that should be addressed to preserve individual dignity and self-governance; and where the limit of that decision making is reached, they must find the proper orientation to further the patient's best interests through an ethic of beneficent care. Physicians have traditionally regarded their moral responsibility as largely fulfilled in this latter exercise, and while I wish to emphasize the pro-active role of the doctor in identifying choices for their patients and maximizing their individual autonomy, the ethical structure of the doctor's responsibilities requires clarification.

One strategy is to focus on the character of the doctor-patient dialogue, one that should be more comprehensive than a simple focus on a restrictive view of pathophysiology. But what does this really entail? What are the limits of dialogue? Specific answers to these questions cannot be given, but a general orientation may be described. A broadened concept of disease is required to factor in personal factors and a self-reflectiveness on the part of physicians for the appropriate exercise of their professional power (Cassell 1997). These closely aligned goals may be taught and deliberately exercised, but doing so requires a revision in clinical medicine's guiding ethos.

Many critics have maintained that the medical model is insufficient for treating patients, since the biomedical approach is focused on "disease," and persons suffer "illness" (Barondess 1979). The two are not equivalent, inasmuch as patients are objects of disease study and cure, and thus represent the epistemological category in which the doctor-scientist functions. As already discussed in chapter 1, the attempt to seg-regate a fact-dominated science from the individuality of a value-laden illness is fraught with epistemological difficulties and moral implications. Medical science, which seeks general explanations based on universal scientific laws, is still oriented around a specific illness, which may follow some general rules, but is always individualized. Indeed, the epistemo-logical investigation begins with an historical account of the illness, which in itself confers specificity.

The individuality of each case makes the physician a peculiar kind of scientist: "However specialized and fragmented the technical practice of medicine may become, the true physician remains—as he has always been—the person who *takes the patient's history*" (Toulmin 1993, 240). This claim of physician as historian makes several demands. First, vari-ation must be sorted out to discern the universal, which means, simply, that the particular constellation of signs and symptoms must be assigned to a diagnosis. The significance of each datum must be weighed and factored. This requires both certain kinds of scientific assessment and a degree of intuition—what is often referred to as "the art of medicine," or in the terms of chapter 1, value judgments. The intuitive, creative syn-thesis of information is hardly reduced to rigorous scientific assessment, and, indeed, commentators have fashioned many ways of describing medical knowledge and its application, much of which is structured by various kinds of value (e.g., Delkeskamp-Hayes and Cutter 1993).

Beyond the epistemological configuration of the physician as historian is a moral dimension—the ability to *hear* the patient. To truly listen yields an appreciation of the psychological and existential elements of a person's illness. The detached attitude of a natural scientist cheats the physician of a comprehensive understanding of the "whole person," and without that engagement, according to the basic thesis of this book, the physician shirks her full moral responsibility. Stephen Toulmin (1993, 248) puts the case succinctly: "If one does not wish to accept some real psychic involvement with sick people and is not really willing to involve one's whole personality in that interaction—and it is not just a case of the physician treating the patient as a 'whole man,' but rather one of the physician himself, as a 'whole man,' dealing with the patient as a 'whole man'—then, I would ask, *why be a physician at all?*" Indeed.

The Biopsychosocial Model

The contrast between the biomedical and biopsychosocial models divides as follows. The first approaches patients with an "analysis by which symptoms and physical signs—the complex, mostly subjective phenomena known as *illness*—are reduced to a more specific disordered part, the *disease*, to which science can then be applied" (Barbour 1995, 9). This model assumes that analysis of the illness, as described by the patient, indicates a disordered part, or pathology, called the *disease*, which is the cause or basis of illness. The model works very efficiently when the diagnosed disordered part fully accounts for the illness and its treatment restores the person to health. But in most cases, the model is inadequate to the patient's psychological needs. As Allen Barbour (1995, 28) explains, "The disease is not the illness, even when the disease, especially chronic disease, fully explains the disability and there are no other contributory factors exacerbating the illness. . . . No disease is disembodied . . . to understand the illness we must understand the person."

When doctors adhere too closely to the disease model, ignoring the unique characteristics of each person's disease, various problems may result: incorrect diagnosis, inappropriate diagnostic procedures, ineffective therapy, unnecessary hospitalization, prolonged disability, and most importantly, the patient is left dissatisfied that his or her true needs have not been addressed. A more comprehensive biopsychosocial model demands a wider horizon of concern and different resources of inquiry than the commonly appreciated technical skills of clinical medicine (Laine and Davidoff 1996; Frankel, Quill, and McDaniel 2003).

The "biopsychosocial model of illness." was formally introduced by George Engel (1977), whose essential precept was that "emotional, behavioral, and social processes are implicated in the development, course, and outcome of illness." From this standpoint, disease occurs in a complex context that is only in part—sometimes greater, sometimes less—"biological." Accordingly, there is no isolated locus in which physicians might function as applied biologists—geneticists, biochemists, biophysicists, or whatever. In this view, the physician also assumes the mantles of the sociologist, psychologist, priest, and humanist (Chapman and Chapman 1983). Proponents of this patient-centered approach would expand the focus of professional interest from the disease, its diagnosis and treatment, to also encompass the multiple social and psychological dimensions of a person who is ill. This revised responsibility recasts physician identity by advocating a more comprehensive vision of what it means to heal.

Although Engel published his classic paper in 1977, the biopsychosocial attitude had a long prior history. One tributary arose from social medicine,[1] but the Engelian branch grew most immediately from the psychosomatic movement of the 1930s. Engel, an internist with strong leanings toward psychoanalysis and a sensitivity for the psychological dimensions of illness, not only endorsed psychosomatic medicine, he was one of its leading investigators attempting to understand the emotional components of basic physiological processes (Brown 2003). As an academic physician, Engel helped found, at the University of Rochester, a dynamic group of clinicians and investigators, who, through the 1950s and 1960s, promoted a highly integrated psychosomatic approach for treating patients and training physicians (Brown 2003). By the late 1970s, psychosomatic medicine had fallen into disrepute as the result of major changes in the conceptual approach of investigative biomedical science, which were accompanied by a concomitant shift in medical education. In psychiatry, psychoanalysis was rapidly eclipsed by a powerful reductionism in the neurosciences and a biological psychiatry that trumpeted new advances in psychopharmacology. Coupled to devastating critiques of psychoanalysis (e.g., Hook 1959; Grunbaum 1984), a general suspicion of understanding complex emotional etiologies seemed to place this dimension of human biology outside the growing enthusiasm for reductive explanations based in biochemistry and genetics. Departments of medicine became more highly subspecialized as physician-scientists were funded by programs committed to more restrictive models of disease. Engel's 1977 paper was thus written as a challenge to this new orthodoxy by calling for the "adoption of a broadly inclusive, "systems-based, intellectual framework" (Brown 2003, 211).

The crucial *moral* element in this rendering of the medical scenario is that a patient-centered, holistic approach is adopted. By holding onto full personhood, the patient resists the reduction of illness to disease. Instead of unilateral treatment, collaboration between the two parties prompts the patient, guided by the doctor, to take personal responsibility for attaining health (Barbour 1995, 34). And by the criteria discussed earlier, self-responsibility must be the functional definition of autonomous actions. Interestingly, this model of care fosters patient autonomy, and not surprisingly: if the one-way approach of a scientific attitude is adopted, the patient becomes an object of scrutiny; in the biopsychosocial model, the ill person becomes a collaborator and thus intimately involved in his own care. So it is not "what the doctor does *to* the patient" that serves as the therapeutic goal, but rather an expanded agenda that includes the doctor's capacity to help the patient understand the specific personal sources of the problem and the effects of the disease. Accordingly, care is not simply the performance of necessary services, but also entails "interest, concern, and understanding. *Taking care of* and *caring for* are not the same, but in medicine they are interdependent. . . . *Taking care of* patients by *taking over* is not necessarily *caring for* them. The patient often needs a doctor who is more guide than therapist" (Barbour 1995, 43–44). Person-centered care medicine sets different criteria for care, and for our purposes provides the moral framework in which patient autonomy and physician responsibility might easily coexist side by side to achieve the same ends, the attainment of health. In the end, this is an ethical pursuit: "The proper application of knowledge to individual human beings demands an accurate appreciation of their particular needs and conditions; so that the task of medicine—however 'scientific' it may become—remains fully *ethical*" (Toulmin 1993, 238).

This revised role of the physician would require a major revision in medical education, indeed, in the very conception of medicine that is so enamored of the power of biochemistry and genetics. Doctors know how to ask questions pertinent to their biomedical mission, but not necessarily how to listen to their patients. Person-centered evaluation requires a broadened approach to determine relevant factors in an individual's illness beyond abnormal clinical data. The initial dialogue is crucial, for not only does it establish the ground rules for the doctor-patient relationship, but the all-important task of attaining trust is approached. Critical to the successful navigation of these often troubled waters is to listen to the patient discuss her illness, and approach the problem from her perspective before a translation is made to understanding the symptoms and signs as manifestations of disease. This takes some time, and for economic reasons, efficiency primarily, interviewing is usually curt. For instance, in one small study, the mean elapsed time from the moment patients began to express their primary concern to the doctor's first interruption was eighteen seconds (Beckman and Frankel 1984) and in another study performed fifteen years later, twenty-two seconds (Marvel et al. 1999). Following the interruption, the doctors took control of the interview by asking increasingly specific, closed-end questions. By so structuring the fact gathering, only certain kinds of information become available. Indeed, when patients are allowed to tell their full story uninterrupted, the time spent is hardly excessive, even by the most structured time analysts. In a large Swiss study of 335 patients referred to a tertiary care center, the mean spontaneous talking time was ninety-two seconds; 78 percent of the patients finished their initial statements in two minutes, and only seven patients talked for longer than five minutes (Langewitz et al. 2002). The doctors thought the time was well spent.

In one review of the status of biopsychosocial medicine, the exhortation for this approach is made primarily on pragmatic grounds of patient satisfaction, physician competence, and general promises of increased effectiveness. Indeed, proponents might take some satisfaction in recognizing that while the evidence is still rudimentary, by the early 1990s, the biopsychosocial model of disease had a firm place in many medical school curricula (Sperry 1991), and more recently it has found a place in some resident training programs (Schmidt 1998). But a ripple effect is evident throughout American medical school education, inasmuch as interviewing skills have become an almost universal component of preclinical education and explicit training in Engel's formulation occurs in a significant proportion (Novack et al. 1993).

Strikingly, the moral basis for its adoption is rarely invoked by its champions! (e.g., Frankel, Quill, and McDaniel 2003b), and when they do note the ethical dimension, they avoid making their case on that basis and choose, instead, to "hold the approach and its adherents to the highest standards of evidence" (p. 260). In other words, the compelling moral justification yields to clinical efficacy, that is, practical results, and to a scientific rationale. To be sure, these are worthy criteria, but ethics makes its own legitimate claims. I would argue that if for no other reason than highlighting the moral dimension of care, the biopsychosocial approach effectively addresses a responsibility that need have no other justification than the complex psychological and social requirements of the patient.

I justify this claim by turning to a literary genre, "pathography," which offers an important clue for understanding this arena of experience. Myriad testimonies of illness, disability, mental disease, death, and recovery have poignantly revealed the world of illness with a frankness and clarity hitherto reserved for high literature and drama. These personal accounts have made the phenomenology of illness an important source for reevaluating how students should be instructed to deal with patients, and, perhaps, awakened some experienced doctors to dimensions of suffering they might not otherwise have appreciated (Hunter 1994; Nelson 1997; Charon and Montello 2002). Given the popularity of such books, the public has obviously seized the opportunity to reclaim disease from exclusive scientific scrutiny (with its inherent power relationships) to the domain of personal experience. Thus, beside the growing self-consciousness about medical ethics and judicial requirements of care, popular culture now expresses a need to understand (and perhaps control) disease within a broader context than orthodox medicine allowed. Pathography taps into a widespread discontent with biomedicine's ethos, a perspective that shuns the personal dimension for objectivity, and thus the stories may be seen as purging an older paternalism and thereby redress the values that have guided health care for a century. Some regard this genre as an articulation of a major shift from "biomedical" to "biocultural" medicine—from a clinical science directed to repairing a broken machine composed of genes, regulated by biochemistry, and studied by x-rays to a biopsychosocial complex revealed by various kinds of cultural, familial, emotional, and biological narratives (Morris 2002). "Reading" this array of stories expands the physician's obligations to a far wider scope of concerns than traditionally taught.

At the very least, pathography is an indicator of changing expectations. As an expression of a deep-seated disaffection, this genre reflects the widespread sentiment that physicians must couple the imperative of technological advance with more personalized, humane interaction. Accordingly, patient narratives have been studied from various perspectives (e.g., psychiatry, sociology, literature, theology), not only to reconstruct medical histories, but also to define the value structure within which disease is perceived (Cousins 1979; Cassell 1991). Such phenomenologically based stories often dramatically portray the complexities of illness that were hardly apparent within traditional medical case-study methods (Toombs 1992; Barbour 1995). The disturbing, but hardly startling conclusion: objective characterizations of disease are inadequate to address what are often the central concerns of the ill person. Only a more global assessment captures the complexity of disease as experienced, and when appropriately explored, patients might eloquently, and too often surprisingly, offer insights that would add new requirements to care. In the patient narrative setting, comprehensive care takes on new dimensions and new meanings.

From this perspective, more comprehensive history taking offers the opportunity for moral attunement as well as providing potentially useful information. By becoming more responsive to the patient's needs, the doctor is likely to be more creative in formulating the full scope of concerns that impact on the patient's disease. And the goal is not solely a humanistic one, but also serves the ends of the pathological model as well, because clinical judgment ultimately depends on how *all* the data, subjective and objective, past and present, are assembled and integrated to effectively regard the problem in its full ramifications and to better account its causes. A dialogical model for the doctor-patient relationship asserts that only by abandoning a constricted mode of discourse, and instead embracing a broadened mutual interaction, can sound medical decisions be reached (Katz 1984, 163).

Following this course requires a major reorientation of how we train doctors to think of themselves and the responsibility and authority they exercise. Let us follow the wise lead of James Oliver: "Conversation, however, will protect the integrity of the physician-patient relationship only if doctors are willing to confront and change their views of themselves as sole authority and of their patients as incompetent participants in decision making. . . . An inscription on a Greek temple comes to mind:

'These are the duties of a physician: first . . . to heal his mind and to give assistance to himself before giving it to anyone (else)' " (Oliver 1939; 7 quoted by Katz 1984, 164). And what does this mean? Nothing less than a command for physician self-reflection.

Moving from a lofty authoritative position of scrutiny and judgment to one of more equal standing is not a transition easily made. Authority is hard won and not willingly compromised. Given the disparity of power and the inequality of the knowledge quotient between doctor and patient, the difficulty of meeting on more equal ground requires "a second-order" alignment. I mean by this phrase that the physician must toggle between two states. The first is scientific, one that hardly requires bolstering. The second is what is usually referred to as "humane," where patient and doctor meet, perhaps not as equals, but as collaborators. The doctor, as the authority figure, asks questions and delves into a patient's most personal pool of emotions, social and private problems, and existential predicaments. At the same time, the physician sits in judgment, dressed in a robe (the white coat) and benevolent pose. But where, behind this professional image, is the "humane" doctor? And more to the point, what is his psychic state?

Two approaches to answering this question will be taken here. The first falls under the rubric of empathy: "In clinical medicine, *empathy* is the ability to understand the patient's situation, perspective, and feelings and to communicate that understanding to the patient" (Coulehan et al. 2001). The term was coined by Titchener in 1909 from the Greek *em* and *pathy*—feeling into—and for the next fifty years the psychological literature discussed empathy as a type of emotional response. But empathy is more fairly regarded as a form of "emotional reasoning" (Halpern 2001). Much of our evaluation of the world and others is colored by subjectivity, and, indeed, emotions are evaluative, not in the same way as logical precision commands, but as lenses by which perceptions are refracted by personal experience and temper (Nussbaum 2001; Tauber 2001). So empathy is more than mere emotionalism—it is also a substrate for thought with at least three distinct domains: (1) a cognitive orientation, where the physician enters into the patient's experience, yet maintains a clinical perspective; (2) an emotional focus where emotions resonate between doctor and patient, and (3) an action component, where dialogue establishes enhanced communication and understanding. This last category may foster increased diagnostic accuracy, therapeutic compliance, and patient satisfaction, because patients feel better understood and respected (Beckman and Frankel 1984; Roter et al. 1997; Levinson, Gorawara-Bhat, and Lamb 2000). (Empathy is not sympathy; physicians may be empathetic even when they cannot be sympathetic (Wispe 1986).) Because of its general salutary effects on patient management, empathetic tools are increasingly taught in medical schools and residency training programs (discussed in the next section), and the increased attention to developing these skills highlights the growing legitimacy of this dimension of care (Delbanco 1992; Matthews, Suchman, and Branch 1993; Coulehan et al. 2001).

A second dimension of this discussion concerns the netherworld of the unconscious. Jay Katz, a psychiatrist, alerts us to what I take to be a truism: autonomy assumes that people may be aware of all the forces that influence their behavior; however, psychoanalysis reveals powerful unconscious motivations and influences that render rational understanding incomplete and the notion of making free choices highly suspect. Thus primary and secondary processes, referred to alternatively as irrationality and rationality, respectively, must be considered together and recognized as always present (Katz 1984, 115). Consequently, patient and doctor are consistently subject to their irrationalities: the patient "in an over-evaluation of the physician as healer"; the doctor "in an under-evaluation of the patient as a competent adult" (p. 142). Beset by fears and anxieties, patients characteristically may have increased dependency needs, and physicians should recognize the regressive character of such behavior, compensate for it, and not fall into the empowerment trap of believing that their patients are incompetent as a result of their transference. Countertransference, on the other hand, is the way irrational and unconscious expectations influence physicians as well, specifically the reactions in the physician engendered *by* the patient (Stein 1985, chaps. 1 and 2). While patient suffering may evoke physician empathy and compassion, there is a darker side to this equation. Countertransference may become a double-edged sword. On the one hand, the dependency needs of a patient might evoke responses in his doctor that result in inappropriate assertion of physician control and dominance; on the other hand, dependency needs conceivably might evoke anger, hostility, and disrespect for the suffering person. In either case, physician awareness of these complex psychological dynamics should lead to measured empathy and astute cognizance of the autonomy issues at play. The end point is to protect patients from physicians' unexamined value judgments (Katz 1984, 153–154).

Katz raises the lid of Pandora's box, specifically the relationship of free choice and compulsion, a topic I have considered in previous chapters. It is raised again here, because it remains the central problem in any discussion of free will and autonomy. And although we may never escape determining forces that emanate from our personal and cultural histories, nor the psychodynamics of transference and countertransference, these unconscious forces may be limited by insight and rational review. Although self-knowledge is always partial and imperfect, the moral imperative of self-examination commands that these unconscious factors be limited and *controlled* effectively. Indeed, this is the foundation of autonomy as outlined in the previous chapters: autonomy is attained and freedom experienced by striving for self-knowledge and personal reflection, and thereby gaining insight and perhaps even rational control as to why one decision is better selected than another. In that self-appraisal, in the weighing of alternatives, of measuring other points of view, persons assume responsibility for their choices and actions and thereby enact their highest moral capacity. The act of reflection, the quest for self-knowledge that will balance rational and emotional forces, often represents the exercise of autonomy.

Self-accounting applies to both doctor and patient, for not only must patients be self-reflexive as they exercise their autonomous choices (the Frankfurt-Dworkin model), physicians must also be insightful about their own motivations. Only by such self-appraisal might they attain a perspective on their own professional recommendations, their understanding of their patient's values, and the source of potential antipathy. In short, patient autonomy calls for physician moral (and emotional) self-cognizance.

Doctors cannot prescribe moral reflection and psychoanalytic introspection to all of their patients, but care providers may become more self-conscious themselves of their own drives and needs. In that examination, physicians might attain greater moral maturity by ascertaining more empathetically their patient's needs as opposed to their own. After all, doctors experience the same basic emotional processes as their patients, and it is hardly reasonable to then expect that their medical decision making is determined solely by their claims of objectivity. Judgment, moral sensitivity, and self-awareness are prerequisites to the healing relationship. The question then arises: Can moral traits be learned, or at least reenforced, and what measures might be adopted to fulfill these goals? We will now address those issues by examining how educators are approaching those challenges.

Bioethics Education: Current Status

'Moral competence': the ability to see what is morally relevant in a situation, knowing the point of view from which one sees it, understanding that others may see it differently, and then, with others, responding well to what one sees.
—Verkerk et al. 2004, 37

An "ethos of care" balances the use of science and technology with other humane resources, and these most prominently fall into the domains of medical ethics and the cultivation of physician empathy. While advocates struggle to justify their efforts as both practical and morally *right*, some cynics argue that this newfound attention is due to risk management and the high cost of defensive medicine. And, as already discussed, the very notion that empathy is an important quality is still challenged. I wish to probe further in this dispute over ethics training, which signifies a much broader conflict over the future of medical education and the professional ideals it promotes.

Let us begin with the most pointed objection to providing a more thorough education in medicine's moral philosophy: the entire rationale supporting medical ethics is unfounded. From this point of view, bioethics is not an essential part of medicine, and thus moral philosophy or medical humanities, more broadly, should not be included in medical education. For example, Richard Landau (1993) argues that the aim of the current medical curriculum is to foster objectivity and dispassion, not empathy, in students. This detachment appropriately provides them with the skills required to deal with patients and their diseases. From the first encounter with the cadaver in the anatomy laboratory, the student is introduced to the stark realities of the clinic, a radically altered life from that previously known. This entirely new perspective, where humans are reduced to a scientific scrutiny, is the foundation of modern medicine and cannot be compromised. Indeed, emotional detachment is a value to be encouraged, in order to make sensible, objective choices. Accordingly, the ability to shut out personal and subjective feelings is a potent psychic defense mechanism, allowing physicians to cope with the traumatic aspects of medical care (Landau 1993; Cody 1978, 54). Desensitization is thus both practical and effective. Proper scientific evaluation and diagnosis call for objectivity, and according to this calculus, empathy interferes with professional conduct.

This attitude has a long and distinguished heritage, one that competes with the humanistic image of the doctor: medicine as a science idolizes the physician-scientist, who removes himself from the complexities of emotional attachment in order to achieve optimal objectivity. While compassionate involvement that requires a different kind of psychological commitment may be worthy in another setting, on this positivist perspective, medicine is governed by a different ethos.

I regard this view as myopic in the extreme. Medical competence calls for different faculties. Differing circumstances demand varying degrees of empathy and detachment, and no final prescription is possible beyond calling for both as required. The bedside cannot become a scene of operatic drama. Instead, physicians function in an arena where emotional demands must be controlled and yet also acknowledged. Ideally, the physician will be caring and compassionate, and at the same time objective and scientific. No small demand, and one that calls for individuals with abilities extending from one end of the subjective spectrum to the other. Although the tide is turning, slowly, too much of Landau's sentiment remains, and I worry that while empathy receives a nod of encouragement, too little is being done to foster the countervailing ethos.

Stalwart ethicists are pitched against a well-defended professional tradition, one that emphasizes technical proficiency and expert competence. This older agenda appeals to students, who are largely admitted to medical school for their likely success in a demanding curriculum. To be sure, the care for others is a powerful motive for most students, but it is only one of several intentions, and the selection process provides easy targets for seduction to the power they witness. Studies have confirmed the general impression that students, as they are professionalized, gradually lose their moral sensitivity (e.g., Bissonette et al. 1995; Stern 1998; Patenaude, Niyonsenga, and Fafard 2003).

Sophomores are more likely than seniors to report regard for patients as a central ethical issue, which only confirms the general impression that as the professionalization process progresses, sensitivity toward patients decreases (Self et al. 1993; Bissonette et al. 1995).[2] These findings are attributed to the lessons learned from mentors, inasmuch as the clinical faculty (and the residents who mimic them), instead of serving as moral exemplars, are too often cited as exhibiting insensitivity (Bissonette et al. 1995). Indeed, to simply rely on learning moral sensitivity from the example of senior staff, though essential, is no longer regarded as a sufficient means of ethics training (Johnson 1983, 5).

Mentorship raises the specter of what has been called the "Hidden Curriculum" of medical school (Wear 1998; Goldie 2000). The Hidden Curriculum is a course of study not found in any catalog, but it is, despite its ironic label, plainly visible. It has evolved to teach students and residents how to function effectively in the contemporary environment of health care: doctors in training are shown how to deal with saturated schedules, onerous administrative details, and an incentive system that rewards productivity, not personalized care. Add to these demands, the lurking fear of medical malpractice and the defensive attitudes it spawns, we then readily recognize that powerful and pervasive determinants easily compromise a more humane medicine.

The Hidden Curriculum offers skills that enable the harried physician (or nurse) to effectively navigate in these turbulent waters. Yet all too often, effective only means efficient, and efficiency may easily conspire to rob the best of intentions. Efficiency may define effectiveness in one dimension, but it also may sap the personal resources from which empathy, compassion, and patience are drawn. Of course, compassion and competency are not conflicting values. They are, in fact, complementary, but the practice of "efficient" care does not always discern the quiet questions, "What are we doing?" and "Why?" Again, we discern the powerful influence of the emotional demands made on physicians that heavily contribute to a "defensive" posture, one that recedes from contact, avoids exposure, and acts evasively. "Foreclosure of feeling" (Cody 1978, 46) has many sources, ranging from the reification of illness to the stress of dealing with sick and dying patients. One might well wonder how ethics training can effectively offset the effects of these pervasive influences.

We begin by first considering the claim that ethics training deepens the empathy and moral awareness of medical students and doctors in training—that is, does formal education in ethics assist in promoting an ethical medicine? Not surprisingly, division is split precisely on this crucial question. The advocates for training morally reflective physicians begin with the following assertion: the teaching of ethics and humanities aims to restore, or perhaps rejuvenate, the casualty of professional training, namely, lost empathy. Those who advocate curricular reform to increase ethics education argue that supplementing the traditional program with formal humanities and ethics course work will mold a new generation of physicians, infused with enhanced moral sensitivity (e.g., Kopelman 1995). They argue that the training (or lack thereof) received in medical school shapes the physician as he or she continues through professional practice, and thus the restricted focus on technical skills and scientific expertise minimizes those personal qualities such as compassion and empathy, which play a major role in patient treatment.

Accordingly, students must be armed, from the beginning of their professional training with an awareness of medicine's deep ethical dimensions. This requires reaching down to undergraduate education, instilling the value of such thinking when premedical scientific studies are initiated. After setting the stage, medical students would be poised to learn how to apply this knowledge to medical practice. On this line of argument, treatment of patients requires making "good," virtuous decisions; good decision making requires both scientific and moral knowledge, and how these might be coupled can only be observed in the clinical setting. Ergo, ethical reasoning skills must be learned in tandem with the acquisition of clinical skills. Indeed, to divorce them is to betray medicine's moral mission. On this view, education must help promote (or reawaken) the compassion that inspired (at least in part) students to become doctors in the first place (Pellegrino and McElhinney 1982, 36).

The strongest argument for ethics education, however, does not rest solely on the optimistic opinion that it fosters professional ethics and empathy. Instead, advocates maintain that such training also develops more effective physicians and that clinical performance is linked to moral judgment. Doctors who possess more developed moral reasoning skills may be more competent in the clinic (Sheehan et al. 1980), and this moral awareness is putatively correlated with moral education (Harvan 1993, 361). Accordingly, moral self-awareness presumably spawns real gains in clinical proficiency and performance by fostering increased sensitivity in care, increased self-critical attitudes, and an increased capacity for personal growth. These achievements are in addition to the expected gains for promoting patient autonomy, supporting norms of professional conduct, and finally, producing a doctor-citizen who effectively contributes to public policy debates (Thomasma 1981, 73–74). Can all this be accomplished by *any* ethics curriculum? One might well be skeptical.

A dearth of proper evaluation methods plagues what is already a confused issue (Goldie 2000). Little progress has been made in evaluating the claims made by education reformers. Though standardized vignette exams (Savulescu et al. 1999) and Kohlberg-based tools (a schema that tracks the sequentially sophisticated stages of moral reasoning (Kohlberg 1984)) have been utilized (Sheehan et al. 1980), the goal of making students "more humane" is not easily quantified, and the goals of such education have not been clearly defined (Pellegrino and McElhinney 1982, 37–38). Although some studies suggest that even a relatively short amount of time in ethics-oriented course work favorably influences moral reasoning (e.g., Sulmasy et al. 1990), a more concerted effort on the teaching wards is probably more effective (Carmel and Bernstein 1986). In any case, training ethical sensitivity remains an unresolved issue, at best, and more critically, the empirical basis of correlating ethics training with clinical effectiveness is hardly impressive (Arnold, Povar, and Howell 1987; Self, Wolinsky, and Baldwin 1989; Goldie 2000).

Even some of those sympathetic to medical ethics' larger agenda, contend that ethics and moral views are "caught," not "taught." In other words, students have acquired their values by the time they reach medical school through family, church, and societal interaction. Consequently, formal teaching will be unable to modify these preestablished beliefs (Pellegrino and McElhinney 1982, 35). Following this line of reasoning, critics of humanities education in medical school almost scoff at the notion that such course work will have a salutary effect on physician behavior. They maintain that compassion and empathy spring forth from the child's earliest socialization and is supported or altered by the vast cultural influences of a society that may or may not foster such precepts. Even the most ambitious humanistic education cannot alone promote increased moral self-consciousness (Roochnik 1987).[3]

Although disturbing misgivings remain, ethics education is easily defended and, brushing aside rearguard opposition, various forces have converged to create a new consensus. The first is in response to the clamorous demands of a public increasingly frustrated by depersonalized health care, which is closely coupled to the general appreciation that patients require "protection" from the medical establishment. The bioethics movement was fueled by the patient-rights movement arising from these concerns. And the profession responded, perhaps sheepishly, perhaps belatedly, but nevertheless acknowledged that enhancing moral sensitivity is the *right* thing to do. After all, the argument over teaching ethics is not won or lost on data, but on the widely appreciated perception that ethics has been too long neglected and redress is now required. Specifically, given the current search for compassionate care and heightened ethical awareness of patient autonomy, ethics education is no longer seen as optional, but has become a necessary component of medical education. With 58 percent of all U.S. medical schools undergoing major curricular reform in 2001 (Barzansky and Etzel 2001), rethinking on this matter has been active.

But nagging questions persist about bioethics education: How much? What kind? To what end? Is educational reform the correct way to encourage more empathy, and if so, how would success be measured? Is increased empathy even the proper goal? Is medical education the appropriate venue in which to attempt basic reform of the profession? So, despite a general consensus about the importance of teaching ethics, the actual details as to how and what are disputed, since the purpose, content, teaching methods, and means to measure the success of ethics education are each contested.

For instance, should neutrality be embraced or a particular moral orientation adopted? Indeed, some have argued that it is impossible for teachers and students to remain neutral in this endeavor. Yet, the "neutral" goal of teaching ethics without expecting students to become more ethical and thereby embrace a moral perspective is fundamentally contradictory (Kopelman 1999, 1309). Instead of efforts to remain impartial and avoid discussion about values, which are unavoidably present even in the choice of the material and cases presented, teachers should be willing to recognize and discuss these values (Kopelman 1999, 1309). Acknowledging that to teach any one moral standing as superior to others already assumes a set of values, which in turn must be scrutinized (Goldie 2000). The exercise is directed toward developing a sensitivity to the ethical domain, not to impose a moral order on another (Levi 1999).

A pluralistic society exposes students to numerous viewpoints, and they must be able to think critically about them in order to achieve the widely accepted goal of cultivating compassion and moral sensitivity. Although students enter medical school with a well-established set of values and moral sensitivities, it can hardly be assumed that these necessarily will be consonant with those values that foster humane care. In liberal society, diverse moral beliefs contend with each other, and while the law might adjudicate some common practice, in the netherworld of interpersonal relations and life-directing decisions, no prescribed moral code necessarily prevails. Because ethics is a formal philosophical discipline that fosters the examination of fundamental moral presumptions, ethics training putatively allows students to critically reflect on their own values, a vital skill in the fair consideration and treatment of patients whose personal values may not coincide with those of the physician. Accordingly, the first priority of ethics education is to provide students the opportunity to actively scrutinize their own moral assumptions, something that they may have never previously done. One hopes this leads to moral growth and the opportunity to fully assimilate one's passively attained beliefs (Pellegrino and McElhinney 1982, 36; Levi 1999). The point is to develop a critical attitude in regards to ethics, just as in the clinical sciences.

If we reject the notion that ethics education should indoctrinate students, what should we accept as a more proper goal? In general, a reasonable aspiration is "to develop physicians' values, social perspectives, and interpersonal skills for the practice of medicine" (Miles et al. 1989, 705). In addition to these general aims, a chief priority of ethics education is to provide practical decision-making skills to be used in the clinic (Miles et al. 1989; Goldie 2000). Thus, a rather neutral view holds that ethics education should provide physicians with

1. An awareness of the humanistic and ethical aspects of medical careers.

2. The capability to evaluate and affirm their own personal and moral commitments.

3. A proper foundation of philosophical, social and legal knowledge.

4. The ability to use the aforementioned knowledge in clinical reasoning.

5. The interpersonal skills necessary to apply this insight, knowledge, and reasoning to humane clinical care.

The basic objective is to hone the practical ability of moral reasoning for application in the clinical setting so that the physician will be aware of not only the fundamental ethical concepts governing care, but also the dynamic of physician and patient values determining what and how care is administered (Pellegrino and Thomasma 1981; Goldie 2000). Of these fundamental skills, the ones that emerged from a consensus group of leading bioethicists include (Culver et al. 1985, 254–255):

1. The ability to identify the basic moral aspects of medical practice. This includes the routine explanation of risk, ascertaining whether the patient understands the risk, and the validity of the consent given.

2. The ability to obtain a valid consent or a valid refusal of treatment is fundamental to patient autonomy. Knowing the basis of consent and what constitutes adequate information, the ability to appropriately communicate such information, and the ability to distinguish persuasion from coercion are critical moral (albeit interpersonal) skills.

3. The ability to determine the competency of patients to give consent or refusal of therapy. Students must understand that competency is a murky area where legal and psychiatric determinations are at play. Standards should be reviewed.

4. Knowledge of how to proceed if a patient is only partially competent or incompetent to consent or refuse treatment—that is, understanding the clinical (psychiatric) and legal (administrative) procedures for dealing with a compromised patient.

5. Knowledge of how to proceed if a patient refuses treatment. The issues of health-care proxy and the valid appointment of such an individual must be understood as legal matters.

6. The ability to know when it is morally justified to withhold information from a patient or breach confidentiality. Although these are rare problems, physicians in understanding justification of breaking normal practice are concomitantly aware of routine standards.

7. Knowledge of the moral aspects of the care of patients with poor prognosis or who are terminally ill. This vast area requires training in effective interaction skills, the propriety of sharing of such information (confidentiality issues), determining when it is morally justified to forgo or discontinue treatment, and defining the role of "Do not resuscitate" orders.

Despite a general acceptance of these basic goals, agreement has not coalesced on the content of instruction. One topic of much dispute relates to whether ethics should be taught in general or in specific terms. The recent shift toward context-based, specific ethical training has been challenged; some say that the training should be more generalized, in hopes of providing students with a foundation for recognizing ethical issues. Among the "content areas" suggested are "ethical theory and humanities," "professional ethos," "multidisciplinary issues," "patient autonomy and clinical dilemmas," "student physicians," "academic medicine," and "social issues" (Miles et al. 1989; Goldie 2000). The content of ethics courses may vary depending on the area of medicine, the perceived purpose or founding philosophy, and the specific approach adopted, for example, principalism (autonomy, beneficence, and so on), decision theory (analyzing the decision-making process as a model to provide the skills for investigation and resolution of moral dilemmas), or "topics" (clinical moral problems, such as professional codes of ethics, human experimentation, informed consent, resuscitation status, withholding of information, refusal of treatment, allocation of resources, and confidentiality) (Layman 1996, 153).

Not surprisingly, a uniform curriculum evades adoption. In recent surveys of U.S. medical schools, at least thirty-nine different topics are covered, and only six content areas were taught in a majority of schools: informed consent (85 percent), health care delivery (75 percent), confidentiality and privacy (67 percent), quality of life/futility/provision of treatment (67 percent), death and dying (66 percent), and euthanasia and physician assisted suicide (60 percent) (DuBois and Burkemper 2002). Of the 1,191 ethics readings used by U.S. medical schools, only eight are used by more than six schools, and no reading is used by more than ten schools, which dramatically illustrates that there is no consensus on the relevant literature! (DuBois and Burkemper 2002).

The heterogeneity of the content of ethics courses only reflects a portion of the deep imbroglio about medical ethics education. Of even greater concern is how to effectively integrate ethics in the curriculum (Myser, Kerridge, and Mitchell 1995; Lehmann et al. 2004). Most agree that ethics should not be taught in one course alone, for this will convey the message that ethics are separate from the day-to-day practice of medicine. The more sensible choice is that of "a single, discrete course and integrated modules across the curriculum" (Layman 1996, 154). This method of integration, popular in allied health education, shows students that ethics are not optional, but rather occupy a central position in professional medicine. Another popular approach in medical schools is that of offering several courses or seminars supplemented by clinical rotations (Layman 1996). This practical method allows students to employ the skills learned in the classroom to the real life situations of the clinic. Corresponding to the desire of integrating medical ethics with daily practice is to limit the lecture hall as the setting for ethics education. In its place, small groups, the customary clinical setting and also the easiest place for students to voice their opinions about specific dilemmas, is favored to promote role-playing, casuistry, decision analysis, and Socratic questioning (Layman 1996; Johnson 1983; Goldie 2000). But the bare facts reveal that medical ethics education still comprises a small segment of the curriculum, and in a recent survey of U.S. medical schools, educators largely agree on one thing: inadequate time is allocated to medical ethics training throughout the four years of medical school (Lehmann et al. 2004).

The selection of faculty to teach medical ethics poses another critical problem. Who is equipped with the proper qualifications to impart such important material to future physicians? Furthermore, what are the pertinent qualifications? The greatest challenge in finding the best instructors lies in the few number of people trained to teach this subject. The chicken-egg conundrum stymies progress. Piecemeal solutions have been offered: the "competent amateur" and group teaching, the most popular choices. Neither is optimal, nor a third option that calls for an intermingling of faculty from nonmedical fields, such as law and theology. The "solution" is begging for resolute leadership. Until institutional assets are committed to medical ethics, this field, like any other, will only be able to patch together elements that can only approximate the required resources (Layman 1999, 155).

And, finally, critics rightly ask, How is ethics education evaluated? After all, of what benefit is adding ethics to the curriculum if educators have no way to determine success and thus improve their programs? Several problems are glaringly evident. First, because of the numerous and ambiguous purposes of ethics education, it is difficult to devise any dependable measure of success. In order to assess progress, specific goals must be identified; which are appropriate? Second, since the basic structure of moral development has already taken place prior to a student's entrance to medical school, how can discernment be made as to the extent medical ethics education has modified or expanded moral reasoning, and whether success, or lack thereof, is due to the curriculum or other factors embedded in the medical culture? Third, which test best measures development? The widely used Defining Issues Test is based on the moral development theories of Kohlberg, which, if anything, measure an ethics at odds with the moral sensitivity sought for caregivers (Gilligan 1982; Baier 1994a). Fourth, the impact of ethics education may not surface until many years have passed, for ethical sensitivity may develop with growing maturity. One final point: many options for the evaluation of ethics education exist, such as tests, interviews, simulations and peer review, and it may be necessary to employ more than one approach to determine accurate assessments of moral sensitivity (Layman 1996, 156).

These confusing pedagogical issues explain only in part why medical ethics education has had difficulty in asserting itself as an equal member of the medical school curriculum. At least at my medical school, medical ethics remains a distant cousin to other disciplines taught and thus it remains subordinated to other agendas. The reasons are complex, and in some sense, daunting.

The most obvious explanation at the level of clinical training pertains to time and money: the demands of an overburdened health-care system make time-consuming efforts at attaining doctor-patient intimacy an impractical venture, displacing professional time and effort better placed elsewhere. Improvement yes, real change, no. And at the level of pre-clinical education, to trade precious resources from basic or clinical sciences to teach ethics, which is poorly supported by outside agencies and foundations, and not at all by reimbursement schemes, is simply cost ineffective, whether measured by accountants or by the academic establishment committed to bioscience. The harsh verdict: medical ethics just does not pay.

Reforming Medical Education

The troubled status of bioethics education reflects a much deeper and pervasive understanding of medical education, one that resists more serious attention to the moral domain. Although considerable effort has been devoted to reforming the curriculum, changing its fundamental commitments have not been addressed. Most effort has been directed toward practical extensions, such as health promotion, disease prevention, interdisciplinary teams, multidisciplinary collaboration, evidence-based medicine, quality improvement, informatics and system-based practice. Teaching techniques have also evolved, with a greater use of interdepartmental courses, problem-based learning, standardized patients, small group discussions and ambulatory sites. Attempts have also been made to foster mentoring and to strengthen students' skills in

areas such as communication, interpersonal relationships, professionalism and the habits of lifelong learning. Pedagogical techniques have also
improved, including interdepartmental courses, problem-based learning,
standardized patients and the greater use of small-group discussions and
ambulatory sites (Regehr 2004). While measures such as these advance
the current commitments of medical education, they do not seek to better
balance scientific competency *with* the principles of humanistic care.
While well intended, an assessment of such efforts, unfortunately yields
dismissive terms such as "marginally effective," or "clinically irrelevant"
(Benbassat et al. 2003).

This is not surprising. From one side of the aisle, I might say, "Why
apply a Band-Aid to a hemorrhage?" and from the other side, "Enough
of the warm, fuzzy stuff." Indeed, as I lobbied for increased ethics training at my medical school, a faculty member complained, "Our students
did *not* come here to attend Sunday School." And my experience is
hardly unique (e.g., Anonymous 2003). To be generous, the detractors
are correct in noting the discordance between such efforts and the prevailing mode of practice. And from my point of view, none of these
efforts are effective in shifting the ethos of medicine from a positivist orientation to a more complex one that encompasses *both* scientific competency and the values of humane care.

Despite new directives from various medical education governing
boards, the failure to adequately address ethics education or more comprehensively consider the ethical dimension in day-to-day activities continues to plague clinical practice despite repeated calls for reform over
the past three decades (Carlton 1978, 171). Although it may be possible
that an active interest in medical humanities will revive atrophied moral
and emotional sensibilities (Cody 1978, 46), I agree with Shimon Glick
(1985) that curricular reform restricted to teaching "medical ethics," by
itself, is unlikely to be effective. (He argues that although the humanities have historically played an important role in heightening sensitivity
and facilitating self-expression for physicians, "they were not, however,
expected to provide ethical direction" (p. 12).) So, if formal ethics
instruction, *alone*, can only play a limited role in the student's ethical
growth, what remedy is at hand? Basically, positivism's strong hold on
medicine's self-identity will continue to effectively skew priorities from

ethics and the acknowledgement of the value-laden character of clinical practice unless a major reorientation is adopted (Cooper and Tauber, forthcoming). Therefore, I believe a much more radical reorientation is required, no less than a sea change, as quixotic as that appears.

As chapter 1 detailed, medicine's quandary is, in large part, due to the metaphysics of a scientific orientation that determines *what* constitutes bona fide knowledge and the kinds of thought processes that legitimate it. Narrow positivist commitments have effectively shaped the ideals of medicine—the allure of a molecular science that will define disease and cure it. Whether such a program will ever be accomplished is not for us to predict. Here and now, we must admit how distant medicine is from its own self-proclaimed goals. The vast majority of illnesses, ailments, and afflictions remain ill-defined, and when clearly demarcated, usually only "cured" in part. If medicine's scientific agenda remains only partially filled, then *care of the ill* (not *disease* which effectively limits ethical concerns) turns to its moral relationship with patients and the values and uncertainties that such relationships entail. Current educational goals are more restricted, despite the demands that students must gain both a deeper social and moral vision and an enhanced capacity to understand the value-laden characteristics of clinical information and decision making. These goals can best be understood in terms of three intertwined paths: content, thought, and values.

The basic science curriculum has compressed massive amounts of new knowledge into the existing time constraints, not only tipping the balance toward its own agenda, but largely precluding the inclusion of other subject matter that, like the basic sciences, has evolved in content and importance over time. Subjects such as sociology, epidemiology, anthropology, philosophy, ethics, economics, and law have acquired new importance in contemporary medicine. These lessons also must be taught, and, indeed, a thorough grounding in the basic sciences need not exclude other subjects and experiences that expand students' breadth of knowledge. Because of medicine's holistic character, balance in curricular content is sorely needed.

The void that is created by insufficient attention to the social sciences is not simply one of content. The need to teach the social sciences has as much to do with how they equip the mind to evaluate and integrate

knowledge. Clinical facts are just the beginning of the decision tree—
solutions lie beyond in a forest of ambiguity and values. The problem in
current medical education is that its emphasis on certitude sets up paradigms of thinking that work in the laboratory but too often fail at the
bedside. As a result, physicians tend to be comfortable with facts and
adept at clinical decisions based in the biomedical perspective, but they
tend to be uncomfortable with values and uneasy with the vicissitudes
of their own emotion, whose expression as empathy should be regarded
as a salutary form of emotional reasoning (Halpern 2001).

Teaching the place of values and emotion in clinical practice is the
most significant void in medical education. After applying the scientific
and technological tools of clinical medicine, physicians must be able to
act in the context of the social, spiritual and cognitive elements that are
at play as patients experience illness. As already discussed, they must see
their patients not simply as organic entities but as individuals with psychological, social, and historical natures. Participation in this personal
drama requires that physicians not only possess a capacity for empathy
and an ability to blend scientific information with issues of autonomy,
they must also appreciate the value-laden qualities of clinical information and medical decisions.

In short, physicians of the twenty-first century require a keen dual
intelligence. On the one hand, they must be conversant with science and
able to adopt the positivist stance of objectivity. On the other hand, they
must be responsive to patients' needs and values and effectively engage
in dialogue and negotiation. This latter, self-reflexive stance is the one
that is least developed in our current educational paradigm and the one
most in need of redress. The Institute of Medicine's recent report on
medical education moves the discussion in this direction (Cuff and
Vanselow 2004). It calls for a more patient-centered perspective, a focus
on the behavior of both patients and physicians, and increased attention
to the social and cultural issues in health care. But the problem is much
larger (Cooper and Tauber, forthcoming).

Returning to the original question as to why bioethics is not more
prominent in the educational agenda, I believe that the mindset of what
constitutes a "good" doctor simply obstructs the implications of placing
medical ethics in a central position of education and patient care. The

goals of curriculum reform cannot rest at adding a layer of humanism to a mountain of facts if we are to take seriously the need to change the current paradigm. Rather, the education process must be reoriented to one that gives primacy to the interplay of values, ethics and facts in order to foster the complex calculus of their proper integration. Reorienting medical education in this manner means that students must be trained to become scientifically competent within the context of a deep understanding of the psychological and social elements of illness and of the ethics of care that frame the clinical encounter. The details of accomplishing such a reorientation will vary, but the underlying principles include the following (Cooper and Tauber, forthcoming):

1. *A radical assertion of medical ethics as foundational to medical education.* Medical education must begin by communicating an understanding of the principles of ethics, the moral theory that gives them meaning and the application of such theory to clinical encounters. The legal and regulatory focus of most current ethics courses must be transcended by a deep commitment to understanding what constitutes ethical medicine. Identification of moral choice, protection of patient autonomy, the nature of professional responsibility and the articulation of beneficent care must serve as the core of such training.

2. *An understanding of the modes of assessing clinical science.* Students must gain a comprehensive appreciation of how value is embedded in clinical decision making and how uncertainty can be accommodated amidst a plethora of scientific and clinical facts. While evidence-based medicine and decision analysis are important tools for sorting out concrete spheres of knowledge, it is uncertainty that plagues clinical decisions and that must be mastered.

3. *A thorough grounding in the ethos of humane care.* Most students are naturally empathetic. Yet the curriculum does not encourage these tendencies nor equip students with ways to exercise them. Approaches to accomplishing this include teaching emphatic standards for interviewing patients throughout the continuum, from freshman student through residency; rewarding successful clinical educators, a practice already followed in many schools; and as proposed here (next section), devoting a section of the patient's clinical chart to ethical concerns.

Ultimately, the goal is to training the next generation of empathetic role models.

4. *Selecting medical students with a broadened vision of medicine.* As the medical curriculum is broadened to create a better balance between scientific and ethical concepts, admission policies must emphasize not only a strong quantitative aptitude but personality characteristics that display a commitment to the moral and social dimensions of patient care (Antonovsky 1987).[4] Both quantitative skills and humane traits may be strengthened in school, but the absence of either portends failure to educate a clinically competent, morally reflexive physician.

These proposals are threatening to those who hold a different vision of medicine's fundamental character. But sometimes choices are made that seem cost-ineffective or even contrary to more immediate aspirations and the values upon which they are based. Perhaps ironically, bioethics will attain a more important place in education and patient care because of biomedicine's own success ... not because ethics will directly promote the prospects of that program, but because the dominant focus on biomedicine is self-defeating to medicine writ large. Being realistic, a middle path must be found.

The question looms as to how dual faculties—positivist and empathetic—may be effectively promoted. If the root of the problem is physician ignorance, education could indeed be the answer. Yet any attempt at curricular reform is plagued by simplistic optimism and naïveté. It does not address the greater problem of the established mentality of the physician, which is systematically passed from generation to generation through informal mentorship and explicit instruction (Carlton 1978, 4). The reforms sought cannot be the product of a simple directive by those who seek a more comprehensive moral education. Indeed, as discussed in the preceding section, a significant reorientation is required to make a patient-centered approach to medical-care imperative. This requires deliberate education reform, as outlined above, as well as revising the narrative structure of the medical record, which so plainly reflects the positivism embedded in contemporary medical care.[5]

The next section presents a way of putting medical ethics into the center of clinical practice, now. We need not wait for curriculum reform, and, instead I am willing to opt (as a temporary strategy!) for a more restricted change. For now, the scope and aims of medical ethics training should be understood as fulfilling the same educational goals as those of any other preclinical course of study. Ethics instruction should provide the basic vocabulary and essential concepts for application at the bedside, so that moral sensitivity may be better exercised in the day-to-day routine of health care. Specifically, my modest proposal explores a practical way in which patient-centered care would be facilitated by providing a place in the routine evaluation of patients for establishing doctor-patient intimacy. Such attention to "ethics" upgrades communication among all participants involved in a case, improves understanding by physicians of patients' and families' expectations, and thereby increases the overall quality of care. In this sense, ethics becomes "leaven in the dough" (Dan Dugan, personal communication, 2004), as the inherent empathy of health care givers would achieve better expression. If widely adopted, this proposal would reflect a significant acceptance of a change in the ethos of care. Once tilted to a better alignment with patient needs, we might proceed with more comprehensive reform.

Taking Medical Ethics Seriously: Reform at the Bedside

"The patient is a 51 y.o. [year old] Hispanic man with a chief complaint of weakness. He is a poor historian, but claims onset of general fatigue about 6 months ago. He has a weight loss of approximately 20 lbs. over this period with loss of appetite. No medical record. Denies any G.I. symptoms, fevers, night sweats, cough, lumps, bumps, or neuro signs.

    PMH [past medical history]. Appendectomy age 14; fractured nose age 20; hepatitis age 32.

    FH [family history]. Mother—diabetic, hypertensive; father— unknown. 6 sibs—A & W [alive and well].

    SH [social history] Born in Puerto Rico; unemployed; divorced; 3 sons; lives alone; smokes 2 ppd [packs per day]; drinks wine and beer, ? amount." ROS [review of systems]. . . .

The ongoing debate concerning the role of medical ethics in medical education, and more broadly in daily practice, reflects its perception as occupying a peripheral place in medical reasoning. Most physicians have a general awareness of medical ethical concerns, but these are generally subordinated to the other more pressing immediate issues of efficiency and the competent application of medicine's tools of care. We require a vehicle by which medical ethics might be centered into the routine of daily practice. To do so, I suggest that physicians, doctors in training, and nurses apply an analogous evaluative model to the ethical dimension of patient care as they do to diagnosing and treating organic dysfunction. In short, I suggest that an ethics workup become a required standard part of the clinical evaluation of *every* patient. That assessment should be routinely documented in the medical record, as are findings concerning the heart, the lungs, and the abdominal organs.

Rationale

The rationale is simple: To place medical ethics more firmly into medical practice, we must devise an *explicit* focus of attention on moral concerns by the entire health-care team. To redress the missing input of ethics, a separate section of the medical chart devoted to identifying and dealing with ethical issues should be established. Fully integrated with various clinical evaluations and ongoing progress notes, this section would become the identified site in which health-care providers would clearly articulate both the obvious and the less apparent ethical issues pertinent to each patient. This so-called *Ethical Concerns* section is designed to proactively identify such problems and thereby raise these issues as part of ordinary evaluation and care. This section of the medical record would then join the open forum for the communication of findings and opinions that is crucial for the effective treatment of a patient's illness in all of its dimensions. I have previously outlined this proposal (Tauber 2002b, 2002c), and here I more fully explain its rationale and the context of its need.

"Ethical" in this instance encompasses all those matters related to the value-based decisions, which are constantly made when caring for a patient. Broadly speaking, there are two domains where value judgments are prominently at work. The first concerns the implementation of knowledge: In considering and applying the scientific and technological tools of clinical medicine, the question arises, "What should be done for a patient in the context of the personal and social contexts of the illness?"

The second domain concerns how physicians, beyond the exercise of their clinical science, participate in the patient's life story. These issues, as crucial as they can be, are rarely voiced in the medical record and thus remain conspicuously muted. Discerning and integrating them into medical treatment may be implicitly achieved, for better or for worse, or explicitly articulated and thus available for scrutiny and discussion. The latter approach would seem more effective in protecting patient dignity and rights. After all, an evaluation that addresses the ethical dimension of care is prima facie evidence of such an effort.

An *Ethical Concerns* section of the medical record would provide for a recognition and synthesis of personal, social, and ethical issues related to the effective care of the individual patient. There, medical students, physicians and other health care providers would address problems, which range from decision making in crisis to more mundane details of support for the ill during the hospital stay and after discharge. In making deliberate efforts to identify such issues in the context of the patient's life history and future goals, the heath-care team might more effectively deal with those concerns closest to the patient's own experience of illness. More than a scientific and legal document, the medical record might then become a more comprehensive construction of a person's illness.

Why the Medical Record?
Because the medical record is a narrative of a particular sort (see note 5), it tells a story—in its current format, a story of disease. What is included in that story formulates, structures, and thereby interprets. Standardized along prescribed lines, the medical chart may be perused quickly by anyone conversant with current practice. Such a document displays information uniformly, and (perhaps more subtly) the logic and ethos underlying practice—how care is thought of and ultimately delivered. But the record is more than a *reflection* of practice and thought, it is also a *determinant* of what kind of care is given, because the record functions in structuring clinical thinking. Doctors are trained to fulfill the template of the record's divisions and subdivisions, to obtain data relevant to the particular problems that require attention, as well as to address unsuspected disease. If questions are not asked, answers cannot be given. If tests are not performed, the best-intentioned scrutiny will not

suffice. Similarly, if inquiry is not made into the welfare and support of a patient, the physician will not identify potential or present problems. And while there is an increasing sensitivity to gleaning such insight in the clinical interview (the "patient profile"), there is as yet no formal place in which to situate and organize such information. By specifically addressing the moral or value-based concerns of the patient as part of the medical encounter, physicians will have a straightforward means to consider such matters. By demanding that the busy physician attend to this dimension of his patient, ethics will be given appropriate standing for attending to the concerns of the ill that too often are bypassed or forgotten.

What are the goals of this proposal? First, this proposal is supplementary and complementary to the current medical record, and not "radical" in any sense. Evaluating a patient's social history and psychological state, as well as identifying patient's prior decisions and current values regarding health care are already important elements in patient evaluations. I am advocating a reorganization plan, albeit somewhat expanded. As a reform of data gathering and organization, what is already *implicit* will become *explicit*. In systematizing the ethical concerns of patient care, all members of the heath-care team will have a template for the ethical reflection often required for comprehensive, empathetic care. Doctors, medical students, nurses, social workers, clerics, and others undoubtedly will supply complementary information that reflects their particular professional orientation; in their combination, a portrait of the ethical status of the illness will emerge. This effort is designed to better perform patient-centered care and may thus be regarded as a contribution to enacting a more comprehensive biopsychosocial approach to medicine (Frankel, Quill, and McDaniel 2003b).

Second, to take medical ethics seriously in current practice, namely, to treat the ethical issues of patient care as a crucial component of evaluating and treating illness, the medical record is the natural home for that evaluation. Informal understandings, silent consensus, assumed discussions do not suffice for management of disease (the pathophysiological domain), and they cannot suffice for the care of the ill.

Third, the medical record is the only locus for assembling this assessment, for the chart depicts health care and also has a role in structuring that care and its governing logic. In its narrative, the chart identifies clinical problems and the efforts to diagnose illness, and records therapeutic interventions. The medical record also proscribes the ways each of these processes is performed and ultimately records the rationale for the decisions which are made. In short, the record reflects the structure of clinical thought and action, and less obviously expresses the values embedded in clinical practice. We seek clarity.

One might well wonder why an ethics section has not already been incorporated in everyday assessments. Considering the widespread attention in health care organizations to respecting patient dignity, privacy, autonomy, and rights, one cannot but be struck with the incongruity of paying homage to such precepts while simultaneously ignoring them as part of the medical record of care. If the record indeed records the clinical encounter, why are organic concerns separated from the moral ones? Why does the current chart carefully record the former and only in an ad hoc fashion acknowledge the latter? The moral dimensions of care are constitutive of that care. So why not make an effort to identify how that domain is understood for each patient, and why not explicitly record how the patient as a person (as opposed to a disease) is understood and treated?

History provides useful insight to answer these questions. When the format for keeping medical records was last revised about thirty-five years ago, an effort led by Lawrence Weed (1969), reform was largely in response to a new appraisal of how physicians thought about their patients. The problem-oriented medical record was a deliberate attempt to reorganize the chart according to clinical problems. Because of the explosion of medical technology in the 1960s, the patient's comprehensive health needs risked being lost among the competing interests of one subspecialty perspective or another. The revised chart helped the doctor to identify all the medical issues at hand, assess each individually, and then integrate them to ensure that the patient received comprehensive care.[6]

But the aspiration of integrated care remains unfulfilled in a health-care system too often seen as dehumanizing. Weed was writing in the late 1960s, so his vision and point of view predates the emergence of patients' rights and bioethics. His efforts to better articulate the purposes of the medical record, to "organize" medical care around "all of the patient's problems," to be a tool of communication, and to provide a basis for quality improvement, are still valid. Indeed, Weed's fundamental thesis seems commonplace now: the obligation to address all the patient's problems, and to enlarge the patient profile in service of treating problems in their full context, serves the goal of being a "whole physician" in service to the "whole patient." But what is different today is that the scope of clinical care now encompasses newly articulated patient rights. Indeed, the emergence of patients' rights and bioethics during the past thirty years requires an enlarged definition of *all* of the patient's problems. The medical chart must be revised to address this expansion.

In addressing the ethical concerns of patient care, both routine and exceptional, a systematic approach is required. As in the evaluation of disease, a stepwise protocol provides a basic template in which to gather data, structure its evaluation, and organize decision making. What might such an ethics-workup section of the medical record entail? Should a series of specific questions be asked or a prescribed format followed? What, indeed, are the limits of such an inquiry? Or better, How comprehensively should one attempt to address such concerns? Where should it appear? Clearly, different patients have different requirements and different questions dominate different clinical settings. But no matter what the particularities of any given case may be, a self-conscious consideration of the patient's values must be considered. No less important, the physician's self-awareness of the values guiding his or her own choices and actions also must be understood. Defining the value structure of both the patient and the doctor, and making them explicit, provide the basis by which the clinical encounter remains a consensual and cooperative effort.

Because the "moral space" of clinical decision making is constructed by a complex confluence of values, sometimes in perfect alignment, and sometimes not, an ethical work-up must describe and ultimately encompass the values of the patient *and* the values of the clinician in the setting in which he or she operates. In other words, there is an ongoing negotiation as to what *can* be done, what *should* be done, and *who* decides those choices for each patient (Pellegrino and Thomasma 1981). In making this deliberation explicit—articulating the basic ethics, which will guide and inform clinical decision making—the doctor is enacting what might otherwise remain a silent dialogue.

Under this scheme, doctors and nurses would fully explain therapeutic options to their patients (already routine), and in doing so, make more apparent the ethical norms and the meta-ethical assumptions underlying those choices. To determine mutually agreed upon therapeutic goals, the physician must be aware that the decision integrates perspectives, where embedded values often silently determine what is seen, what is believed, and what is advised. The point of the exercise is to deliberately address potential conflicts of value *before* they arise, and, as in any negotiation, to understand both points of view to arrive at some consensus.

Surprisingly, scant attention has been given to formulating a comprehensive ethics workup, although both general guidance (Lo 1995), as well as specific protocols have been devised for certain problems, such as palliative care (Lo, Quill, and Tulsky 1999; Karlawish, Quill, and Meier 1999). This is due in part to the competing systems of medical ethics (e.g., axiomatic, consequentialist, consensual, or pragmatic ethics (Murphy, Butzow, and Suarez-Murias 1997, 23ff.)), the sheer complexity of the issues involved, and the restrictions imposed by the particularities of individual cases.

Several practical approaches have been devised to offer a deliberative procedure for arriving at the patient's social and moral profile.[7] This appraisal is aimed at protecting the patient's free choice, or at the very least, establishing a basis for further discussion. I am not advocating a specific method here, and instead emphasize that the point of the exercise is to highlight moral self-reflection and proceed with an orderly procedure to understand a patient's wishes. The detail of inquiry will varying depending on the ethical complexity of the issues at hand, but without probing, those ethical concerns will as likely remain buried as not. Thus, whatever format is adopted, the evaluation should provide a framework in which to understand the basic parameters of the patient's social and psychological life, which will provide a body of information that will direct the process of decision making to maximally include the patient or his or her surrogate.

Fact gathering of relevant information concerning the psychosocial and moral features of the case is key. The critical modification of current practice is both obtaining more comprehensive information, and placing the deliberative process on a coordinate system that includes both the patient's values and those of the health care provider. Thus the ethics workup is directed toward understanding the patient's needs, resources, and values, and coordinating these elements with the clinician's efforts, which are themselves guided by a set of values and priorities, both personal and institutional. The self-reflective elements of the ethics workup make this portion of the clinical portrait different in kind from the rest of the chart, which is oriented from the examining doctor or nurse toward the patient. In the *Ethical Concerns* section, a true dialogue is encouraged.

Objections and Rebuttal

Since medical practice already addresses the psychosocial setting of the patient's experience of illness, why is this modification in record keeping required? Simply stated, the clinical priorities as a function of the wider life concerns of the patient are rarely described in current chart documentation. Perfunctory notes about marriage status and employment typically constitute an acceptable social history, and only ancillary psychiatric or social worker narratives provide a more comprehensive picture of the patient in the home setting. By deliberately addressing this aspect of care, the clinician must define the moral space within which care is administered. In so doing, ethics will be firmly placed in the chart, thereby powerfully directing and self-consciously justifying the mode of professional behavior.

As usually considered, most cases require little or no ethical reflection or problem solving. Certainly ethics discussions, conferences or consultations to assist with and resolve questions and decisions for those facing end-of-life decisions, code status determinations, interpretations of living wills, autopsy requests, and uncertainties or disagreements about health-care proxy authority are frequent features of current health care. The dramatic issues of transplantation, in vitro fertilization, abortion, and prenatal genetic testing hardly need comment here, because the ethical concerns of such decision making are integral to these clinical problems.

The "ethical extremes" of the medical practice spectrum are not my primary concern.

What needs attention is the more ordinary case, where determination of choices must be made in the context of a patient's values that are not easily articulated, and are frequently overlooked. In one report, almost one in seven patients suffered a moral dilemma unrecognized by the ward team (Lo and Schroeder 1981). While much depends on the patient population examined and the moral "index" adopted, I suspect further study will reveal this figure is conservative. However, these fractions do not address the essential challenge: *Every* patient demands an ethical response, because of the primary moral character of care (Tauber 1999a). Whether acute and demanding, or minimal and subtle, the specifics of clinical care are fundamentally shaped by ethical considerations; the science and technology follow.

I acknowledge that significant objections to this proposal may be raised (indeed, I have heard them!). The primary dissension arises from the "economic" realities of contemporary medical practice—the economics of time and professional priorities. In this view, physicians are already over-taxed in their commitments and do not have the time to obtain the information called for here. A second objection (one already described) comes from a deeper source and is more difficult to address: While physicians may wish to be humane, they, by and large, function as technocrats and thus are rarely called upon to exercise moral sensitivity. Consequently, the patient in the typical setting does not expect to discuss values and beliefs, and only in the most pressing of circumstances do such deliberations take place, or even should take place.

As for the first concern, the economics of time and commitments currently divide the professional day according to certain expectations and standards of conduct. If physicians were expected to devote more professional effort in getting to know their patients, then the time it took to accomplish that objective would be acknowledged as important and factored in. The skeptic will not be calmed by reassurances that the increased work this new activity will command is manageable. Admittedly, I have avoided discussing implementation, but whether this effort is worthwhile or not must be decided after we concur that the merits of the case are worthy of study and trial. That justification rests on a painful admission: patients are correct that too often their personal concerns are not identified, their fears are not appropriately addressed, their true opinions are not sought. Only in alerting the professional and lay community alike to the short-changing that is obviously occurring, can the profession begin to adopt formal standards that will eventuate in change.

As to the second objection, perhaps more effort devoted to establishing the moral relationship between doctor and patient is unnecessary. Why should the physician move beyond serving as technocrat to a more complete caregiver? After all, is not medicine ultimately a scientific discipline, ever more beholden to technological applications? In this view, technical proficiency is paramount and attention to humane values will come into play only as required, and in a minimal expression. Others on the health-care team—nurses, social workers, clergy, administrators, psychiatrists, ethics committees—can deal with ethical complications as they arise. The rebuttal begins by observing the fundamental difference between the physician and the other members of the health-care team: The doctor holds a privileged position. In concert and collaboration with the patient, physicians yield an authority that has a more powerful influence than other health-care providers. The decision-making calculus is hardly simple, but suffice it to say here that the doctor cannot abdicate responsibility for defining, at a minimum, the various options for care and advising the selection of one or another. To perform that task adequately, physicians must *know* the patient beyond a biomedical description, for in the end, clinical choices are made within a more complex universe than described by clinical parameters divorced from the patient's individual personal reality. The goal is the individual's *health*, not simply disease elimination. On this critical point, I end my argument.

Although medicine's moral calling is compelling enough to demand more attention to ethical concerns (Pellegrino and Thomasma 1988, 1993; Tauber 1999a), I believe an even better argument arises from understanding medicine's epistemological construction. After all, we may reasonably disagree about moral beliefs, but there is less room for argument about the character of the clinical enterprise in which we all share. Note, I might have rested my rebuttal on the tenet that scientific (positivist) ideals must be *balanced* with the humane values of empathy and compassion (the values residing at the foundation of medical care), but I do not. That strategy has proven weak against those who argue that medicine is a technocratic enterprise, because their underlying understanding leads to a predicted outcome: They begin by falsely separating clinical facts and values into separate domains. Once divided, some (doctors) will address the facts and others (ethicists, social workers, clerics) will deal with the values. Split the problem and split its solution between specialists for each. But this configuration, as already discussed, may only be defended by distorting the character of medical practice. The "facts" of care disallow the severe distinction in which the divided formulation begins. So instead of seeking better "balance" between (scientific) facts and (human) values, I argue for acknowledging their inextricable linkage. And in light of that understanding, we possess a powerful rationale for taking medical ethics seriously by *all* health care providers.

My goal is to make ethics more explicit in the day-to-day practice of clinical medicine, and thereby enact the precept that medicine is fundamentally ethical (Tauber 1999a). To enact that understanding, we physicians must remind ourselves that clinical science and its applications are tools for fulfilling our fundamental and self-defining moral responsibilities to patients; further, we must better balance the claims of a nineteenth century scientific ideal of objectivity with a twenty-first century appreciation that clinical science in service of patients is value-laden. Values have a wide expanse: clinical decision making is a dialectical process of doctor recommendation and patient understanding and choice; respect for patient autonomy is more than informed consent and demands from us an ever-present effort to preserve patient dignity; and the economies of practice must balance efficiency with efficacy, which in turn depends on some measure of empathetic, personalized care.

Not only must mentors *teach* the skills requisite for such behaviors, they must *practice* them and thereby *show* doctors in training that professionalism includes certain humane behaviors. The lasting lessons are learned at the bedside, not in the classroom. The tools for practicing an ethical medicine may be obtained in lecture; the enactment must occur with the patient. (In fact, empirical research has amply shown that students are more deeply influenced by the behavior of role models than by the material presented in course work (Glick 1993; Goldie 2000).) In short, the moral encounter occurs in the intimacy of the doctor-patient relationship. Contemporary practice needs a directive and a means to enhance that relationship.

In espousing a deliberate emphasis on ethics in daily practice, I seek to strengthen doctor-patient intimacy that many find lacking. While an invigorated standard of patient autonomy signifies one aspect of the changed social and economic climate in which medicine finds its own place, neither informed consent nor regulations can substitute for primary trust. Both remedial and proactive responses are required to strengthen the weakened personal bond between doctor and patient. I contend that placing medical ethics firmly into the heart of the medical chart, as a constituent part of the medical evaluation, is a mechanism that represents an important step in that process. The routine articulation of ethical concerns may provide the most direct way of pulling medical ethics from the periphery of the medical landscape into its very center where it belongs.

In the end, I make this proposal not to argue for more recognition of "medical ethics" as an area of knowledge and skill. Ironically, I regard the expert character of the field as part of the "problem." As important as this discipline has become, and as much as it still requires support, I seek to "democratize" bioethics. As long as medical ethicists are perceived as practicing another "subspecialty," medical ethics itself will be regarded as "somebody else's" expertise and responsibility, and, consequently, the discipline and its practitioners are easily marginalized until dire circumstances call for rescue. But if the discussion is raised to the moral plateau it deserves, the pursuit of an ethical medicine then encompasses not only bioethics, but also includes the wide constellation of patient-centered activities that contribute to a humane medicine.

Teaching ethical principles, moral theories, medical jurisprudence, and the other components of medical ethics may be seen as the tools of this enterprise. A robust curriculum is required, but put the horse before the cart: make identifying and addressing ethical concerns a part of the routine clinical evaluation through an ethics workup. Just as the student learns to use a stethoscope to auscultate the heart, he or she should learn the basics of moral reasoning and apply them to the clinical scenario. I suggest that only by a self-conscious effort will moral sensitivity be highlighted in a way that will tilt the doctor-patient relationship toward the empathetic ideals most would endorse. The time constraints and other difficulties in establishing more intimate relationships between doctors and patients is a testament to what is *not* being done, what is left in the interstices of care to be noticed or not by chance and circumstance. The encumbrances we face in bringing forth the full panoply of a patient's illness is a challenge to be met, not effaced or ignored. So, instead of seeing the difficulties as insurmountable, I prefer to regard them as providing an opportunity for individual moral attunement. If we cannot directly change the system in which care is administered, at least we can resist conformity to its strictures and demands.

In this diffusion of moral self-consciousness, I advocate the *Ethical Concerns* section of the medical record as a means to better ground an *ethical medicine*. Enhancing awareness of medical ethics as belonging to the core of day-to-day practice is the means toward that larger moral agenda. More than judicial directives, risk management, and academic debate, the morality of medicine defines the very foundation of practice, the moral substrate on which clinical care is built. One might see most choices and actions—even the most mundane—as enacting some underlying value system, but such awareness is not ordinarily part of clinical practice. In adopting serious efforts to ensure that medical ethics does not become another subspecialty, but rather flourishes as an integral component of every physician's training, conduct, and practice, clinicians should begin to embed moral reflection, as an *explicit* exercise. Establishing an *Ethical Concerns* section highlights how ethics is the business and responsibility of every clinician. Toward that ethical ideal is where I believe we should direct our energies, and medical ethicists should be able to help in that effort, and perhaps even lead the venture.[8]

Conclusion

This book has sought to understand and redress medicine's moral foundations. It is part of bioethics' larger agenda of retrieving and then protecting medicine's moral mandate from those extrinsic complex political, economic, and social forces that have seemingly shaped it into just another industry. Most would agree that health care is like education, fundamentally different from the industries committed to making cars and cereals. But we are caught in a web of competing interests, confused priorities, and contested ideologies, which impede reform toward a more humane and just ideal. The inequality of health care delivery, the scandalous number of uninsured and underinsured citizens, and the huge siphoning of the health-care budget for administration and profit are only the most obvious examples of a profound dereliction. Only at the microlevel of the patient's encounter with the doctor might a moral intimacy offset the insidious effects of a health-care system organized by principles that often have little correspondence to the patient's primary concerns.

To effectively deal with the deepest issues with which bioethics grapple (namely, the loss of trust and the search for more humanized care) may well require nothing less than a revolution in health-care organization. Perhaps the emergence of bioethics thirty-five years ago heralded only the beginning of an ongoing battle over the character of our medical system. The "battle lines" constantly shift, so it is difficult to clearly see how rationing of resources represents one "front," while protecting patient autonomy is another part of the same conflict. Indeed, a communitarian approach is required to equalize care and provide the justice now so obviously absent (Tauber 2002a, 2003c). (That agenda, I see as linked, but resides outside the scope of this book.) But as I write, at the beginning of a second George W. Bush administration, this seems far-fetched, because such an orientation would be organized on social and political principles radically different from our present temper.

Nevertheless, I regard bioethics as a vehicle for change. To that end, I have claimed that with a better understanding of medicine's philosophical infrastructure, we possess an indispensable insight as to what needs repair and the direction in which we should proceed to best protect individual dignity. I have followed a twofold strategy: raise moral self-awareness and integrate moral reasoning with the other, more inclusive cognitive skills governing medical practice. Here a patient-centered, biopsychosocial medicine complements the ethics of care I have advocated. Integration requires both an acceptance of the value-laden nature of clinical science, and the commitment to an ethics that endeavors to humanize patients as well as their caregivers. Powerful forces may conspire against these goals, but we must begin with them clearly in sight. So, while I readily admit the limits of my argument to significantly change the deepest sources of our unrest, I modestly hope that this analysis offers a basis for directing our individual efforts. I seek nothing less than a "return to the future" in order to find the patient in the bewildering maze of contemporary health care in which we are all entrapped.

Epilogue
On Praxis and an Ethics of the Ordinary

To be a philosopher is not merely to have subtle thoughts, nor even to found a school, but so to love wisdom as to live by its dictates. . . . It is to solve some of the problems of life, not only theoretically, but practically.
—Thoreau [1854] 1971, 14–15

Much of modern philosophy swirls around the question, What is philosophy? The agonized debates, especially in the twentieth century, about what constitutes bona fide problems and approaches ultimately fractured the discipline. There are many ways of characterizing philosophy, sometimes divided by technical interests and sometimes by deeply held opposing metaphysical visions: by schools (existentialism, pragmatism, analytical philosophy, phenomenology, and so on); by subject matter (ethics, political philosophy, philosophy of science, aesthetics, history of philosophy, metaphysics); by orientation (idealism, rationalism/ empiricism, skepticism, realisms/antirealism, and so forth); and, for our purposes, by the theoretical versus the ordinary or the practical. In this last opposition, and through its incomplete resolution, we find the origins of medical ethics and its sustained vitality.

Beginning with the romantics, a philosophy of the ordinary has gained momentum and analytical acuity. Notable twentieth-century philosophers have extended earlier critiques primarily through the philosophy of language (Wittgenstein and John Austin), pragmatism (Dewey), and phenomenology (Husserl, Heidegger, Merleu-Ponty). And these traditions are actively pursued today by Richard Rorty, Stanley Cavell, and Stanley Rosen, among others. They answer the question what is philosophy? with surprising modesty: most directly, philosophy attempts to capture "the elusiveness of the ordinary" (Rosen 2002), a tradition with a venerable heritage (see chapter 5, note 8). These philosophers share a concern with replacing a deconstructive skepticism with a constructive understanding of pretheoretical, everyday experience. They obviously differ as to how this goal might be achieved, but all are part of the movement against philosophical formalisms.

Instead of constructing a theoretical structure on which to hang the messiness of the world to order it and to penetrate the bewildering swirl of the mundane to the deeper reality or significance of human life, philosophers of the ordinary seek to grasp everyday life on its own terms. This approach to the prosaic requires more than theoretical constructions. Philosophical formalisms, with their carefully crafted definitions, rhetoric refined over centuries of debate, and various kinds of logic, are replaced with an orientation that combines theory and practice. In a sense, this movement is an attempt to recover philosophy's original intent. Whereas the pre-Socratics like Heraclitus and Parmenides devoted themselves to theoretical speculation on nature, ignoring or belittling day-to-day concerns, Socrates tied together the theoretical and the practical as the two dimensions of philosophical reflection. More to the point, "The dramatic form of the Platonic dialogue exhibits the tacit thesis that theory and practice are not so much two distinct lives as two aspects of human life. . . . They are not ways of understanding life so much as ways of living" (Rosen 2002, 3). In other words, for philosophy to attend to its full agenda, the theoretical and the practical must be synthesized, for in their sundering, the point of theory is lost.

For Socrates, philosophy begins in the everyday, but the "erotic ascent" allows the enlightened to witness the perfect Ideas and return to the ordinary with an insight that helps direct human behavior. So philosophy both transcends and remains deeply rooted in ordinary life, beginning and ending at the same spot, so to speak. The key for a philosopher like Rosen (2002, 10) is to see that ordinary experience is saturated with the extraordinary and that philosophy's present task is to recover "the origins of human experience, that is, to remove the sediment deposited by traditional rationalism" (p. 6). In this view, philosophical formalisms, with their meticulously argued precepts and rules, enable the philosophical edifice to be built on carefully laid layers of argument, but the process becomes self-absorbed and too easily loses sight of philosophy's true goal. Rorty, in reviewing Cavell's *In Quest of the Ordinary* (1988), succinctly captures the problem of why philosophers kick up the dust and then complain that they cannot see:

[Certain philosophical] problems could only be stated in a particular jargon, in Philosopher's Talk. They cannot arise if we speak Ordinary Language. Descartes and Ayer had discussed, for example, whether the external world was real. Real? Austin asked. As opposed to what? A plywood stage set? A hallucination? A computer simulation? In the ordinary, human world these are the sorts of alternatives that give the word "real" its use and its force. In the philosophers' world, there is nothing to do the same job. That is what Wittgenstein meant when he said that Philosopher's Talk is language "on holiday." (Rorty 1989, 39)

Cavell, claiming Wittgenstein and Austin for support, and enlisting Rorty, wishes to overcome skepticism and renounce the quest for purity to recover the human dimensions in which we live as the site for philosophical discussion.

This "metacritique" of contemporary philosophy has direct relevance to our own concerns here. Lurking behind every corner of the hallway in which medical ethics finds its various "rooms" of thought (here the principles of autonomy, beneficence, justice), reside the questions of applicability and relevance: What are the limitations of any system of philosophical ethics in addressing the practical concerns of patient care? Each philosophical approach is curtailed by its own perspective. Ethical theories—utilitarian, deontological, liberal individualistic, casuistic, coherent, pragmatist, communicative, existentialist, and so on—each restricts in its own way by framing ethics in its own characteristic fashion. Building on certain axioms—for instance, the standing of rationality if one is a Kantian, or the bias of gender if one is a feminist—allows the moral philosopher to develop his or her argument toward some end. Again, if a Kantian, the primacy of autonomy and freedom, or, if a feminist, the correction for gender prejudice serves as the telos of the entire argument. Along the way, these contending ethics slip past their detractors and other contestants in seeking dominance. There may be active debate within a Kantian or feminist group, but when contested by those holding a different point of view, discourse rarely engages the core issue separating the disputants. After all, no final arbiter or gold standard exists. In short, theories, for all their power to structure debate and persuade skeptics, have inherent limits: they refract the world and human behavior in their own characteristic fashion.

So, for all the hope, and conceit, of providing comprehensive accounts of ethics, reality, knowledge, and so on, the project always fails. No doctrine, no school, no titanic intellect can overwhelm other views, and while philosophy has an enormous influence on human life, few would be so bold as to claim that philosophy is "comprehensive." Suffice it to admit that no system is hegemonic, and while each contributes to constructing our notions of the Real, the True, and the Good, none—either singly or in concert—captures it all.

These truisms point to a cardinal admission: at a simple level, I have been dissatisfied with any singular approach to understand the ethics of clinical medicine, and so I have mixed various elements—most prominently, utilitarian, feminist, communitarian, and virtue ethics—to define an ethics of responsibility. The "vocabulary" has been principles (Beauchamp and Childress 2001); the strategy, pluralistic; the mode of justification, reflexive equilibrium (Rawls [1971] 1999); the overriding metaphysics, a Levinasian variant of phenomenological and existentialist orientations (Tauber 1999a)—heavily sprinkled with a relational understanding of selfhood (Mackenzie and Stoljar 2000), and governed by a broadly humanistic conception of virtue (Pellegrino and Thomasma 1993) and beneficence (Pellegrino and Thomasma 1988; Frankena 1988). Perhaps only by creating this web of interlocking components could I reveal my understanding of the "structure" of moral medicine. And so after placing each of these components into the net that I am calling the "ethics of responsibility," one might well ask, What orders or orients that structure? The short answer, moral self-reflection.

I have called on doctors to become more self-reflective, more aware of the moral dimensions of everyday care, more keenly aware of their respective roles and degrees of freedom. This perspective offers physicians a way of seeing themselves as having, beyond certain functions as actors in the clinical drama, a group of obligations and responsibilities that arise from their *ordinary* encounters with their patients. We need not, indeed, should not articulate the ethics of medicine exclusively in response to acute crisis, but rather draw the parameters of moral conduct by examining the structure of physician commitment and identity in the setting of the everyday life of the hospital or clinic. The utility of this orientation is to make explicit the social currency of ordinary interactions and their rules of exchange. Finding the meaning of this ordinary experience (i.e., engaging in a hermeneutic analysis) hopefully offers enhanced self-awareness.

Physicians would do well to look about themselves and more fully recognize the value-laden world in which they function. Bedazzled by the power of machines, drugs, and techniques, rushed through the hubbub of hectic schedules, answering to diverse professional calls and demands, beholden to, and restricted by, external economic and political forces, doctors require an ethics of the ordinary, an ethics seeped in a cognizance of the *Mitsein* (Olefson 1998) of social interactions. There I believe they will find a moral mandate of care, an abiding sense of responsibility for another, and the professional demand for excellence in the *techne* of clinical practice. Here is where trustworthiness must be established and enacted. It is the basis of their patient's trust, which is the essential ingredient of the healing arts.

Inescapable and overdetermined, clinical medicine is governed by its ethics, and when mentors and their students better recognize the complex moral reality in which they live, the more likely their craft will be transformed from its technocratic and bureaucratic obsessions to a more humanized life form. When thus understood, the conclusion is inescapable: clinical medicine is, among other competing agendas, a moral exercise. Framed by the standards of care, by empathy, by cost-effectiveness, and so on, some hierarchy of interests prioritizes clinical choices in answer to patient needs, and each health-care provider is governed by a particular set of standards and the morality that legitimates them. The medical crisis dramatically reveals this process. What I have emphasized is the ordinary moral character of the healing praxis.

On this reading, some form of ethics is implicit in all that doctors optimally do in their daily performance. Why then is medical ethics a specialty field? Why is risk management too often the substitute for ethical reflection? Why, indeed, does moral self-consciousness wane under the glare of the objective stare? Undoubtedly, reasonable responses appear effortlessly, but the dictum remains that in the clinical universe, values structure all facts so that their meaning and significance only take form when they are sorted, organized, prioritized, and acted on as determined by the rules governing the value-based choices optimizing patient care. In this sense, the medical world is, indeed, "startlingly moral" (Thoreau [1854] 1971, 218).

I turn to a philosophical novelist to make a final comment in support of medicine's moral locus in the ordinary.[1] Leo Tolstoy retells the story of the painter Bryullov, who corrected a student's sketch:

"Why, you only touched it a tiny bit," the student exclaimed, "but it is quite a different thing." Bryullov replied: "Art begins where the tiny begins. . . . That saying is strikingly true not only for art, but for all of life. One may say that true life begins where the tiny bit begins—where what seem to us minute and infinitely small alterations takes place. True life is not lived where great external changes take place—where people move about, clash, fight, and slay one another—it is lived only where these tiny, tiny, infinitesimally small changes occur." (Tolstoy, "Why Do Men Stupefy Themselves?"; quoted by Morson 1988, 521)

Such awareness has immediate moral consequences: because intentions are shaped continually by small, usually imperceptible influences, every moment of our lives has moral value (Tauber 2001). Each action has potential effects we cannot predict, but for which we still remain responsible. We must be morally alert, because decisions, far from being reduced to a set of rules to follow, require that attentiveness be marshaled for deliberate action. Rules, principles, and maxims may guide our choices and deepen our understanding, but in daily life traditional philosophy typically ends and prosaic ethics begin (Morson 1988).

This orientation relies in large measure on Aristotle, whose fundamental question is not "What ought I *do*?" but "What should I *be*?" In other words, "Morality is internal. The moral law . . . has to be expressed in the form, 'be this,' not in the form 'do this.' . . . The true moral law says, 'hate not,' instead of 'kill not.' . . . The only mode of stating the moral law must be as a rule of character" (Leslie Stephen, *The Science of Ethics*, 1882; quoted by Thomas and Waluchow 1998, 38). In many ways, the moral reality of the clinical encounter is well served by including this depiction, for it captures the "ether" in which we live our moral lives. In the confusion of everyday life, the process of ordering the unique interactions with particular people in particular settings demands that we make unique ethical choices, *constantly*. The Aristotelian perspective captures this state, for moral behavior expresses virtues or qualities of character, and these are expressed at every moment of consciousness.[2] This fidelity to ethical behavior is the demand of caring for another, an ongoing, unwavering responsibility. I maintain that this obligation is the ethical heart of medicine. Responsibility does not end with signing an informed-consent agreement or mollifying a family about terminating care of an aged relative, because the legalities of care shape, but hardly define, the ethics of physician responsibility. Ultimately, care for another is a question of character.

A moral philosophy based on character emphasizes how we are held responsible for even the most mundane actions. But more, to be self-consciously moral in the context of the prosaic also provides the potential for one's ordinary choices to produce meaningfully different outcomes. And this is an individual accomplishment, one integral to a creative, productive, and morally responsible life. As Bakhtin wrote (with Nietzsche looking over his shoulder), "That which can be accomplished by me cannot be accomplished by anyone else, ever" (quoted by Morson 1991, 218). This is not some narcissistic conceit, but rather the acceptance of moral accountability, which for the health-care provider, is the fundamental moral maxim of caring for another. This has been the theme of my earlier work (Tauber 1999a) and it remains central here. Patient autonomy offers no challenge to this formulation, because respecting individual dignity is a fundamental precept of an ethics of responsibility. The practical task remains how to heighten such moral vigilance and couple it to vitalized, humane health care. We have begun by excavating to the foundations of our predicament. On that understanding, we can proceed with confidence toward a renewal of an ethical medicine.

Notes

Prologue

1. None of the issues swirling in this discussion is more charged than those directed at reducing physician options for the care of their patients, yet surveys offer confounding data and some show that the extent of patient complaints is exaggerated (Weinstein 1999). Nevertheless, physician disaffection is more widely appreciated, and the model of an intimate, long-standing doctor-patient relationship has suffered grievously over the past twenty-five years (Stoeckle 1987, 54ff.). Interestingly, trust as a subject of inquiry has been largely ignored by philosophers until recently (Baier 1994b). Such topics as the character of moral agency, the nature of social cooperation, and the meanings of contracts and laws are more typical topics for philosophical discussion, and although related to trust, they remain quite distinct subjects. (These issues are discussed in detail in chapter 5.)

2. Elsewhere (Tauber 2002a, 2003c), I have sought to place the intimate world of the doctor and patient in its broadest social context: American health-care social policy is disproportionately aligned with individual choice (autonomy's label in the marketplace) as opposed to communal responsibility for providing comprehensive health care to all citizens. A rights-based culture condones inequality, and thus compromises social justice. This inequality, in its insidious discrimination against the less affluent, compromises the autonomous integrity of all. This argument extends the philosophical construction of the doctor-patient relationship considered here with an eye toward distributive justice. If we continue the present unequal system, then our current fragmented policy suffices, if not economically, at least as an expression of certain moral choices. In arguing for an equitable distribution of medical resources, I have affirmed universal health-care coverage as an ethical position, from which a certain set of economic and political parameters follow.

3. But medical ethics is making its own contribution to philosophy by offering the mother discipline an important opportunity to refashion itself. Stephen Toulmin (1982) has cogently written of "How Medicine Saved the Life of Ethics," by which he means that medical ethics has made an important

contribution to what he calls "the recovery of practical philosophy" (Toulmin 1988). Toulmin is pointing to a shifting of interest in the abstract and theoretical concerns of mainstream philosophy to now include—in respectable academic circles—"applied ethics," or what he refers to as "practical philosophy." An increasingly intimate relationship between philosophy and its offspring is potentially a critical development for the continued growth of medical ethics and must be regarded as a promising alliance.

4. Michael Walzer's *Thick and Thin* (1994), a work of sociopolitical philosophy, adopts "thinness" from George Orwell's *Coming up for Air* ("There is a thin man inside every fat man, just as . . . there's a statue inside every block of stone") and "thick description" from Clifford Geertz's *The Interpretation of Cultures* (Walzer 1994, xi), while John Evans (2002) borrows the dichotomy from another sociological source (Hart 1995). The thick-thin distinction is also used by Bernard Williams in his discussion of how facts and values are conflated (1985, 129) and John Sadler in his discussion of values (1997). Undoubtedly used in many other contexts, the thick-thin distinction in reference to philosophical discourse seems to have been first introduced by William James in *A Pluralistic Universe* ([1909] 1987, 691), alas, from an unidentified critic: "Among the philosophic cranks of my acquaintance in the past was a lady all the tenets of whose system I have forgotten except one. Had she been born in the Ionian Archipelago some three thousand years ago, that one doctrine would probably have made her name sure of a place in every university curriculum and examination paper. The world, she said, is composed of only two elements, the Thick, namely, and the Thin. No one can deny the truth of this analysis, as far as it goes . . . and it is nowhere truer than in that part of the world called philosophy."

Adopting this trope, my own book moves in deeper currents than those currently carrying medical ethics along. For instance, in his article "Recent Advances in Medical Ethics" (2000), Peter Singer focuses on what I would regard as "thin" questions: end-of-life care, medical error, setting of priorities or rationing, acceptability of stem cell research, medical ethics education, and global health. As important as each of these topics is, and no matter how much "progress" has been made by clinical ethics as a discipline (Singer, Pellegrino, and Siegler 2001), these discussions must be firmly grounded in "thicker" philosophical deliberations if they are to have intellectual merit and robustness.

5. For Ramsey (1970), Edward Shils (1968), and Daniel Callahan (1969), the sanctity of life—essentially a religious principle—was secularized into the moral principle of autonomy, where it joined a rich political tradition (Jonsen 1998, 338).

6. For instance, my colleague at Boston University, George Annas, an acknowledged expert on the relation of the law to bioethics, has made the following remarks in this regard: "American bioethics has been driven by the law. . . . The stress on autonomy and self determination comes from our Bill of Rights, our Declaration of Independence and the whole common law tradition. And law's primary contribution to bioethics is procedural. Lawyers are expert at procedure.

The common law itself is based on deciding individual cases and using these cases as the basis of creating law. Bioethics has adopted this technique. In the United States, with its pluralism of beliefs and people, the law is what holds us together. There is no other ethos. Thus, the law—procedural, autonomy based and case focused—came into bioethics" (quoted by Jonsen 1998, 343).

7. The imbalance between the legal articulation of physician fiduciary responsibilities and patient autonomy is illustrated with how we deal with involuntary hospitalization of the insane (Tauber 2003a). The commonsense notion of physicians possessing fiduciary authority has been displaced in favor of a legalistic assertion of patient "free choice," sometimes with dire consequences. My argument here supports the general portrait of autonomy's role in medicine much as in a Picasso painting, where critical elements—though all present—are at times distorted and misplaced.

8. Medical ethics accommodates empathy under the banner of "beneficence," but this hardly does justice to the moral imperative empathy commands, and the very language of medical ethics is too often inappropriate for *moral* discourse: "The law is the *lingua franca* of bioethics. The language in which bioethics is discussed revolves around largely quasi-legal notions such as consent, competence, rights to refuse treatment, to have an abortion and so on. Many writers have targeted the language of rights and autonomy for special criticism, suggesting that we need to develop an alternative vocabulary. This is an understandable suggestion, but I also think the law's influence on bioethics has been much deeper and more subtle. It has given us a picture of morality as somehow like the law in structure—for example, as a set of rules that govern interactions between strangers. This picture of morality may work adequately as long as we are in fact talking about interactions between strangers, especially strangers whose relationship is adversarial. But it overlooks many kinds of questions that are crucial to morality, and it distorts many others" (Elliott 1999, xxviii).

Stephen Toulmin (1981) reminds us that authentically moral relations exist only between intimates, and consequently the discourse designed for controversy is not adequate or appropriate to relations governed by rules of intimacy and commitment. This is a telling critique of the conduct of medical ethics and of the language it has appropriated.

9. Critics with differing perspectives have exhaustively debated the utility of "principlism" (Gillon 1994b). Some have propounded this approach as a foundational (but hardly sufficient) basis for doing medical ethics (Beauchamp 1994), while others have decried this approach as inadequate to the task. These disparagers range over a broad philosophical territory: from a general resignation to postmodernity's nihilistic conclusion about systematic ethics (Engelhardt and Wildes 1994) to the inability of principles to "systematically relate to each other by an underlying theory," making them incapable of doing the work required (Clouser and Gert 1994, 251). Some of the disagreement stems from an in-house argument between philosophers who embrace a top-down strategy for moral philosophy (a comprehensive theoretical construct ordering all the components within it) and those who advocate a bottom-up approach (where the bottom

begins and ends is another matter!). The sociological critique takes another tack (Wolpe 1998): principles are too often poor guides for the micromoral dilemmas involved in everyday clinical decisions, they give scant attention to the socially constructed and historically situated meaning of such concepts as self-determination, and perhaps more broadly, the discourse based on principles ignores how values on which the principles themselves rest are socially constructed and thus relative to individual contexts of culture, psychology, and religion. From such a sociological perspective, "The background assumptions of the common medical morality, both medico-cultural . . . and structural . . . should be the subject of ethical inquiry, not the basis on which ethical judgments are weighed. Principles based on a common morality cannot be used to critique that common morality" (Wolpe 1998, 42–43). Despite the severe limitations of the language employed, the strictures of the constructions utilized, and the admittedly narrow purview of the principles-based approach to medical ethics, that orientation remains dominant.

Chapter 1

1. From this brief overview, it should be obvious that what constitutes a fact depends on the metaphysics, epistemology, theory of truth, and semantics that determine its definition. Insofar as facts are what make true statements true, inquiries that do not distinguish the metaphysical nature of truth from epistemological concerns or from the linguistic use of truth will hopelessly muddle important distinctions. Notwithstanding debates about correspondence theories of truth and the empirical status of facts (scientific realism versus social constructivism), it is apparent that descriptive medical science encompasses a wide variety of facts, whose epistemological status and linguistic uses vary (Stempsey 1999).

2. Medicine, of course, was never monolithic, and well into our own century renewed challenges to reductive orthodoxy have appeared, even within mainstream conventional medicine: constitutionalism, psychosomatic medicine, neo-Hippocratic medicine, neohumoralism, social medicine, Catholic humanism, and, in Europe, homeopathy and naturopathy (Lawrence and Weisz 1998). These "holistic" systems have been espoused not only by various kinds of practitioners, but in noteworthy instances, championed by "legitimate" basic scientists, for example, Henry Head, Walter B. Canon, and Alexandre Besredka (Lawrence and Weisz 1998). Through historical reflection, we can see that the discussions of today are directly linked to similar debates held between 1920 and 1950, which in turn were reframed arguments dating to the nineteenth century.

3. For instance, disputes about the extent to which alcoholism and schizophrenia are genetically determined illustrate the extension of the biological-determinism debate to complex behaviors. This is not the place to explore this complicated issue, but it is important to note that much of the impetus for defining the human genome has come not only from a desire to cure disease, but also

to control "aberrant" human behavior, which, now in this broadened biological model, extends beyond clearly organic processes such as infection or diabetes, to include violence, homosexuality, and depression. Sahotra Sarkar and I have called this the "ideology" of genetic reductionism, and its import extends from understanding the evolutionary character of organic disease, to complex emotion, the character of human social structures, and the morality governing them (Tauber and Sarkar 1993).

4. This moral concern is distinct from those recent attempts to criticize the bio-medical model as epistemologically too narrow. For instance, Laurence Foss and Kenneth Rothenberg (Foss and Rothenberg 1987; Foss 2002) argue for a "new psychobiological" approach that endeavors to bridge the mind-body divide they see plaguing contemporary medicine. They seek to reformulate bioscience into a new "infomedicine," which, by their account, is a "top-down" approach (emergentist as opposed to reductionist) that integrates the "mental" and the traditionally configured "physical." Overlooking some grandstanding and simplistic interpretations of recent findings, I find their position, notwithstanding my general sympathy, poorly developed and lacking in compelling argument. There are important interfaces between the neuroendocrine system and the immunological (Ader, Felten, and Cohen 2001), and elucidating those relationships is critical for understanding how each functions, but we are far from developing a new paradigm to account for how "the mind" functions with "the body" from these early insights. Suffice it to acknowledge that new frontiers beckon and we must patiently await their exploration.

5. Beneath this level of discussion, we are facing an intimidating limit, one perhaps best summarized by William James in 1902: "[Nature] is a vast *plenum* in which our attention draws capricious lines in innumerable directions. We count and name whatever lies upon the special lines we trace, whilst the other things and the untraced lines are neither named nor counted. There are in reality infinitely more things 'unadapted' to each other in this world than there are things 'adapted;' infinitely more things with irregular relations than with regular relations between them. But we look for the regular kind of thing exclusively, and ingeniously discover and preserve it in our memory. It accumulates with other regular kinds, until the collection of them fills our encyclopedias. Yet all the while between and around them lies an infinite anonymous chaos of objects that no one ever thought of together, of relations that never yet attracted our attention" (James [1902] 1987, 394). If this "selection" argument is applied to medicine, and to do so we must cast our conceptual net widely, truth claims operating in different therapeutic contexts may be championed on the basis of cultural diversity, folk belief, spiritual values, and diverse (multicultural) communal standards for objectivity. Indeed, from these deep reservoirs alternative medicine draws its potions to effectively challenge biomedicine (Callahan 2002). Include the psychological dimension (of even the most erudite Western sophisticate!) and we begin to perceive the bewildering complexity of the healing engagement.

When David Eisenberg finally told the secret about the appeal of complementary and alternative medicine (CAM) in America, it sent shock waves through the biomedical establishment (Eisenberg et al. 1993). Conventional medicine had enjoyed a hegemony since World War II but suddenly appeared to be dangerously complacent. Its sanctimonious authority was being disputed not within the medical schools or clinical journals, and not even in Congress, but through the persistent walking of patients to other kinds of practitioners. This social revolt has gained momentum, because by 2002, CAM had exploded into a $21-billion-a-year industry, with about one-third of Americans visiting its practitioners at least once a year (Bushnell 2002). Here we come face to face with patient autonomy exercised in its full authority. Not only are patients rejecting orthodox medicine's sovereignty and prestige, they are invoking a belief system at odds with it. Yet both conventional and alternative medicine make effective claims to treating illness, and the quandary is in finding their common ground, or perhaps their distinctive playing fields (Tauber 2002b). No consensus has been reached as to how this might be done (Jonas 2002; Kopelman 2002; Schaffner 2002). At stake are basic issues about how disease is defined and therapy assessed (Hrobjartsson and Gotzsche 2001; Hrobjartsson and Brorson 2002; Jonas 2002). Certain underlying precepts frame any comparison of health-care systems, and these precepts may not only conflict, but be incommensurable. Many examples come to mind. Disease and human suffering cannot be understood solely from a single perspective—medical, personal, or cultural. The experiences of being sick and of caring for the ill are different. There are multiple systems of meaning that confer significance and an ordering to such experience. Biomedicine, for all of its explanatory power and therapeutic triumphs, is an approach to care that admittedly stresses certain positivist criteria and ignores others. And perhaps more to the point: the clinical scientist is as absorbed by her worldview as the acupuncturist is by his.

Despite the NIH mandate to explore alternative therapies in a serious and systematic fashion (Stokstad 2000), the problem is daunting. Not only is there disagreement about the character of such studies (considering the difficulty of defining psychosocial factors), it is difficult to prioritize among the competing alternative systems being actively pursued by the public. And when one considers the state of evidence-based conventional medicine, it is easy to understand the laments of those who see the attention to acupuncture or homeopathy as misplaced as compared to efforts to assess more "rational" approaches. But the case for measuring the effects of CAM remains compelling. Like Janus, we must peer simultaneously in two directions. On the one hand, alternative medicine challenges orthodox medicine to examine its own assumptions, its methods of evaluation, its outcomes, and its truth claims. In short, a crucial element of biomedicine is its own critical self-evaluation and scrutiny of its claims—exactly the same judgments orthodox medicine claims to place before its contenders (Hufford 2002; Jonas 2002). The out-of-hand dismissal of claims simply because they do not appear consistent with current dogma is myopic in the extreme. Such a "know-nothing" position seems to me untenable, both practically and philosophically. On the other hand, even if CAM proves to have placebo effects, these do not in themselves exclude the efficacy of the therapies. Indeed, efficacy and veracity are different and do not necessarily map onto each other perfectly, for they measure different things. Ultimately, given the limits of knowledge, we must be satisfied with efficacy and aspire to veracity. Controlled clinical trials are mandatory, but they will fail to address the basic issue: the legitimacy of belief systems seemingly incompatible with Western biomedicine.

6. Putnam (1990, 141) elaborates: "If values seem a bit suspect from a narrowly scientific point of view, they have, at the very least, a lot of 'companions in the guilt': justification, coherence, simplicity, reference, truth, and so on, all exhibit the *same* problems that goodness and kindness do, from an epistemological point of view. None of them is reducible to physical notions; none of them is governed by syntactically precise rules. Rather than give up all of them . . . and rather than do what we are doing, which is to reject some—the ones which do not fit in with a narrow instrumentalist conception of rationality which itself lacks all intellectual justification—we should recognize that *all* values, including the cognitive ones, derive their authority from our idea of human flourishing and our idea of reason. These two ideas are interconnected: our image of an ideal theoretical intelligence is simply part of our ideal of total human flourishing, and makes no sense wrenched out of the total ideal, as Plato and Aristotle saw."

7. The question of what patients value in their medical care is conflicting and notoriously biased by research methodology, but I was struck by a recent survey, which showed that 27 percent of those polled switched doctors because of perceived incompetence, whereas 76 percent left because of a failure to foster a strong interpersonal relationship, which included assessments of physician respect and honesty (Bright 2004). When ranking professional qualities, 85 percent regarded physicians' treatment of patients with respect and dignity as extremely important, whereas only 54 percent thought "a lot of experience treating patients with your medical condition" was extremely important. This is only one study and its limits are obvious, but I believe that patients are increasingly dissatisfied with health care they perceive as regimented, impersonal, and ultimately inhumane. The vulnerability of the ill lowers the threshold for complaint. These issues are explored in chapter 5.

8. An entire discipline is now devoted to understanding clinical data, so-called evidence-based medicine (Evidence-Based Medicine Working Group, 1992). In the early 1990s a growing self-consciousness about the spotty nature of medical knowledge became widespread, not only on the part of an increasingly skeptical public, personified by third-party payers who were aghast at medical costs with no obvious criteria for success, but also on the part of the medical profession itself, which was being challenged by its own members to justify its interventions. That academic champions have emerged as self-appointed guardians of a more vigilant clinical science might seem surprising, since for over a century, the dominant model of clinical care has claimed to be based on sound scientific information and its objective application. Indeed, that claim is the rationale for discrediting all other practitioners (see note 5 above; Eisenberg et al. 1993).

9. The philosophical literature on the definition of value is extensive (e.g., Brandt 1996; Stempsey 1999; Railton 2003). *Value* has at least three uses (Najder 1975): quantitative (what something is worth), attributive (that something *has* value), and axiological (a criterion or principle that ascribes value). This last sense is the most difficult to describe and apply, though philosophers have attempted to distinguish the various dimensions in which values might be recognized— for example, linguistic, causal, and descriptive (which in turn falls under various guises, including aesthetic, ethical, epistemic, and pragmatic values) (Sadler 1997). Values, whether understood as arising from moral realism (Sayre-McCord 1988) or in response to certain needs (Putnam 1985), come into play at both the level of scientific knowledge, in assessing what constitutes a scientific explanation and scientific fact, and at the level of clinical judgment—in the process in which medical facts are used to decide actions on the basis of an array of value judgments. In the above example of treating sickle cell disease, pain is no less a "fact" than the abnormal hemoglobin, because the *meaning* of each is determined by the patient's report of illness. The patient's illness, whether described in scientific terms or in personal ones, is the ultimate "fact."

10. A good case in point is the attempt in Oregon to rank medical procedures for Medicaid benefits, given the state's insufficient resources to cover all medical exigencies (Bodenheimer 1997; Ham 1998). In 1989, Oregon passed legislation to provide increased access to health-care insurance by increasing eligibility for Medicaid. To increase enrollment, cost control of a basic health-care package was sought, which required a prioritization of services. That ranking was conducted in public hearings and generated widespread debate. The plan, launched in 1994, provided funds for 565 out of the 696 treatments on the final priority list, which included the bulk of preventive and curative services (Ham 1998). Controversy about the ranking process resulted partly from a lack of data with which to make rational analyses of cost-benefit ratios. Moreover, even if the data was available—let's say in QALY units—the moral judgment as to who might be more deserving of a higher rank generated considerable discussion.

QALY—Quality Adjusted Life Year (Normand 1991)—is a measurement to assess how much it costs to provide the same quality of life for each patient in a health-care system for a given period of time, that is, one year. So, irrespective of the disease any patient might suffer, calculations are made to determine the cost for each to maintain the same quality of life. Once that is determined, policymakers faced with limited resources are then in a position to decide whether, for instance, an older woman with diabetes and hypertension or a child with diabetes is more deserving of the scarce resources. This is of course a rigged example. But it highlights what is increasingly becoming apparent: we need rational planning for the health-care budget; this requires formal quality-control measures; and, finally, we must have a basis for determining allocations utilizing some common denominator for cost comparisons. When this calculation is completed, choices must be made. For instance, in this example, the probability of hospitalizing the woman with health complications must be gauged against all the expenses and possible dire complications of the child with diabetes, whose life span is in all likelihood shortened. This is rationing at the bedside, and the moral difficulties it entails are clearly shown whenever the debate about rationing becomes public. In most cases, insufficient data allows for uninformed decisions. When available, ethical decisions stratify the population at risk. In either case, the role of values is too apparent to warrant further comment.

Chapter 2

1. Relative to this fourth characteristic, Paul Root-Wolpe (1998, 50) makes a cogent observation: "The paradox of our church-state separation is that it ultimately denies the religious voice a role in the process of policy formation. In the absence of unified moral communities, pluralism is translated into a radical individualism where all moral voices have equal valence. Autonomy as a guiding principle of American public life is meant, in part, to ensure freedom of religion and religious expression, but, ironically, it tends to silence the religious voice in policy formation, which is often the strongest voice in defending other values, such as justice."

2. The alienation between physicians and patients was intensified after World War II: "In the post–World War II period, a social process that had been underway for some time reached its culmination: the doctor turned into a stranger, and the hospital became a strange institution. Doctors became a group apart from their patients and from their society as well, encapsulated in a very isolated and isolating universe. The familiarity that had once characterized the doctor-patient relationship gave way to distance, making the interactions between the two far more official than intimate. By the same token, the links that had tied physicians to their communities . . . were replaced by professional isolation and exclusivity. Finally, the bonds of neighborhood and ethnicity that once had made the hospital a familiar place for its patients became practically severed, giving to the institution an alien and frightening atmosphere" (Rothman 1991, 108–109).

3. Preston (1981, 93) comments as follows: "Professionalization is the social mechanism by which physicians institutionalize themselves as the ultimate source of healing power, and unite with other physicians in an effective and profitable social and economic organization. . . . According to the basic contract, the medical profession is surrogate protector for the public, and public interest becomes easily confused with self-interest. The change occurs in the development of the physician with the unrecognized, unspoken, and barely perceptible transition from being patient-oriented to being profession-oriented."

4. In his words, "Perform all this calmly and adroitly, concealing most things from the patient while you are attending him. Give necessary orders with cheerfulness and serenity, turning his attention away from what is being done to him; sometimes reprove sharply and emphatically, and sometimes comfort with solitude and attention, revealing nothing of the patient's future or present condition" (Hippocrates 1923, 297–299).

5. It is noteworthy that John Locke, despite his magisterial standing in defining the self, has virtually nothing to say about medical ethics per se. This is surprising inasmuch as he was trained as a physician, and he may fairly be regarded as fusing his philosophical endeavor with that of medicine: "To Locke at least, the concerns of morality are but those of medicine on a larger scale: Morality as the proper business of mankind in general coincides, in ideal of practicality, with medicine as the proper business of physicians in particular. If there is one field of human endeavor that is thoroughly practical, and vitally so at that, literally, medicine is definitely it, life and death being its daily concerns" (Romanell 1984, 18). Locke's commitment to medicine as essentially pragmatic might be construed as the basis of his ignoring the ethical component of care, but if so, he was guilty of a positivism that was to plague medicine in our own era (see chapter 4).

6. Indeed, the key architects of early modern science, most notably Galileo and Francis Bacon, were self-consciously philosophical in their studies. In particular, Bacon wrote much about the link between ethics and science, and he differentiated between a general and a respective ethics. Bacon called the professional duty a "respective duty" (Haakonssen 1997, 22), and in his contemplation about "who, ideally, should write a professional ethics or system of duties," the practitioner or the "disinterested spectator," concluded that it should be the former. Nevertheless, "he must not only describe the duties of his profession, he must also be able to describe its vices" (p. 23). Bacon's ideas inspired all three men, and also sparked a great deal of medical reform in the Enlightenment. According to Bacon's rules for a practitioner-moralist, Percival, Gregory, and Rush were all well qualified, for they had achieved a proper balance between the practical and the speculative or theoretical aspects of their science.

7. According to Wallace (1998, 548), "Moral sentimentalists grounded human autonomous moral faculties not in reason, but in the so-called 'moral sense.' The moral sense was interpreted as an innate susceptibility to feel sentiments of approval when confronted with morally virtuous character traits. . . . Virtuous traits were understood primarily in terms of benevolence [or justice]; and later proponents of the approach took the moral sense that approves of those traits to rest on a mechanism of sympathetic identification with others" (i.e., empathy).

8. That these pursuits were motivated by Scottish political aspirations and driven by certain economic necessities is beside the point here (Howe 1997, 50ff.). Suffice it to note that education, civility, a new vision of the human sciences, and a complex moral philosophy were all invoked to support Scottish politico-economic development in a venture that had repercussions well beyond the rocky highlands. The founders of the American Revolution were heavily indebted to Scottish thinkers (Bailyn [1967] 1992), and in the context of this discussion, medical ethics assumed two new tacks as a result of this Scottish influence.

9. Baker, Porter, and Porter (1993, 6) provide the following historical background: "The word 'professional' was pejorative, inasmuch as it was linked to the guild, an association predominantly marked by self-interest. Indeed, many commentators of this period noted how it was imprudent (crudely, bad for busi-

ness) for doctors to be identified in the public mind too closely with tradesmen. The status, dignity, and authority necessary for a distinguished profession would accrue not from following the laws of the market . . . but from adopting the mien of a gentleman. . . . Indeed, prior to the publication of Thomas Gregory's *Lectures on the Duties and Qualifications of a Physician* in 1772 . . . at least in the English-speaking world, recommendations as to the proper behavior of doctors were often hard to distinguish from the much broader genre of *advice to gentlemen* purveyed in general conduct manuals."

10. All duties were reciprocal in this contractual relationship between patient and physician. For instance, in the case of malpractice, since the primary duty of a physician was the honest exercise of his skills, malpractice was a breach of duty. In 1767, the famous malpractice case of *Slater vs. Baker and Stapleton* placed emphasis on the necessary minimal consent of a patient as part of this professional contract and of "customary practice" (Haakonssen 1997, 31–33).

11. Accordingly, the candid physician must "not only . . . be able to give a rational account of his treatment or prescription, he must also be able to accept criticism from his colleagues and patients and "be ready to acknowledge and rectify his mistakes'" (Haakonssen 1997, 76). Morals and manners in the patient-physician relationship were also subject to Gregory's analysis. According to him, the patient had both rights and duties to his physician, thus permitting, if not encouraging, the patient's "right to speak where his life or health is concerned." And, appropriate to the genteel custom of the day, the patient must "do so with politeness and deference to the judgment of the physician" (p. 76). In turn, the physician should be candid and listen attentively, considering the suggestions of the patient. Further, "If he agrees with the patient, he should say so and, if not, he should explain carefully the reason for his disagreement" (p. 76). In short, as conceived by Gregory, civil dialogue was to mark the doctor-patient relationship, with mutual respect and consideration guiding that discourse.

12. Regarding the doctor-patient relationship, for Percival the family became a model for the hospital and the physician became in loco parentis—the head of that household. Hospital officers were responsible "for the overall physical and moral welfare of the patients who, by implication, were like children and servants" (Haakonssen 1997, 132). Percival carefully described the appropriate role for each: the patient must show gratitude, patience, and forbearance, while the two most important tools for the physician in this affiliation are condescension and authority, which were thought to "inspire confidence and respect . . . that was in the end the most effective medicine a physician had to offer" (Haakonssen 1997, 152). Like Percival and Gregory, Rush based his ethics on the doctrine of sympathy, an innate capacity essential to human bonding. Accordingly, the physician should also "ignore the peevishness of patients," which was thought to be merely a stage of illness that would eventually lead to recovery (Haakonssen 1997, 217). But sympathy had limits in Rush's view, and he shared none of Gregory's more empathetic considerations for patients. After all, Rush believed that patients were inferior to their physicians, and their duties were carefully prescribed. The patient must (1) properly select a qualified physician; (2)

avoid the habit of trying to escape higher fees by not consulting with a physician at the onset of a disease; (3) dutifully be honest in reporting his past health and current habits; and (4) closely follow physician orders. Rush then outlined a series of minor duties, such as prompt fee payment! From our vantage point, he was not only self-serving, he was unapologetic by claiming all this in the patient's best interest. In his view, sickness had a practical function in life, for "illness was a visitation providentially provided for" (Haakonssen 1997, 132), and just as in every other "office" in life one must embrace its related duties, sickness is no exception, having "duties as well as rights" (p. 132). This attitude is all the more jolting considering that Rush was a prominent member of the founding Fathers!

13. For instance, although Mark Twain ([1899] 1992) was highly skeptical of the growing dominance of allopathic medicine, he was adamant about the sanctity of individual choice. In reacting to a licensing scheme to elevate what was to become orthodox scientific medicine, Twain ([1867] 1992, 228) wrote, "There has always been a variance of choice under which system a citizen preferred to find his way across the Styx, and he enjoyed in this State till now the privilege of choosing the rower who was to aid in ferrying him over in Charon's boat." He went on to decry government influence in medicine, expressing sentiments that would please the most ardent proponents of laissez-faire, market-based health care: "The mania for giving the Government power to meddle with the private affairs of cities or citizens is likely to cause endless trouble, through the rivalry of schools and creeds that are anxious to obtain official recognition, and there is great danger that our people will lose that independence of thought and action which is the cause of much of our greatness, and sink into the helplessness of the Frenchman or German who expects his government to feed him when hungry, clothe him when naked, to prescribe when his child may be born and when he may die, and, in fine, to regulate every act of humanity from the cradle to the tomb, including the manner in which he may seek future admission to paradise" ([1867] 1992, 230). As Twain testified, whether written as political or social history, the nineteenth century was a celebration of the individual and of new notions of individual freedom.

14. Martin Salgo, a fifty-five-year-old man, underwent a surgical procedure after which he awoke to find himself paralyzed in both legs. He claimed that his paralysis was due to the negligent performance of a translumber aortography, and claimed that the physicians negligently had failed to warn him of the inherent risks of paralysis in the procedure. Justice Bray coined the phrase "informed consent" after pondering the difficult questions regarding physician disclosure to apprehensive patients, and while his decision left the law of disclosure and consent still unresolved, subsequent civil court cases served to shape and further define the doctrine.

15. The most recent formalized code of professional behavior is the 2002 Charter on Medical Professionalization, whose three fundamental principles are (1) primacy of patient welfare, (2) patient autonomy, and (3) social justice (Blank et al. 2003). Accompanying these basic precepts are ten professional responsi-

bilities, which include commitments specifically designed for individual patients (i.e., maintenance of honesty, confidentiality, and appropriate relations with patients), and a second group addressing a physician-advocacy role for improved quality and access of care, just distribution of finite resources, and maintaining trust by managing conflicts of interest. This charter, jointly sponsored by American and European medical academic societies, has been widely endorsed (Blank et al. 2003) and criticized (Reiser and Banner 2003). In seeking to improve patients' welfare, the charter reflects the growing concern about advancing the well-being and dignity of patients (an indication of the self-consciousness about patient autonomy) and a newer response to a social and economic reality: physicians no longer dominate health-care delivery policy and have instead become subordinate partners to corporate health institutions such as insurers, managed-care providers, and government-run health systems. Physician identity is changing as a result of split responsibilities to patients and corporate employers, with resulting challenges to the trust characterizing the doctor-patient dyad. The charter thus reflects a dual professional agenda for physicians: a traditional role of healer and, firmly placing professional allegiance with the patient, a new assignment of agent for social change.

Chapter 3

1. As a pragmatist and a liberal, Mead was in step with his colleague, John Dewey, whose own writings on the subject of social identity follow a similar line. For instance, in "The Ethics of Democracy," an early essay on political philosophy, Dewey draws a portrait of society as an organism consisting of individual units. None of the units has any significance apart from its integration in the whole: "Society in its unified and structured character is the fact of the case; the non-social individual is an abstraction arrived at by imagining what man would be if all his human qualities were taken away. Society, as a real whole, is the normal order, and the mass as an aggregate of isolated units is the fiction" (Dewey [1888] 1997, 187).

Pragmatism's liberal attitude toward social responsibility rests on this basic premise about the character of selfhood—that is, because people are constituted only in society, the group is ultimately responsible for the welfare of the individual. Indeed, by 1930 Dewey wrote of rugged capitalist individualism: "It is not too much to say that the whole significance of the older individualism has now shrunk to a pecuniary scale and measure. The virtues that are supposed to attend rugged individualism may be vocally proclaimed, but it takes no great insight to see that what is cherished is measured by its connection with those activities that make for success in business conducted for personal gain" (Dewey, *Individualism Old and New* (1930); quoted by Diggins 1994, 378).

The communal welfare espoused by Dewey, Mead, Jane Addams, and other pragmatists during the high tide of American liberalism derived its philosophical bearings from their understanding of the social character of the self (Diggins 1994). The pragmatists' emphasis on the collective is a radical break from earlier

American religious philosophies that emphasized the individual self as the bedrock of personal responsibility (i.e., the individual might rise in grace through his own personal efforts for salvation) and as the sole source of conscience and guilt (Shain 1994). But the pragmatists denied any such entity as "the self": "In pragmatism the self is a product created in social interaction, a "process" that becomes an object of its own awareness. With such awareness, we can know how our selves have come to be formed. The rest is history, the story of the self's development beyond itself, by situations, systems and structures within which the self resides, thinks, and acts" (Diggins 1994, 374). Instead the pragmatists posed moral authority as the question, not the answer: "One recalls Lippmann's definition of liberalism as the overthrow of authority and the search for its sub-stitute. In America the search ended with pragmatism, which promised to take the place of traditional authority. . . . [For pragmatism] authority is functional rather than foundational, what works, or, as Dewey put it, whatever "will do" in satisfying human need" (Diggins 1994, 374).

2. Emerson championed a mystical communion with Nature, which was achieved through a jealously guarded personal isolation. In claiming privacy to achieve a heightened religious experience, he set the punctual self alone in the universe: "Standing on the bare ground [in pristine woods],—my head bathed by the blithe air, and uplifted into infinite space,—all mean egotism vanishes. I become a transparent eye-ball; I am nothing. I see all. The currents of the Universal Being circulate through me; I am part or particle of God" (Emerson [1836] 1971, 10). Here we see Emerson adding mystical communion with Nature to self-reliance and personal perfectionism as the third component of a New American personality, one uniquely created from the promise of an unconquered natural frontier. In *Nature* ([1836] 1971) and also in the essay "Experience" ([1844] 1983), he described an essential interior identity that exists in intimate union with the rest of nature, unaware of its own singularity (*Nature*)—a metaphysical assertion—or shockingly disjointed from human experience ("Experience")—an existential observation (Tauber 2003b).

3. My favorite anecdote characterizing the political difference between Thoreau and Emerson is the apocryphal story of an encounter between them in 1846: Emerson visited the jailed Thoreau (incarcerated for a night for not paying a poll tax that he regarded as supporting the unjust Mexican War) and asked him, "Henry, what are doing in there?" Thoreau answered, "The better question is, What are you doing *out* there?"

4. When Emerson ([1841] 1979, 186), in a famous line from "Circles," says "cause and effect are two sides of one fact," he describes the twofold character of human divinity. On the one hand, the divine resides within us (and is, indeed, the basis for our discovery of Spirit), and at the same time delivers a moral lesson: do not mistakenly assert self-reliance as some kind of autonomous, or freed, effect, and thus break the divine unified cause-effect relationship that unites us to the eternal. As Emerson wrote in his journal: "And what is God? We cannot say but we see clearly enough. We cannot say, because he is the unspeakable, the immeasurable, the perfect—but we see plain enough in what direction it lies.

First we see plainly that the All is in Man. . . . That is, there is no screen or ceiling between our heads & the infinity of space/heavens, so there is no bar or wall in the Soul where man the effect ceases & God the cause begins. The walls are taken away; we lie open on one side to all the deeps of spiritual nature, to all the attributes of God. . . . Again; because the All is in Man we know nothing arbitrary, nothing alien shall take place in the Universe, nothing contrary to the Nature in us" (Emerson 1965, 229–230).

5. These observations are based on Max Weber's classic study, *The Protestant Ethic and the Spirit of Capitalism* ([1904–1905] 1958), which argued that in response to the doctrine of predestination, Calvinism developed a strong emphasis on independent achievement. Salvation was to be achieved through self-reliance, the active pursuit of individual perfection afforded to the elect marked for redemption. In short, God aided those who helped themselves, and thus individualism achieved its religious justification. Although Puritanism began with a strong communitarian ethos, as these ties were eroded, individualism forged from these religious tenets remained as the relic of a more complex social morality (Shain 1994). According to Kirschner (1996, 45), "Protestantism exemplifies 'religious individualism' with its doctrines of the priesthood of all believers (highlighting the individual's personal unmediated relationship with God, and the inner life in general) and the respect for individual conscience (emphasizing the individual's right to his own spiritual practice and responsibility for his own spiritual condition)."

6. The movement of this core idea was hardly novel, for as David Walsh says about the early modern period more generally, "The [historical] picture that emerges . . . is not of a world increasingly separating itself from God, but of a world progressively absorbing the divine substance into itself" (Walsh 1983, 9). This particular translation is but one chapter in the evolution of theological ideas into a more secular world: "It is an historical commonplace that the course of Western thought since the Renaissance has been one of progressive secularization, but it is easy to mistake the way in which that process took place. Secular thinkers have no more been able to work free of the centuries-old Judaeo-Christian culture than Christian theologians were able to work free of their inheritance of classical and pagan thought. The process—outside the exact sciences at any rate—has not been the deletion and replacement of religious ideas, but rather the assimilation and re-interpretation of religious ideas, as constitutive elements in a world view founded on secular premises" (Abrams 1973, 13).

7. Kant explains: "The consciousness of oneself in accordance with the determinations of our state in internal perception is merely empirical, forever variable; it can provide no standing or abiding self in this stream of inner appearances, and is customarily called **inner sense** or **empirical apperception**. That which should **necessarily** be represented as numerically identical cannot be thought of as such through empirical data. There must be a condition that precedes all experience and makes the latter itself possible, which should make such a transcendental presupposition valid" (Kant [1781, 1787] 1998, 232 [A107]; emphasis in the original). Hume's view of this matter is not dissimilar from Kant's

skepticism. Whereas they begin with the same general orientation, Kant goes further in offering a transcendental structure consistent with his idealism.

8. Hume articulates his position as follows: "There are some philosophers who imagine we are every moment intimately conscious of what we call our *self*; that we feel its existence and its continuance in existence; and are certain, beyond the evidence of a demonstration, both of its perfect identity and simplicity. . . . Unluckily all these positive assertions are contrary to that very special experience which pleaded for them; nor have we any idea of self, after the manner it is here explained. For from what impression could this idea be derived? This question is impossible to answer without a manifest contradiction and absurdity; and yet it is a question which must necessarily be answered, if we could have the idea of self pass for clear and intelligible. It must be some one impression that gives rise to every real idea. But self or person is not any one impression, but that to which our several impressions and ideas are supposed to have a reference. If any impression gives rise to the idea of self, that impression must continue invariably the same, through the whole course of our lives; since self is supposed to exist after that manner. But there is no impression constant and invariable. . . . It cannot therefore be from any of these impressions, or from any other, that the idea of self is derived; and consequently there is no such idea" (Hume [1739] 1978, 300–301).

9. The critical philosophy Kant developed in the *Critique of Pure Reason* ([1781, 1787] 1998) offered a scaffolding by which the natural world might be known. The mind, according to Kant, had certain categories whereby sensory data were organized and given various forms of order. The forms of order are not externally imposed on the mind, but are an aspect of the laws of natural phenomena, that aspect that make the experience lawful. These laws are "pure" or devoid of any empirical content in themselves, yet they contain the "structure" by which the mind discerns their order. Analogously, Kant sought a structure by which our behavior might be explained as he understood human perception, that is, through an organizing faculty. This parallel cognitive faculty—"practical reason"—directs and organizes human action through its own structure, analogous to how pure reason organizes experience (Kant [1788] 1996). The perfect will, determined by its own inner lawfulness, is inherently good and perfectly rational, but unfortunately humans suffer from imperfection, driven by desires whether they are rational or not. We feel the perfect will's operation, however, as a constraint against the pull of desire. Like natural law, the categorical imperative is contentless (empirically empty) and is only the form of lawfulness itself.

10. As Rawls ([1971] 1999, 225–226) puts it, "Kant's main aim is to deepen and to justify Rousseau's idea that liberty is acting in accordance with a law that we give to ourselves. And this leads not to a morality of austere command but to an ethic of mutual respect and self-esteem. . . . The person's choice as a noumenal self I have assumed to be a collective one. The force of the self's being equal is that the principles chosen must be acceptable to other selves. Since all are similarly free and rational, each must have an equal say in adopting public princi-

ples of the ethical commonwealth. This means as noumenal selves, everyone is to consent to these principles."

11. Here are Mill's words: "The only purpose for which power can be rightfully exercised over any member of the community, against his will, is to prevent harm to others. His own good, either physical or moral, is not sufficient warrant. He cannot rightfully be compelled to do or forebear because it will be better for him to do so, because it will make him happier, because in the opinions of others, to do so would be wise, or even right. These are good reasons for remonstrating with him, or reasoning with him, or persuading him, or entreating him, but not for compelling him, or visiting him with any evil in case he do otherwise. To justify that, the conduct from which it is desired to deter him must be calculated to produce evil to some one else. The only part of the conduct of any one, for which he is amenable to society, is that which concerns others. In the part which merely concerns himself, his independence is, of right, absolute. Over himself, over his own body and mind, the individual is sovereign" (Mill [1859] 1972, 78).

12. Communitarians do not believe Rawls and company have gone far enough in espousing a social ethic. Communitarians are linked by their program against what they regard as a pervasive and insidious culture of rights, where (radical) political and judicial protection of the individual is seen as eroding those social values that must operate for communities to effectively cohere (Etzioni 1995, 1996; Tam 1998). They seek a more balanced emphasis on an ethos of shared values, which emphasize the needs of the community at large. Interestingly, health care and medical ethics have not played a prominent role in these discussions (despite efforts to the contrary; see, e.g., Walzer 1983; Emanuel 1991; Nelson 1992; Tauber 2002; Callahan 2003), but it seems to me that it is precisely in this arena that the issues raised by communitarians become especially cogent.

Communitarianism has been associated with the philosophers Alasdair MacIntyre (1984), Michael Sandel (1982), Charles Taylor (1985), and Michael Walzer (1983), who may be broadly understood as engaged in a sustained argument with John Rawls (Mulhall and Swift 1992). Rawls (certainly the "earlier" Rawls) follows traditional liberal individualism, which celebrates themes of individuality, autonomy, and disengaged rationality, so that the self is understood as ideally rational and capable of free choice as a self-aware and assertive individual (Rawls [1971] 1999). To express these capacities, the individual must be allowed to act as independently as possible, both within his or her local social group, and within the larger state. Hence protective rights are enacted and enforced to limit the power of the state, and it is at this point that the political debate has ensued.

Philosophical critiques begin as to how important communitarian themes are represented in liberal philosophy, and more specifically, how clear a distinction must be drawn between liberalism and individualism (Frazer 1999, 19). Rawls himself, in later writings, denies any bias toward individualism, and emphasizes the values of reciprocity and associational life, stressing the importance of communal values to liberal politics (Rawls 1993, 190, n. 221; [1971] 1999). Putting aside the specific debate between Rawls and his critics, the argument in fact is a reiteration of criticism directed at certain interpretations of Kantian autonomy. The communitarian version, like other social-based theories, deemphasizes atomistic autonomy, and instead formulates moral agency within the context of the social relations of individuals, who play multiple social roles, enact diverse social responsibilities, and engage in various social discourses. The settings in which citizens develop and live are conceptualized as "nonnatural" (i.e., culturally constructed), and thus individual choices, reasons, and actions are conceptualized as contingent but sociologically or historically explicable (Frazer 1999, 15–23). In short, atomistic autonomy is "encumbered" with social identities and commitments to class, gender, race, education, religion, and local community. This conception of the person as essentially social is associated with values that sustain social order—trust, reciprocity, mutuality, substantive equality, and community (Frazer 1999). In this regard, communitarianism is an application of the basic sociological tenet concerning the primary social identity of persons (Mead 1934).

Contemporary communitarianism is philosophically based on three theses:

1. Communities are not reducible to individuals and their rights.
2. It follows then that community values are not simply the extrapolated values of the autonomous individual, but must encompass the values of the social individual, which are derived from community-sustaining values. These include the values of reciprocity, trust, solidarity, and tradition.
3. Derived from the above two tenets, the concluding position is that the individual does not, indeed cannot, stand in a direct unmediated relationship with the state and society. There are, to be sure, degrees of choice and independence, but the notion of strict social, political, or ethical autonomy is regarded by communitarians as not only a conceit, but also distorting of the social reality. Most importantly, the moral relation of the individual and the state demands a reciprocity of responsibility that places those values sustaining the community as paramount.

In short, the debate swirling around communitarianism has focused on the political strain between atomistic individualism and the view of the subject as assuming his or her identity as a *result* of identification or membership in a group or community. Issues such as the responsibility of the group to the person and the reciprocal question of the individual's relation to the group assume quite a different character when approached from these disparate points of view. Although utilitarianism seems to dominate characterizations of communitarianism, this is an oversimplified reduction. In a communitarian ethic, the communal structure determines not only how choices are made, but more particularly what those choices might be when driven by concern for the community at large. These *may* be utilitarian, but they may also be driven by other goals or ideals. Whatever the communal ethic, the position of the individual is balanced within and against social needs. These contemporary discussions reiterate debates dating to antebellum America. Communitarians see the social fabric as Tocqueville did in the 1830s, skewed toward citizens seeking their greatest individual advancement at the expense of investing heavily in the social capital of their communities (Mulhall and Swift 1992; Etzioni 1995, 1996; Tam 1998).

13. Kierkegaard wrote that "the self is a relation which relates itself to its own self, or it is that in the relation which relates itself to its own self, or it is that in the relation [which accounts for it] that the relation relates itself to its own self. . . . Man is a synthesis of the infinite and the finite. . . . A synthesis is a relation between two factors. So regarded, man is not yet a self. . . . Such a relation which relates itself to its own self (that is to say, a self) must either have constituted itself or have been constituted by another. If this relation which relates itself to its own self is constituted by another, the relation doubtless is the third term, but this relation (the third term) is in turn a relation relating itself to that which constituted the whole relation. Such a derived, constituted, relation is the human self, a relation which relates itself to its own self, and in relating itself to its own self relates itself to another" (Kierkegaard [1849] 1955, 146).

14. Generally, *alterity* refers to the post-Hegelian understanding of the self as defined in opposition to, or engaging with, an "other"—God, man, nature, self-reflection, society—and in the self's response to the other, identity is configured. Briefly, the self, to the extent that it can be actualized, is, from this general perspective, defined by the other. Discussion has focused on whether, and how, in response to an encounter, the self articulates itself or is altered as a consequence of that engagement. Also considered is how the engaged self might change its object and their shared world. In short, the phenomenological approach explores how the self lives in its world, inseparably in a universe of others. The self alone is either alienated—that is, alienated in its selfness—or it actively engages the world and becomes actualized. The debate revolves about the contingency of this process, and its problematic opportunities for success (Tauber 1994, 201ff.).

But even the contingency of the self's construction has been attacked in more recent poststructuralist arguments. From this perspective, there is nothing "natural" about cultural structures (e.g., language, kinship systems, social and economic hierarchies, sexual norms, and religious beliefs), and there is no transcendental significance to limit "meanings." Only power explains the hegemony of one view over another. Similarly, "the self" may be regarded as constructed by arbitrary criteria, and thus occupies no natural habitat. Indeed, as an artifact of social and historical contingencies, the phenomenological insistence on the self's dependence on the other has been radically challenged: not only has the self's autonomy been rendered meaningless, *any* construction of the self is regarded as arbitrary. Late twentieth-century voices spoke of the self's "indeterminacy"—a "decentered" subject. No longer an origin or a source, it becomes only the contingent product of multiple historical, social, and psychological forces (see Mauss 1985 and the commentaries in Carrithers, Collins, and Lukes 1985; Rose 1990, 1998). So what began in the romantic period as a trial of self-examination, culminated in postromanticism (what is usually referred to as postmodernism) in finding only an empty "space" where personal identity once was grounded (Tauber 1994).

15. Twentieth-century proponents of naturalistic approaches have taken up the challenge again in the form of neuroscientific accounts (e.g., Skoyles and Sagan 2002; Metzinger 2003; Kircher and David 2003), but those who did not regard the self as an object (and thereby incapable of scientific assessment) shifted discussion of personal identity into other arenas, most notably to phenomenological, existential, analytical, and moral discourses.

16. The "ethics of caring" has a complex history, but in its contemporary formulation, perhaps it is most directly traced to Carol Gilligan's *In a Different Voice* (1982). (In some respects, Nel Noddings's *Caring: A Feminist Approach to Ethics and Moral Education* (1984) is more focused and thus more directly applicable to the medical setting. Empirical studies with direct implications for the doctor-patient relationship have also been published (Gilligan and Pollak 1988).) The feminist critiques have influentially realigned the debates about moral philosophy along a new continuum between a masculine rights-based justice model and a feminist relational model of ethics (summarized by Baier 1994a). Gilligan's target was the Kantian tradition (i.e., Rawls) that espoused justice as the "first" moral principle, and in her attack she also focused on the psychological schools of Piaget and Kohlberg, whose studies supported the moral ideal of individual rational will or autonomy. In her own empirical studies, Gilligan discovered that the standard of *what* was moral determined moral development, and if those standards followed a particularly masculine trajectory, women fared less well when assessed. She argued that perhaps another standard of ethics might be applied, one that stressed different values—connections, relationships, and reciprocity—and within such a moral system, women prevailed over men. Thus the ethics of caring was contrasted with the ethics of justice along a continuum that was, in large part, embedded in deep roots of gender identity and cultural values.

By contrasting this feminist moral compass with a male ethos stressing independence and separateness, Gilligan presented a strong challenge to older versions of individualism. The response to dependency and to the need for interconnections between people portrayed a social universe characterized by interrelated actors, not atomistic ones. Thus the "ethics of caring" was born as a product of an understanding about persons in a social web designed to create harmonious interactions. The arguments presented here about relational autonomy stem from this intellectual tradition.

17. In the justice model, from which atomistic autonomy derives, obligations are understood within a contractual scheme, or as arising out of voluntary consent, while the ethic of care accounts for obligations to which we have not deliberately consented and consequently requires that we expand our account of obligations beyond a specified contract (Clement 1996, 113). This contrast of a contract versus a so-called covenant model of care is extensively discussed in chapter 6.

Chapter 4

1. In the procedural, or content-neutral, accounts, the *content* of a person's desires, values, beliefs, and emotional attitudes is irrelevant to the issues of whether the person is autonomous with respect to those aspects of her motivational structure and the actions that flow from them. What matters for autonomy is whether the agent has subjected her motivations and actions to the appropriate kind of critical reflection (Mackenize and Stoljar 2000, 13–4). Catherine Mackenzie and Natalie Stoljar make this claim based on the following: "First, the idea that hierarchical views involve an ontological commitment to a metaphysically distinct true self . . . misrepresents the process of critical reflection . . . [which] should be understood as a process of self-constitution. As Frankfurt makes clear . . . the self is not a static, deep metaphysical entity but is constantly being reconstituted through the process of reflection, deliberation, and decision, by means of which we define our cares, commitments, and values. Second, as Susan Wolf has argued convincingly, the metaphysical problem conflates the moral responsibility for the self with metaphysical responsibility for the self" (2000, 29).

2. Gary Watson (1975) depicts the regress problem as follows: What ensures that higher order desires are in fact freely selected and thus autonomous? The only way to stratify desires is to impose higher orders, which in turn must be scrutinized as free or determined. How, indeed, can one determine with confidence what is socially or psychologically determined, as opposed to values derived from some source of "inner value" or self-actualization? The distinctions are hopelessly blurred, and consequently the ability to prioritize one set of desires over another depends on some *rationalizing* process, but not necessarily a rational, independent one. Similarly, Irving Thalberg (1978) has questioned the hierarchy itself, namely, why and how does one assign higher value to certain desires and not others? On what basis is the ontological status of one versus another achieved? Each of these critiques alludes to the problematic status of the self—some true metaphysical identity by which a hierarchy of desires might be established or whose desires reflect such a self (Friedman 1986). Does autonomy require acting in accordance with such a true self? If so, how is that self formed and does free agency require it to be free of the determinants discussed above (i.e., the socialization process)? Without some firm construction of selfhood, these critics argue that there is no foundation or resting place from which to accomplish a sorting by criteria that may claim some final legitimacy. Again we see, as in chapter 3, how constructions of selfhood and autonomy have gone hand in hand.

3. Offering an alternative to mandatory positive autonomy, Carl Schneider (1998, 174) describes "selective autonomy" as the choice to make only the truly important decisions and to delegate the rest: "Indeed, for many people in much of their lives, the problem is not the absence of choice, but its abundance. . . . In sum, the obligation to make all one's decisions . . . states an unattainable and unwise standard." This view follows the Frankfurt-Dworkin formulation that

choice is made in a hierarchical fashion, where some choices are reserved and others are delegated.

4. Schneider (1998, 85) elaborates: "For many patients, medical decisions are both above and beneath their attention. Above, because patients are concentrated on day-to-day coping. They try to perdure with their lives despite their disease, to make it work. . . . They do not ignore their illness. But their attention is concerned with adapting to it, not treating it. . . . On the other hand, medical decisions fall beneath patients' attention because illness urgently presents the largest kinds of questions to them, questions about their religious faith, about whether their lives have been well led, about what a good life is."

5. As Joel Feinberg (1986, 117) observes, "It may not always be possible, even in principle, to say of one act that it is more voluntary or closer to being voluntary than another. . . . Still, we can conceive clearly of completely involuntary end points, and of some choices near the high end of the scale, and we can talk, with appropriate caution, of higher and lower standards of voluntariness. . . . We should treat voluntariness as a variable concept, determined by higher and lower cut-off points depending on the nature of the circumstances, the interests at stake, and the moral and legal purposes to be served."

6. Schneider (1998, 177) observes that "the autonomy paradigm has triumphed on the field of principle partly because it embodies an ideal with rich contemporary appeal. The model patient is strong, competent, intelligent, aggressive, and self-reliant. . . . The model patient brings to medical decisions a well-considered life plan that is the product of long reflection on the kind of person the patient truly is. These characteristics have their merits. But they do not state all the virtues we might hope for, and they are conducive to some vices. . . . They offer little help to, and even lead astray, patients who cannot achieve control and independence."

7. The best-studied case of disputed competency concerns the involuntary hospitalization of psychotic patients, which clearly illustrates how beneficence (more specifically, fiduciary responsibility) has been trumped by patient autonomy as a governing medicolegal principle of medical care (Tauber 2003a). In the progressive era of the 1960s and 1970s, the insane acquired civil rights previously blocked because of the stigmatization of their illness. Intrusive mental health treatment, violations of due process, and invasions of privacy have repeatedly been asserted as violations of fundamental constitutional rights of the mentally compromised (Winick 1997, 256ff.). In short, the hitherto implicit fiduciary responsibilities of psychiatrists were usurped by a widely expanded understanding, and application, of patient autonomy.

Involuntary hospitalization is based on the police power of the state to protect citizens and the individual against harm—only against harm to self or others—and sometimes in the interest of promoting the health and welfare of those who cannot care for themselves. Society may not impose its police powers on those who are simply nonconformist. While this principle protects the fringe elements, it also promotes the welfare of all, for "the greatest harm [of oppression] done is to those who are not heretics, and whose whole mental development is cramped, and their reason cowed, by the fear of heresy" (Mill [1859] 1972, 101).

Modern law presumes competence unless proven otherwise, and in this setting the assessment of competence is restricted to the *potential* of danger; it cannot simply be based on a diagnosis of insanity. However, there is no general agreement concerning the appropriate standard for determining competency even in this restricted sense (see, e.g., Winick 1997; Sedgwick 1982; Appelbaum and Grisso 1988; LaFond and Durham 1992; Griffiths 1994). And when data is sought on the effectiveness of involuntary detention—that is, or how accurately it identifies those truly in danger—studies are beset with design problems that make such information difficult to gather and then assess (Chodoff 1976; American Bar Association 1977, 87; Culver and Gert 1982). If empirical data do not help identify those truly in danger, then competency tests, despite their problems, are most often employed. Competency requires the ability to make and carry out a decision, to understand information disclosed, to arrive at a decision in a rational manner, and to make a reasonable treatment decision (formulated in the 1982 President's Commission Report; cited in Winick 1997, 347ff.). Several tests have been used to determine whether these criteria are satisfactorily met, but both the standards and their application are hardly uniform. Although mental illness sometimes impairs competency to process information and make rational choices, it often does not do so (Grisso and Appelbaum 1995; Winick 1997, 257ff.). Even the best studies are flawed and not easily extrapolated to individual cases (Tauber 2003a), but the best approximation is that somewhere between a quarter and a half of schizophrenics have "substantially impaired decision making" (Appelbaum and Grisso 1988, 172). Is the glass half full or half empty? Perhaps more salient for the champions of autonomy, even in the midst of a psychotic episode, patients may function normally some of the time due to the intermittent nature of their impairment (Rosenhan 1973). Despite persistent confusion, two general points may be made: (1) the task of assessing rational impairment based on a psychiatric diagnosis is fraught with uncertainty and must be carried out on a case-by-case basis (that is, mental illness per se cannot be equated with incompetency), and (2) a significant number of psychotics, especially in acute decompensation, have greatly impaired ability to make rational choices.

But note that the issue is not "rationality" writ large—for example, the ability to solve certain kinds of problems or think abstractly—but rather the narrower question of whether one is able to think logically during a sustained period *about oneself*, both as an agent of action and as a member of a larger social and natural universe. So, if one accepts that "competence" is not a global characteristic, but is composed of several complex mental faculties, then the mentally ill are best understood as possessing some rational functions that are intact and others that are not.

But in practice, such a nuance is not recognized by current legal practice. Insanity per se is not at issue. Either one is competent or not, and the only criterion with legal standing that can determine competence is danger to others or oneself.

Note that judges are not asked to measure competence, but only to assess danger under the auspices of competence. A ruse is at play here: the insane are by definition not competent in an ordinary sense, but they are given this designation to secure their rights as citizens. The judicial authority thus determines whether to sustain autonomy based on one set of criteria (danger), whereas the medical authority, in making a determination of "insane," uses a different set (delusions) to argue that an individual is no longer autonomous—that is, competent. The latter determination, the one employed to demarcate the sane from the insane, is superseded by the former in deciding involuntary confinement and treatment. While these approaches may overlap, they need not. In short, judges deal with individual rights; psychiatrists deal with insanity and its treatment. The crucial point: citizen and patient are not necessarily the same social agent governed by the same moral concerns.

Apparently the judiciary follows the philosophy of Oliver Wendell Holmes, who was well aware of the practical demands made on the moral standards governing the courts. He understood that because the law possessed conflicting tenets and was applied within changing social contexts, judges must interpret the law for what they perceived as the best outcome for society as a whole (Menand 2001, 423–431). When Holmes ([1881] 1963, 5, 63) wrote, "The life of the law has not been logic: it has been experience. . . . The law did not begin with a theory. It has never worked one out," he meant that the law has no essentialist aspect—neither formalist, utilitarian, nor historicist—and he thus regarded moral principles as amenable to manipulation in order to address the best interests of the community. In short, while the law seeks universality, the pragmatic application of legal principles cannot be uniform. The context of behaviors is crucial.

Chapter 5

1. For instance, economic analysis has shown a correspondence between economic success and trust, which is understood as a precondition for prosperous economic activity (Gambetta 1988). When characterizing the function of civil society and politics, a legion of commentators have heralded the centrality of trust in determining the character of democracy (e.g., Sandel 1982; Walzer 1983). And in the realm of personal interactions, trust has increasingly figured as a central trope in understanding psychological (e.g., Erikson 1968; Giddens 1992; Brothers 1995) and sociological (e.g., Misztal 1996; Govier 1997; Cook 2001; Hardin 2002) relationships. Indeed, it is impossible to think of society in any dimension independent of trust. But the issue assumes its urgency because we are in the midst of dramatic changes that are altering basic social relationships. In seeking to comprehend the basis and significance of these transformations, commentators I have focused on the meaning and significance of trust.

2. While quantitative scales seem to be improving (Kao et al. 1998b; Hall et al. 2002), we are left largely with impressions: "Despite a relative avalanche of information about patient satisfaction, the paucity of empirical research on trust has

provided little data pointing to clear correlates of patient-physician trust. Moreover, there is not a single published study to date [2000] of a successful intervention that has measurably improved patients' trust in their physician" (Pearson and Raeke 2000, 512). The changing practice environment with a particular focus on the ethics governing the relations of doctors and patients is reviewed by Campbell (2000).

3. The term *social capital* was invented or reinvented at least six times in the twentieth century and refers to the benefits of social ties: "Whereas physical capital refers to physical objects and human capital refers to properties of individuals, social capital refers to connections among individuals—social networks and the norms of reciprocity and trustworthiness that arise from them. In that sense social capital is closely related to what some have called 'civic virtue'" (Putnam 2000, 19).

4. Surveys measuring trust consistently show a significant decline. For instance, in 1998, Americans, by a margin of three to one, believed that our society was less honest and moral than it used to be. This is not nostalgia for a more innocent time. In studies that compare present responses to those made a generation or two ago, the evidence yields a striking result: "Most, if not all, of the decline in American social trust since the 1960s is attributable to generation succession" (Putnam 2000, 140), a finding confirmed by others using different, and in some ways more sensitive, scales (Robinson and Jackson 2001). As an older trusting generation (those born before 1940) declines demographically, a cynical post-1960 generation now comprises almost one-third of the population. If one surveys how these generations respond to the question of whether "most people are honest" (and therefore trustworthy), the older generation affirms their confidence at a rate of 75 to 80 percent, while their mistrusting grandchildren are less optimistic, agreeing at a rate of 50 percent (Putnam 2000, 141). The cohort responses remain constant at the generational level (growing age does not increase the group's trust level), and the net result is a general decline in social trust.

5. Notwithstanding their current standing, since 1977, according to Gallup polls conducted nearly every year to measure the perceived honesty and ethical standards of numerous occupations and professions, public opinion of physicians has remained steady. Generally in the top five, medical doctors range from 47 to 58 percent of those surveyed who believe that doctors maintain high ethical standards (Gallup Poll 1977–1997). Note, about half have a more circumspect opinion.

6. Seligman aligns himself with Luhmann in regarding *trust* in persons and *confidence* in institutions as encompassing different social expectations. He derives this position from his definition of trust: "Trust is something that enters into social relations when there is role negotiability, in what may be termed the 'open spaces' or roles and role expectations. Another way of saying this is that trust enters into social interaction in the interstices of system, or at system limit, when for one reason or another systematically defined role expectations are no longer viable. By defining trust in this way we manage to 'save' the phenomenon

sociologically from either a reduction to faith or belief on the one hand or to confidence in the fulfillment of role expectations on the other. We also cut through many of the current philosophical debates on trust which in the main, turn on either the viability (or rationality) of belief or the existence of sufficient (verifiable or not) bases for confidence" (Seligman 1997, 25). According to Seligman, trust then becomes a rare phenomenon, exercised when role expectations either break down or are unknown. And more relevant to my own concerns, the doctor-patient relationship, he would argue, is governed by confidence, not trust, because the roles are so well prescribed. I think a theoretical distance separates Seligman's construction from the reality of the clinic, and the distinction between trust and confidence, originally made by Luhmann, is not useful.

7. Sociological critiques typically follow culturalist, functionalist, symbolic-interactionist, and phenomenological lines. None of these specific approaches will be discussed here, but it is useful to understand where the concept of trust resides in the edifice of sociological theory. As Piotr Sztompka observes, sociology has two competing approaches: a focus on social collectives versus one emphasizing social agents. The first studies social structures or systems and their operations; the second characterizes persons and their actions. The latter is more concerned with describing how agents interact—the matrix of their relationships and the meanings, symbols, rules, values, codes, modes of discourse, and trust that govern their interactions (Sztompka 1999, 2). Within this agent-centered approach, again there are two competing agendas: on the one hand, actions may be seen from the point of view of choice theory (how choices are made to maximize gain and minimize risk), and on the other hand, behaviors are understood as reflecting humane values—emotions, social bonds, loyalties, identities. And again a division occurs within this last group. One path of research pursues psychological meanings (motivations, reasons, intentions, attitudes) to elaborate sociopsychological theories of action. The other course follows cultural meanings (rules, norms, values, symbols) to produce a culturalist sociology of action. This last approach allows "various qualitative, interpretative, hermeneutical procedures, suitable for unraveling the cultural aspects of action. It is also marked by the reversal of perspective: from treating action as the dependent variable to be explained by rational appraisal of circumstances, toward treating action as an independent, creative variable, involved in constructing, shaping, and modifying all other social objects, including social wholes of all sorts: groups, communities, societies" (Sztompka 1999, 3). This general orientation seems most suitable for characterizing trust as a moral category.

8. The question of how philosophy is situated in the ordinary world is hardly a new problem. For instance, the Roman rhetorician, Quntilian (30–100 CE), in his *Institutio Oratoria* (about 96 CE), lamented how philosophers had abdicated their input into the actual practices and experience of life: "Philosophy no longer moves in its true sphere of action and in the broad daylight of the forum, but has retired first to porches and gymnasia and finally to the gatherings of the

schools" (book 12, chap. 2; quoted in Leitch 2001, 168), leaving to the lawyers and rhetoricians the work of common discourse.

9. A key challenge is how to recover the "patient" in the corporate setting by a reexamination of how fiduciary responsibilities apply in the managed-care context (Jacobson and Cahill 2000). Yet we must note that the law does not address beneficence as a guiding professional principle: patient recourse for bad outcomes, by and large, is limited to malpractice, not breach of fiduciary responsibility. In other words, the law has directed complaint away from the general protections offered by fiduciary law to damage rewards for technical incompetence and malexecution.

10. The commentary summarized here on the conditions of moral bonds and moral community has a history dating to the mid-nineteenth century, and follows at least five related themes (Sztompka 1999, 6–8): (1) alienation (associated most closely with Marx) emphasizes the distancing of the individual from his work and political life, which leads to loss of identity, dignity, and purpose; (2) anomie (originating with Durkheim); (3) "revolt of the masses" (Ortega y Gasset); (4) "iron cage" (Weber) themes emphasize the isolated character of modern life resulting from urban mass society, depersonalized bureaucratization of social organizations, and mass government; and (5) the "lonely crowd" theme describes the inward turning of persons as a result of the individualization of social life and the resulting atrophy of moral communities. Such concepts as civic culture, civic society, cultural capital, and social capital have been used to characterize what has been lost and why.

11. Adam Smith's "interactive sympathy" replaced republican "virtue" as the foundation of his vision of the moral community. He separated himself from Ferguson and Hutcheson, whose notion of "mutual sympathy" was a particular type of emotion, by arguing that sympathy was a function of a practical virtue, "propriety," which was assessed by an inner "impartial spectator": "We endeavor to examine our own conduct as we imagine any other fair and impartial spectator would examine it. If, upon placing ourselves in his situation, we thoroughly enter into all the passions and motives which influenced it, we approve of it, by sympathy and with the approbation of this supposed equitable judge. If otherwise, we enter into his disapprobation and condemn it" (Smith, *Theory of Moral Sentiments*, 110; quoted by Seligman 1997, 112). Smith thus established a means by which to tap into common standards, while at the same time creating an independent moral standpoint. As Knud Haakonssen (1981) has observed, the continued search for this neutral third-party position is the cornerstone of the eighteenth-century liberal enterprise.

12. Misztal (1996, 7) also sees vast social forces at work in the articulation of the trust issue, not the least of which is the construction of selfhood in its various guises: "Any attempt to integrate society as a system of trust relationships is faced with new tensions between universalism and particularism, duties and rights, autonomy and community, market and state, integration and fragmentation, local and global. The search for a new balance between these tensions has

re-opened debates about the fate of modernity and the meaning of progress, about the principles of integration, about individual freedom and collective responsibility, about the modern political identity and the construction of the modern self."

Chapter 6

1. An important antecedent to Engel's efforts was that of Milton Winternitz, dean of Yale Medical School (1920–1935), who envisioned an Institute for Human Relations for the comprehensive study of the patient as a biopsychosocial being. The institute was designed to integrate various university departments and schools, and his critics rallied against him on the charge that such an interdisciplinary structure would severely compromise the scientific agenda of the medical school faculty. His efforts were effectively resisted by those committed to a strict biomedical research agenda, and the institute collapsed with Winternitz's resignation (Spiro and Norton 2003).

2. My own experience confirms these observations. As a second-year medical student, I wrote a letter of moral outrage (published in: *The New England Journal of Medicine*) directed at another medical student (Mark Newman), who had inveighed against humanistic pursuits and anything less than a Victorian dedication to duty. I countered with "we have been taught that certain humanistic values and skills, which Newman neither can measure nor, apparently, esteems, are essential in our development as physicians." This lesson I embraced, and then I went on with a circumspect view of the accomplishments of modern medicine, concluding with an eye toward the empathetic physician I still hoped to be: "Possibly, a physician who takes the time to look and even see beyond his stethoscope might discover basic maladies affecting his patient's world that are also in need of attention" (Tauber 1971). In this account, I was a typical sophomore medical student, whose "empathetic index" was still high. By the time I was an intern, I had learned another lesson, and this has been amply confessed elsewhere (Tauber 1999a; see especially 1–2, 75–76, 91–92). Fortunately, I regained my earlier sensibilities (Tauber 1999a).

3. Artists, philosophers, and poets lead lives intimately connected with the humanities. Yet as history confirms, they have been no more compassionate than others, and have often been profoundly inhumane. Some, in fact, are just as detached from their human subjects as are our much-criticized modern-day physicians. In the contemporary world, there is no ethical consensus, and art cannot substitute for such a concordance. Thus the study of literature or art will not necessarily make us more virtuous, and it may in fact contradict values that might be espoused in the medical setting. In short, the humanities may, at best, only indirectly impart the desired values of compassion and morality (Glick 1985, 12).

4. Such an educational orientation was formally adopted by the health science faculty of Ben Gurion University (Be'er Sheva, Israel) during the 1970s when

they sought to combine orthodox medical education with a new emphasis on teaching empathy. The opportunity to create a new medical school in a socialized medicine environment at a time when medical ethics was being born combined to allow a unique experiment. This curriculum may well serve as a model for reform directed at developing empathetic physicians by specifically addressing four problematic areas of medical education, which have conspired to maintain the positivist status quo: student selection (Antonovsky 1987), the educational process, the overemphasis on technical skill at the expense of compassion and caring, and finally, the lack of appropriate role models in the clinical setting (Glick 1993). Evaluations of the curricular reform have been encouraging (Benor et al. 1984; Glick, Naggan, and Prywes 1987), but aside from the symbolic gesture of the White Coat Ceremony inaugurated there, American medical schools have not adopted the Ben Gurion philosophy.

5. William Donnelly (1997) has shown how the medical record employs language that obscures or even ignores the personhood of the patient and his or her experience of illness and medical care. The physician typically describes the sick person as a biological specimen, uses rhetorical devices that enhance the credibility of clinicians and laboratory data against the patient's own testimony, and subordinates the patient's subjective perspective and wishes relative to the doctor's value structure. Building on a rich literature, Donnelly recommends several revisions of the clinical language used in record keeping: personalize the clinical narrative; relate some of the case history in the first-person singular; compose a two-perspective history—one of the illness, the other of the disease— since neither perspective alone is the whole story and each complements the other; and include the patient's perspective as an integral part of the case history.

Another angle of criticism is offered by Todd Chambers in *The Fiction of Bioethics* (1999), where he argues that medical case histories are narratives like any other literary text and consequently open to a self-reflexive analysis. In this view, at one level the story itself structures the meaning of the case, but at a deeper level, the ultimate interpretation of the case is subject to the kind of analysis offered. So, on this second-order examination, the interpretation of "the text" is open to the same kind of scrutiny contemporary literary theorists engage in when discussing novels or poems (Leitch 2001). Thus a structuralist approach may yield a different understanding of the case *and its interpretation* than one employing, for example, semiotic, poststructuralist, New Critical, or reader-response theory. In short, the analysis itself is open to interpretation, and in what might appear as a dangerously steep recursive spiral, such criticism might easily leave the bioethicist miserably self-conscious and even ineffective as he subjects his own analysis to analysis. If one wants to study bioethics as a discipline, Chambers's insight might be of interest, but it is not what I have in mind for being morally self-conscious.

6. In the face of the rising subspecialty culture, Weed (1969, vii) endeavored to design a chart, which was to be a "scientific manuscript" and a "creative instrument for facilitating comprehensive and highly specialized medical care." There was another salutary effect of this revision for those who saw this structured

approach as a means to combat the fragmentation of care. By listing all of the medical problems, physicians could not be satisfied with pinning Mrs. Smith's hip fracture without treating her arthritis, diabetes, hypertension, and insomnia, which would remain nagging problems long after her hospital discharge. Weed initiated a self-conscious effort to integrate care, albeit in service to a subspecialty-dominated medical practice. Much to his credit, he was successful, but new times demand new solutions and he has continued to be at the forefront of thinking about how to manage medical information and how to empower patients more effectively (Weed and Weed 1994; Weed 2004).

7. The evaluations outlined in table 1 (Jonsen, Siegler, and Winslade 1998) and table 2 (Thomasma 1978) provide an orderly review of factors that characterize the patient's psychological and social identity. With that database, the ethical issues may be extracted, discussed, and acted on. While other, more detailed schemas have been proposed (e.g., Myser, Kerridge, and Mitchell 1995; Fletcher and Moseley 2003), these two examples illustrate the logical development of the ethics evaluation.

I suggest that that ethics workup be placed in an *Ethical Concerns* section, in the hospital admission note, and thereafter in progress notes and in the discharge summary. Because this deliberation requires a comprehensive understanding of the case, I further suggest the section become the penultimate segment of the initial medical admission note or first clinic encounter, placed just before the final Impression and Plan sections. With the growing use of computers for medical record keeping, this section should become more accessible to all members of the health-care team, who should easily be able to make additions to it.

Table 1: Fourfold Ethics Evaluation (adapted from Jonsen, Siegler, and Winslade 1998)
1. Medical Indications   Define clinical problems, goals of treatment, probabilities of success, and plans for therapeutic failure; delineate cost-benefit ratios of care.
2. Patient Preferences   Maintain patient's right to choose by determining preferences for care; assess competence of patient and ability to cooperate with medical treatment; if incompetent, is there health-care proxy or Advance Directives?
3. Quality of Life   Specify prospects, with or without treatment, of patient's recovery; define physical, mental, and social consequences of treatment success; explore plans for care in event of treatment failure.
4. Contextual Features   Clarify family or provider issues that may influence clinical decisions, including allocation of resources, financial restraints, and religious or cultural factors; describe possible legal implications of treatment decisions, for example, clinical research or teaching; establish the scope of confidentiality.

Table 2: Presentation of Ethical Decision Making (adapted from Thomasma 1978)
Step 1   Identify the significant human factors in the case, including demographics (age, occupation, education, family status, home setting, and so on),

behavior history (psychiatric history, criminal record, substance abuse), and religious and political attitudes relevant to health and medical care.

Step 2   Explicitly define related value factors (medical, professional, or human) present for the patient, health-care professional, and others involved in the case.

Step 3   Delineate all ethical choices and major value conflicts.

Step 4   Set priorities for values that are in conflict and give reasons for taking each position.

Step 5   Identify the criteria by which a decision is made, considering underlying ethical norms and meta-ethical assumptions. (How was *this* decision, based on *that* value, moral?)

Step 6   Critique the assumptions underlying the decision made in step 5 and present the final opinion and strategy for dealing with the moral issues identified.

An informal set of questions, for example as developed by William Donnelly (personal communication, 2005), serves as a suitable first approach to address these issues:

• Can you tell me something about yourself? Your work, interests, who's at home, etc.?

• What is your understanding of your condition? (Seek patient's knowledge of condition, beliefs about causation, future course, and role in management.)

• How has your condition (illness or disability) affected your life? Your family and personal relationships? Your work?

• What do you worry (fear) most about your condition or your medical care?

• With regard to your health and your medical condition(s), what are your personal goals? What do you expect (hope to obtain) from medical care here at our hospital?

• How would you like us to share information about your health condition and possible treatments with you? Directly and in private? Directly, with your family? Indirectly, through your family and let them tell you what you need to know?

• Do you feel that you have all the information that you need at this time about your health condition and your treatment plan?

• Do you have a formal advance directive document, such as a Medical Power of Attorney for Health Care, that we should know about or discuss with you? Do you have choices or concerns about particular medical treatments that we should know about? Are there concerns that you'd like more discussion about with your doctor?

• If you become too sick to speak for yourself, who will speak for you? Is she/he here now, so that I can meet her/him? If not, how can I (we) get in touch with her/him should the need arise (name, phone number)?

8. In July 2004, the first specified "Ethics" section of the medical record was inaugurated at Emanuel Medical Center (EMC) in Turlock, California, under the supervision of Daniel Dugan, a medical ethicist consultant, and Tom Johnson, chair of EMC's Ethics Committee. They are preparing a preliminary report of

its function and outcomes; here are Dugan's initial impressions: "Most initial objections concerned 1) time allocations and additional tasks for physicians, and 2) the argument that separating 'ethics' from the rest of the chart might actually fragment rather than integrate the care of the individual patient. The internist who made that objection, by the way, is now one of the most fervent proponents, who recently successfully won the endorsement of the hospital's medical executive committee. For the true facts are that your idea truly organizes important information that people appreciate knowing where to find when the chips are down and time is short; and that 'not enough time' is a smokescreen for an initial thin screen of resistance to re-prioritizing very modest time demands.

The truth is that the current medical record is one-dimensional and centrifugal in scattering information about the patient's moral space throughout the chart. Again and again I go to the chart after a referral and feel like Isis wandering about Egypt trying to reassemble the body parts of blessed Osiris, unable much of the time to find his identifying organs. The initial survey of nurses after a couple of months of use showed overwhelmingly positive response, appreciating that there is ONE place to go to clarify patient's wishes and values, and appreciating an entirely new instrument to use to approach physicians with evidence of the need to clarify miscommunications and misunderstandings when things are happening that are not consonant with patients' expressions of values. The vector of the ethics section in the chart is toward the doctor-patient relationship, toward increasing its depth and sensitivity to the experience of patients, toward promoting more insight, more partnership, and more trust" (Dugan, personal communication, November 12, 2004).

Epilogue

1. Novels often make their business the art of capturing the moral life of the everyday, and they do so in a way complementary to philosophy. The literary critics Gary Soul Morson and Caryl Emerson (1990) have usefully developed the idea of "prosaics" to describe the moral commonplace. Aligning themselves with the "end of philosophy" movement, they argue that the ethics of everyday life is best described in literatures that eschew the formalisms of philosophy. Instead, they argue that while there are many systematic accounts of the historical, of the real, of the true, of the good, no single intellectual account can order human experience: "On the contrary, prosaics assumes that the natural state of the world is a mess, and that it is order, not disorder, that requires an explanation. Order does exist, of course, but it is always the result of work. It is never given, but always made. . . . The philosophers assume that history is a riddle and that it can be solved; but for Tolstoy, as for Ludwig Wittgenstein . . . 'the *riddle* does not exist' (*Tractatus Logico-Philosophicus* 6.5)" (Morson 1988, 516, 518).

2. *Character* has both transitive and intransitive meanings. On the one hand, character *determines* how one behaves—that is, the individual collection of

mores and values that governs conduct and guides ethical judgments. On the other hand, character *reveals* moral identity—that is, it portrays the public persona that others esteem or condemn. Thus, for Aristotle, character and virtue ethics are tied together as one—the good life becomes the ethical life of personal virtue. For a contemporary statement of virtue ethics see MacIntyre 1984, and for a case study see Tauber 2001.

References

Abrams, M. H. 1973. *Natural Supernaturalism*. New York: Norton.

Ader, R., Felten, D. L., and Cohen, N., eds. 2001. *Psychoneuroimmunology*. 3rd ed. San Diego: Academic Press.

Allison, H. 1990. *Kant's Theory of Freedom*. Cambridge: Cambridge University Press.

American Bar Association. 1977. *Mental Disability Law Reporter* 2:73–159.

American College of Physicians. 1990. "Access to health care." *Annals of Internal Medicine* 112:641–661.

American Medical Association. [1847] 1977. "Code of Medical Ethics." In S. J. Resier, A. J. Dyke, and W. J. Curran, eds., *Ethics in Medicine: Historical Perspectives and Contemporary Concerns*, 29–34. Cambridge, MA: MIT Press.

American Medical Association. [1957] 1977. "Principles of Medical Ethics." In S. J. Resier, A. J. Dyke, and W. J. Curran, eds., *Ethics in Medicine: Historical Perspectives and Contemporary Concerns*, 38–39. Cambridge, MA: MIT Press.

American Medical Association. 1981. *Current Opinions of the Judicial Council*. Chicago: American Medical Association.

American Medical Association. 1997. *Code of Medical Ethics: Current Opinions and Annotations*. Chicago: American Medical Association.

Ameriks, K. 2000. *Kant and the Fate of Autonomy: Problems in the Appropriation of the Critical Philosophy*. Cambridge: Cambridge University Press.

Anderson, L. A. and Dedrick, R. F. 1990. "Development of the Trust in Physician scale: A measure to assess interpersonal trust in patient-physician relationships." *Psychology Reports* 67:1091–1100.

Annas, G. J. 1989. *The Rights of Patients: The Basic ACLU Guide to Patient Rights*. Carbondale: Southern Illinois University Press.

Annas, G. J. 1997. "Patients' rights in managed care—exit, voice, and choice." *New England Journal of Medicine* 337:210–215.

Annas, G. J. and Grodin, M. A. 1992. *The Nazi Doctors and the Nuremberg Code: Human Rights in Human Experimentation.* New York: Oxford University Press.

Annison, M. H. and Wilford, D. S. 1998. *Trust Matters: New Directions in Health Care Leadership.* San Francisco: Jossey-Bass.

Anonymous. 2003. "Lessons from a bygone medical ethics program." *Cambridge Quarterly of Healthcare Ethics* 12:102–110.

Antonovsky, A. 1987. "Medical student selection at the Ben-Gurion University of the Negev." *Israel Journal of Medical Sciences* 23:969–975.

Appelbaum, P. S. and Grisso, T. 1988. "Assessing patients' capacities to consent to treatment." *New England Journal of Medicine* 319:1635–1638.

Appelbaum, P. S., Lidz, C. W., and Meisel, A. 1987. *Informed Consent: Legal Theory and Clinical Practice.* New York: Oxford University Press.

Arnold, R. M., Povar, G. J., and Howell, J. D. 1987. "The humanities, humanistic behavior, and the humane physician: A cautionary note." *Annals of Internal Medicine* 106:313–318.

Baier, A. C. 1994a. "The need for more than justice." In A. C. Baier, *Moral Prejudices: Essays on Ethics*, 18–32. Cambridge, MA: Harvard University Press. (Originally published in the *Canadian Journal of Philosophy, Supp. Vol. on Science, Ethics, and Feminism* 13(1987):41–56.)

Baier, A. C. 1994b. "Trust and antitrust." In A. C. Baier, *Moral Prejudices: Essays on Ethics*, 95–129. Cambridge, MA: Harvard University Press. (Originally published in *Ethics* 96(1986):231–260.)

Baier, A. C. 1997. *The Commons of the Mind.* Chicago: Open Court.

Baier, K. 1995. *The Rational and the Moral Order: The Social Roots of Reason and Morality.* Chicago: Open Court.

Bailyn, B. [1967] 1992. *The Ideological Origins of the American Revolution.* Rev. ed. Cambridge, MA: Harvard University Press.

Baker, R. 1993. "Deciphering Percival's code." In R. Baker, D. Porter, and R. Porter, eds., *The Codification of Medical Morality*, 179–211. Dordrecht: Kluwer Academic Publishers.

Baker, R., Porter, D., and Porter, R. 1993. "Introduction." In R. Baker, D. Porter, and R. Porter, eds., *The Codification of Medical Morality*, 1–14. Dordrecht: Kluwer Academic Publishers.

Balint, M. 1964. *The Doctor, His Patient, and the Illness.* Rev. ed. New York: International Universities Press.

Barbour, A. 1995. *Caring for Patients: A Critique of the Medical Model.* Stanford, CA: Stanford University Press.

Barondess, J. 1979. "Disease and illness—A crucial distinction." *American Journal of Medicine* 66:375–376.

Barzansky, B. and Etzel, S. 2001. "Educational programs in US medical schools, 2000–2001." *JAMA* 286:1049–1055.

Beauchamp, T. L. 1994. "The 'four-principles' approach." In R. Gillon, ed., *Principles of Health Care Ethics*, 3–12. Chichester, UK: Wiley.

Beauchamp, T. L. and Childress, J. F. 1989. *Principles of Bioethics*. 3rd ed. New York: Oxford University Press.

Beauchamp, T. L. and Childress, J. F. 1994. *Principles of Bioethics*. 4th ed. New York: Oxford University Press.

Beauchamp, T. L. and Childress, J. F. 2001. *Principles of Bioethics*. 5th ed. New York: Oxford University Press.

Beauchamp, T. L. and McCullough, L. B. 1984. *Medical Ethics: The Moral Responsibilities of Physicians*. Englewood Cliffs, NJ: Prentice-Hall.

Beckman, H. B. and Frankel, R. M. 1984. "The effect of physician behavior on the collection of data." *Annals of Internal Medicine* 101:692–696.

Beecher, H. K. 1966. "Ethics and clinical research." *New England Journal of Medicine* 274:1354–1360.

Bellah, R. N., Madsen, R., Sullivan, W. M., Swidler, A., and Tipton, S. M. 1985. *Habits of the Heart*. Berkeley: University of California Press.

The Belmont Report. 1978. *Ethical Principles and Guidelines for the Protection of Human Subjects of Research*. Washington, DC: Government Printing Office.

Benbassat, J., Baumal, R., Borkan, J. M., and Ber, R. 2003. "Overcoming barriers to teaching the behavioral and social sciences to medical students." *Academic Medicine* 78:372–380.

Bender, C. M., Kramer, P. A., and Miaskowski, C. M. 2002. "New directions in the management of cancer-related cognitive impairment, fatigue, and pain." *Scientific Connections CE Monograph* 2002:2–9.

Benn, S. I. 1976. "Freedom, autonomy, and the concept of a person." *Aristotelian Society Proceedings* 76:109–130.

Benor, D. E., Notzer, N., Sheehan, T. J., and Norman, G. R. 1984. "Moral reasoning as a criterion for admission to medical school." *Medical Education* 18:423–428.

Berlin, I. 1969. "Two Concepts of Liberty." In I. Berlin, *Four Essays on Liberty*. New York: Oxford University Press.

Berlin, I. 1999. *The Roots of Romanticism*. Princeton, NJ: Princeton University Press.

Berwick, D. M. 2003. "Errors today and errors tomorrow." *New England Journal of Medicine* 348:2570–2572.

Bissonette, R., O'Shea, R. M., Horwitz, M., and Route, C. F. 1995. "A data-generated basis for medical ethics education: Categorizing issues experienced by students during clinical training." *Academic Medicine* 70:1035–1037.

Blank, L., Kimball, H., McDonald, W., and Merino, J. 2003. "Medical professionalization in the new millennium: A physician charter 15 months later." *Annals of Internal Medicine* 138:839–841.

Blendon, R. and Benson, J. 2001. "Americans' views on health policy: A fifty-year historical perspective." *Health Affairs* 20:38–46.

Blendon, R. J., Brodie, M., Benson, J. M., Altman, D. E., Levitt, L., Hoff, T., and Hugick, L. 1998. "Understanding the managed care backlash." *Health Affairs* 17:80–94.

Blendon, R. J., Hyams, T. S., and Benson, J. M. 1993. "Bridging the gap between expert and public views on health care reform." *JAMA* 269:2573–2578.

Bodenheimer, T. 1996. "The HMO backlash—righteous or reactionary?" *New England Journal of Medicine* 335:1601–1604.

Bodenheimer, T. 1997. "The Oregon Health Plan—Lessons for the Nation." *New England Journal of Medicine* 337:651–655, 720–723.

Boorse, C. 1977. "Health as a theoretical concept." *Philosophy of Science* 44:542–573.

Brandt, R. B. 1979. *A Theory of the Good and the Right*. Oxford: Oxford University Press.

Brandt, R. B. 1996. *Facts, Values, and Morality*. Cambridge: Cambridge University Press.

Bright, B. 2004. "Doctors' interpersonal skills are valued more than training." *Wall Street Journal Online*, September 28, 2004. http://online.wsj.com/article_print/0..SB109630288893728881.00.html.

Brock, D. 1991. "Facts and values in the physician-patient relationship." In E. D. Pellegrino, R. M. Veatch, and J. P. Langan, eds., *Ethics, Trust, and the Professions: Philosophical and Cultural Aspects*, 113–132. Washington, DC: Georgetown University Press.

Brock, D. W. and Wartman, S. 1993. "When competent patients make irrational choices." In D. W. Brock, ed., *Life and Death: Philosophical Essays on Biomedical Ethics*, 80–92. Cambridge: Cambridge University Press.

Brody, H. 1992. *The Healer's Power*. New Haven, CT: Yale University Press.

Brook, B. 1999. *Feminist Perspectives on the Body*. New York: Longman.

Brothers, D. 1995. *Falling Backwards: An Exploration of Trust and Self Experience*. New York: Norton.

Brown, T. M. 2003. "George Engel and Rochester's biopsychosocial tradition: Historical and developmental perspectives." In R. M. Frankel, T. E. Quill, and S. H. McDaniel, eds., *The Biopsychosocial Approach: Past, Present, Future*, 199–219. Rochester, NY: University of Rochester Press.

Buchanan, A. 2000. "Trust in managed care organizations." *Kennedy Institute of Ethics Journal* 10:189–212.

Burns, C. 1977. "Richard Cabot and reformation of American medical ethics." *Bulletin of the History of Medicine* 51:353–368.

Bushnell, D. 2002. "Demand for alternative care rises." *Boston Globe*, July 14, 2002, pp. K-1, K-6.

Butler, J. 1990. *Gender Trouble: Feminism and the Subversion of Identity*. New York: Routledge.

Cabot, R. C. 1903. "Truth and falsity in medicine." *American Medicine* 5:344–349.

Cabot, R. C. 1931. "Medical ethics in the hospital." *Nosokomeion* 2:151–161.

Callahan, D. 1969. "The sanctity of life." In Donald R. Cutler, ed., *Updating Life and Death: Essays in Ethics and Medicine*, 181–223. Boston: Beacon Press.

Callahan, D. 1990. "Religion and the secularization of bioethics." *Hastings Center Report* 20(July–August):2–4.

Callahan, D., ed. 2002. *The Role of Complementary and Alternative Medicine: Accommodating Pluralism*. Washington, DC: Georgetown University Press.

Callahan, D. 2003. "Individual good and common good: A communitarian approach to bioethics." *Perspectives in Biology and Medicine* 46:496–507.

Camenisch, P. E., ed. 1994. *Religious Methods and Resources in Bioethics*. Dordrecht: Kluwer Academic Publishers.

Campbell, A. T. 2000. "Medical ethics in a changing practice environment: An annotated bibliography." http://www.acponline.org/ethics/map_bibliography .htm.

Canguilhem, G. [1966] 1989. *The Normal and the Pathological*. Trans. C. R. Fawcett. New York: Zone Books.

Caplan, A. L. 1993. "The concepts of health, illness, and disease." In W. Bynum and R. Porter, eds., *Companion Encyclopedia of the History of Medicine*, vol. 1, 233–248. London: Routledge.

Cardozo, B. 1914. Schloendorff v Society of New York Hospital, 211 NY 125, 129–130, 105 NE 92, 93.

Carlton, W. 1978. *"In Our Professional Opinion . . .": The Primacy of Clinical Judgment over Moral Choice*. Notre Dame, IN: University of Notre Dame Press.

Carmel, J. and Bernstein, J. 1986. "Identifying with the patient: An intensive programme for medical students." *Medical Education* 20:432–436.

Carrithers, M., Collins, S., and Lukes, S., eds. 1985. *The Category of the Person: Anthropology, Philosophy, History*. Cambridge: Cambridge University Press.

Cartwright, N. 1999. *The Dappled World: A Study of the Boundaries of Science*. Cambridge: Cambridge University Press.

Cassell, E. J. 1976. *The Healer's Art*. Philadelphia: Lippincott.

Cassell, E. J. 1991. *The Nature of Suffering and the Goals of Medicine*. New York: Oxford University Press.

Cassell, E. J. 1997. *Doctoring: The Nature of Primary Care Medicine*. New York: Oxford University Press.

Cavell, S. 1988. *In Quest of the Ordinary: Lines of Skepticism and Romanticism*. Chicago: University of Chicago Press.

Chambers, T. 1999. *The Fiction of Bioethics: Cases as Literary Texts*. New York: Routledge.

Chapman, C. B. 1984. *Physicians, Law and Ethics*. New York.

Chapman, J. E. and Chapman, H. H. 1983. *The Psychology of Health Care: A Humanistic Perspective*. Monterey, CA: Wadsworth Health Sciences.

Charon, R. and Montello, M., eds. 2002. *Stories Matter: The Role of Narrative in Medical Ethics*. New York: Routledge.

Childress, J. F. 1982. *Who Should Decide? Paternalism in Health Care*. New York: Oxford University Press.

Chodoff, P. 1976. "The case for involuntary hospitalization of the mentally ill." *American Journal of Psychiatry* 133:496–501.

Christman, J. 1989. "Introduction." In J. Christman, ed., *The Inner Citadel: Essays on Individual Autonomy*, 3–23. New York: Oxford University Press.

Clement, G. 1996. *Care, Autonomy, and Justice: Feminism and the Ethic of Care*. Oxford: Westview Press.

Clouser, K. D. 1983. "Veatch, May, and models: A critical review and a new view." In E. E. Shelp, ed., *The Clinical Encounter: The Moral Fabric of the Patient-Physician Relationship*, 89–103. Dordrecht: D. Reidel.

Clouser, K. D. and Gert, B. 1994. "Morality vs. Principlism." In R. Gillon, ed., *Principles of Health Care Ethics*, 251–266. Chichester, UK: Wiley.

Code, L. 1991. *What Can She Know? Feminist Theory and the Construction of Knowledge*. Ithaca, NY: Cornell University Press.

Cody, J. 1978. "The arts versus Agnes Duer, M.D." In D. J. Self, ed., *The Role of the Humanities in Medical Education*, 45–61. Norfolk, VA: Bio-Medical Ethics Program, Eastern Virginia Medical School.

Cook, K. S., ed. 2001. *Trust in Society*. New York: Russell Sage Foundation.

Cooper, R. A. and Tauber, A. I. Forthcoming. "A new physician for a new century." *Academic Medicine*.

Coulehan, J. L., Platt, F. W., Egener, B., Frankel, R., Lin, C. T., Lown, B., and Salazar, W. H. 2001. "'Let me see if I have this right . . .': Words that build empathy." *Annals of Internal Medicine* 135:221–227.

Council of Ethical and Judicial Affairs, American Medical Association. 1995. "Ethical issues in managed care." *JAMA* 273:330–335.

Cousins, N. 1979. *Anatomy of an Illness as Perceived by the Patient*. New York: Norton.

Cuff, P. A. and Vanselow, N. A., eds. 2004. *Improving Medical Education: Enhancing the Behavioral and Social Science Content of Medical School Curricula*. Washington, DC: National Academies Press.

Cull, A., Hay, C., and Love, S. B. 1996. "What do patients mean when they complain of concentration and memory problems?" *British Journal of Cancer* 74:1674–1679.

Culver, C. M., Clouser, K. D., Brody, H., Fletcher, J., Jonsen, A., Kopelman, L., Lynn, J., Siegler, M. and Wikler, D. 1985. "Basic curricular goals in medical ethics." *New England Journal of Medicine* 312:253–256.

Culver, C. M. and Gert, B. 1982. *Philosophy in Medicine: Conceptual and Ethical Issues in Medicine and Psychiatry*. New York: Oxford University Press.

Daston, L. 2000. "Scientific objectivity with and without words." In P. Becker and W. Clark, eds., *Little Tools of Knowledge: Historical Essays on Academic and Bureaucratic Practice*, 259–284. Ann Arbor: University of Michigan Press.

Davis, K., Collins, K. S., Schoen, C., and Morris, C. 1995. "Choice matters: Enrollees' views of their health plans." *Health Affairs* 14:99–112.

Delbanco, T. L. 1992. "Enriching the doctor-patient relationship by inviting the patient's perspective." *Annals of Internal Medicine* 116:414–418.

Delkeskamp-Hayes, C. and Cutter, M. A. G., eds. 1993. *Science, Technology, and the Art of Medicine: European-American Dialogues*. Dordrecht: Kluwer Academic Publishers.

Dewey, J. [1888] 1997. "The ethics of democracy." In L. Menand, ed., *Pragmatism: A Reader*, 182–204. New York: Vintage.

Diggins, J. P. 1994. *The Promise of Pragmatism: Modernism and the Crisis of Knowledge and Authority*. Chicago: University of Chicago Press.

Donnelly, W. J. 1997. "The language of medical case histories." *Annals of Internal Medicine* 127:1045–1048.

Dowie, J. and Elstein, A. 1988. *Professional Judgment: A Reader in Clinical Decision Making*. New York: Cambridge University Press.

DuBois, J. M. and Burkemper, J. 2002. "Ethics education in U.S. medical schools: A study of syllabi." *Academic Medicine* 77:432–437.

Duffy, J. 1983. "American medical ethics and the physician-patient relationship." In E. E. Shelp, ed., *The Clinical Encounter: The Moral Fabric of the Patient-Physician Relationship*, 65–85. Dordrecht: D. Reidel.

Durkheim, E. [1897] 1951. *Suicide*. New York: Free Press.

Dworkin, G. 1988. *The Theory and Practice of Autonomy*. Cambridge: Cambridge University Press.

Dworkin, R. 1993. "Life past reason." In R. Dworkin, *Life's Dominion: An Argument about Abortion, Euthanasia, and Individual Freedom*, 218–242. New York: Knopf.

Ehrenreich, B. and English, D. 1979. *For Her Own Good: 150 Years of the Experts' Advice to Women*. Garden City, NY: Anchor Books.

Eisenberg, D. M., Kessler, R. C., Foster, C., Norlock, F. E., Calkins, D. R., and Delbenco, T. L. 1993. "Unconventional medicine in the United States: Practice, costs, and patterns of use." *New England Journal of Medicine* 328:246–252.

Elliott, C. 1999. *A Philosophical Disease: Bioethics, Culture, and Identity*. New York: Routledge.

Emanuel, E. 1991. *The Ends of Human Life: Medical Ethics in a Liberal Polity*. Cambridge, MA: Harvard University Press.

Emanuel, E. and Dubler, N. N. 1995. "Preserving the physician-patient relationship in the era of managed care." *JAMA* 273:323–329.

Emanuel, E. J. and Emanuel, L. L. 1992. "Four models of the physician-patient relationship." *JAMA* 267:2221–2226.

Emanuel, E. J. and Emanuel, L. L. 1996. "What is accountability in health care?" *Annals of Internal Medicine* 124:229–239.

Emerson, R. W. [1836] 1971. *Nature*. In R. E. Spilles, ed., *The Collected Works of Ralph Waldo Emerson, Vol. 1, Nature Addresses, and Lectures*, 3–45. Cambridge, MA: Harvard University Press.

Emerson, R. W. [1841] 1979. "Circles." In J. Slater, ed., *The Collected Works of Ralph Waldo Emerson, Vol. 2, Essays: First Series*, 177–190. Cambridge, MA: Harvard University Press.

Emerson, R. W. [1844] 1983. "Experience." In J. Slater, ed., *The Collected Works of Ralph Waldo Emerson, Vol. 3, Essays: Second Series*, 25–49. Cambridge, MA: Harvard University Press.

Emerson, R. W. 1965. *The Journals and Miscellaneous Notebooks of Ralph Waldo Emerson, Vol. V, 1835–1838*. ed. M. M. Sealts, Jr. Cambridge, MA: Harvard University Press.

Engel, G. 1977. "The need for a new medical model: A challenge for biomedicine." *Science* 196:129–136.

Engelhardt, H. T., Jr. 1991. *Bioethics and Secular Humanism: The Search for a Common Morality*. London: SCM Press.

Engelhardt, H. T., Jr. 1996. *The Foundations of Bioethics*. 2nd ed. Oxford: Oxford University Press.

Engelhardt, H. T., Jr. and Callahan, D., eds. 1980. *Knowing and Valuing: The Search for Common Roots*. Hastings-on-Hudson, NY: Institute for Society, Ethics, and the Life Sciences.

Engelhardt, H. T., Jr. and Wildes, K. W. 1994. "The four principles of health care ethics and post-modernity: Why a libertarian interpretation is unavoidable." In R. Gillon, ed., *Principles of Health Care Ethics*, 135–147. Chichester, UK: Wiley.

Erikson, E. 1968. *Identity, Youth, and Crisis*. New York: Norton.

Etzioni, A. 1995. *New Communitarian Thinking: Persons, Virtues, Institutions, and Communities*. Charlottesville: University Press of Virginia.

Etzioni, A. 1996. *The New Golden Rule: Community and Morality in a Democratic Society*. New York: Basic Books.

Evans, J. H. 2002. *Playing God? Human Genetic Engineering and the Rationalization of Public Bioethical Debate*. Chicago: University of Chicago Press.

Evidence-Based Medicine Working Group. 1992. "Evidence-based medicine: A new approach to teaching the practice of medicine." *JAMA* 268, 2420–2425.

Faden, R. R. and Beauchamp, T. L. 1986. *A History and Theory of Informed Consent*. New York: Oxford University Press.

Fadiman, A. 1997. *The Spirit Catches You and You Fall Down: A Hmong Child, Her American Doctors, and the Collision of Two Cultures*. New York: Noonday Press.

Feinberg, J. 1986. *Harm to Self* (vol. 3 of *The Moral Limits of the Criminal Law*). New York: Oxford University Press.

Feinstein, A. 1967. *Clinical Judgment*. Baltimore: Williams & Wilkins.

Feldman, S. and Tauber, A. I. 1997. "Sickle cell anemia: Redefining the first 'molecular disease.'" *Bulletin of the History of Medicine* 71:623–650.

Ferguson, A. [1767] 1782. *An Essay on the History of Civil Society*. 5th ed. London: T. Cadell.

Filene, P. G. 1998. *In the Arms of Others: A Cultural History of the Right-to-Die in America*. Chicago: Ivan R. Dee, Publishers.

Fischbach, R. L., Sionelo-Bayog, A., Needle, A., and Delbanco, T. L. 1980. "The patient and the practitioner as co-authors of the medical record." *Patient Counselling and Health Education* 2:1–5.

Fischer, D. H. 1989. *Albion's Seed: Four British Folkways in America*. New York: Oxford University Press.

Fisher, W. 1991. "The development of modern American legal theory and the judicial interpretation of the Bill of Rights." In M. J. Lacey and K. Haakonssen, eds., *A Culture of Rights: The Bill of Rights in Philosophy, Politics, and Law—1791 and 1991*, 266–365. Cambridge: Cambridge University Press.

Fissell, M. E. 1993. "Innocent and honorable bribes: Medical manners in eighteenth-century Britain." In R. Baker, D. Porter, and R. Porter, eds., *The Codification of Medical Morality*, 19–46. Dordrecht: Kluwer Academic Publishers.

Fletcher, J. 1954. *Morals and Medicine: The Moral Problems of: The Patient's Right to Know the Truth, Contraception, Artificial Insemination, Sterilization, Euthanasia*. Princeton, NJ: Princeton University Press.

Fletcher, J. C. and Moseley, K. L. 2003. "The structure and process of ethics consultation services." In M. P. Aulisio, R. M. Arnold, and S. J. Youngner, eds., *Ethics Consultation: From Theory to Practice*, 96–120. Baltimore: Johns Hopkins University Press.

Foss, L. 2002. *The End of Modern Medicine: Biomedical Science under a Microscope*. Albany: State University Press of New York.

Foss, L. and Rothenberg, K. 1987. *The Second Medical Revolution: From Biomedicine to Infomedicine*. Boston: New Science Library, Shambhala.

Foucault, M. [1963] 1973. *The Birth of the Clinic: An Archaeology of Medical Perception*. New York: Vintage.

Fox, R. C. 1990. "The evolution of American bioethics: A sociological perspective." In G. Weisz, ed., *Social Science Perspectives on Medical Ethics*, 201–220. Philadelphia: University of Pennsylvania Press.

Fox, R. C. 1994. "The entry of bioethics into the 1990s." In E. R. DuBose, R. Hammel, and L. O'Connell, eds., *A Matter of Principles? Ferment in U.S. Bioethics*, 21–71. Valley Forge, PA: Trinity Press.

Frankel, R. M., Quill, T. E., and McDaniel, S. H. 2003a. "The future of the biopsychosocial approach." In R. M. Frankel, T. E. Quill, and S. H. McDaniel, eds., *The Biopsychosocial Approach: Past, Present, Future*, 255–267. Rochester, NY: University of Rochester Press.

Frankel, R. M., Quill, T. E., and McDaniel, S. H., eds. 2003b. *The Biopsychosocial Approach: Past, Present, Future*. Rochester, NY: University of Rochester Press.

Frankena, W. K. 1988. *Ethics*. 2nd ed. Englewood Cliffs, NJ: Prentice Hall.

Frankfurt, H. G. 1971. "Freedom of the will and the concept of a person." *Journal of Philosophy* 68:5–20.

Frazer, E. 1999. *The Problems of Communitarian Politics: Unity and Conflict*. Oxford: Oxford University Press.

Freeman, V. G., Rathmore, S. S., Weinfurt, K. P., Schulman, K. A., and Sulmasy, D. P. 1999. "Lying for patients: Physician deception of third party payers." *Archives of Internal Medicine* 159:2263–2270.

Friedman, M. 1986. "Autonomy and the split-level self." *Southern Journal of Philosophy* 24:19–35.

Frost, N. 1976. "Ethical problems in pediatrics." *Current Problems in Pediatrics* 6:3–31.

Fukuyama, F. 1995. *Trust: The Social Virtues and the Creation of Prosperity*. New York: Free Press.

Galaty, D. H. 1974. "The philosophical basis for mid-nineteenth century German reductionism." *Journal of the History of Medicine and Allied Sciences* 29:295–316.

Galen. 1884. *Claudii Galeni Pergameni, Scripta Minora*, Vol. 1. Leipzig: Teubner.

Galison, P. and Stump, D. J., eds. 1996. *The Disunity of Science: Boundaries, Contexts, and Power*. Stanford, CA: Stanford University Press.

The Gallup Poll. 1977–1997. *Public Opinion*. Wilmington, DE: Scholarly Resources Inc.

Gambetta, D., ed. 1988. *Trust: Making and Breaking Cooperative Relations*. Oxford: Blackwell.

Gauthier, D. 1986. *Morals by Agreement*. New York: Oxford University Press.

Gaylin, W. and Jennings, B. 1996. *The Perversion of Autonomy: The Proper Uses of Coercion and Constraints in a Liberal Society*. New York: Free Press.

Geyer-Kordesch, J. 1993. "Natural law and medical ethics in the eighteenth century." In R. Baker, D. Porter, and R. Porter, eds., *The Codification of Medical Morality*, 123–139. Dordrecht: Kluwer Academic Publishers.

Giddens, A. 1992. *The Transformation of Intimacy*. Oxford: Polity Press.

Gilligan, C. 1982. *In a Different Voice: Psychological Theory and Women's Development*. Cambridge, MA: Harvard University Press.

Gilligan C. and Pollak, S. 1988. "The vulnerable and the invulnerable physician." In C. Gilligan, J. V. Ward, and J. M. Taylor, eds., *Mapping the Moral Domain: A Contribution of Women's Thinking to Psychology Theory and Education*, 245–262. Cambridge, MA: Harvard University Press.

Gillon, R., ed. 1994a. "The four principles revisited—a reappraisal." In R. Gillon, ed., *Principles of Health Care Ethics*, 319–333. Chichester, UK: Wiley.

Gillon, R., ed. 1994b. *Principles of Health Care Ethics*. Chichester, UK: Wiley.

Glick, S. M. 1981. "Humanistic medicine in a modern age." *New England Journal of Medicine* 304:1036–1038.

Glick, S. M. 1985. The component elements of physician compassion. *The Pharos of Alpha Omega Alpha* 48:9–14.

Glick, S. M. 1993. "The empathetic physician: Nature and Nurture." In II. Spiro, M. G. M. Curran, and D. St. James, eds., *Empathy and the Practice of Medicine: Beyond Pills and the Scalpel*, 85–102. New Haven, CT: Yale University Press.

Glick, S., Naggan, L., and Prywes, M., eds. 1987. "The Beer Sheva experiment: An interim assessment." *Israel Journal of Medical Sciences* 23(9–10):937–1105.

Goldie, J. 2000. "Review of ethics curricula in undergraduate education." *Medical Education* 34:108–119.

Good, B. J. 1994. *Medicine, Rationality, and Experience: An Anthropological Perspective*. Cambridge: Cambridge University Press.

Good, D. 1988. "Individuals, interpersonal relations and trust." In D. Gambetta, ed., *Trust: Making and Breaking Cooperative Relations*, 31–48. Oxford: Blackwell.

Goold, S. D. 1998. "Money and trust: Relationships between patients, physicians, and health plans." *Journal of Health Politics, Policy and Law* 23:687–695.

Gougeon, L. 1990. *Virtue's Hero: Emerson, Antislavery, and Reform*. Athens: University of Georgia Press.

Govier, T. 1993. "An epistemology of trust." *International Journal of Moral and Social Studies* 8:155–174.

Govier, T. 1997. *Social Trust and Human Communities*. Montreal and Kingston: McGill–Queen's University Press.

Gray, J. 1983. *Mill on Liberty: A Defense*. London: Routledge & Kegan Paul.

Gregory, J. 1998. *John Gregory's Writings on Medical Ethics and Philosophy of Medicine*. Ed. L. B. McCullough. Boston: Kluwer Academic Publishers.

Griffiths, A. P., ed. 1994. *Philosophy, Psychology, and Psychiatry*. New York: Cambridge University Press. Supp. to *Philosophy* 37.

Grisso, T. and Appelbaum, P. S. 1995. "The MacArthur Treatment Competence Study. III. Abilities of Patients to Consent to Psychiatric and Medical Treatments." *Law and Human Behavior* 19:149–174.

Grunbaum, A. 1984. *The Foundations of Psychoanalysis: A Philosophical Critique*. Berkeley: University of California Press.

Guttentag, O. E. 1960. "A course entitled 'The Medical Attitude': An orientation in the foundations of medical thought." *Journal of Medical Education* 35:903–907.

Haakonssen, K. 1981. *The Science of a Legislator: The Natural Jurisprudence of David Hume and Adam Smith*. Cambridge: Cambridge University Press.

Haakonssen, L. 1997. *Medicine and Morals in the Enlightenment: John Gregory, Thomas Percival and Benjamin Rush*. Amsterdam: Rodopi.

Hall, M. A. Forthcoming. "The importance of trust for ethics, law, and public policy." *Cambridge Quarterly of Healthcare Ethics*.

Hall, M. A. and Berenson, R. A. 1998. "Ethical practice in managed care: A dose of realism." *Annals of Internal Medicine* 128:395–402.

Hall, M. A., Camacho, F., Dugan, E., and Balkrishnan, R. 2002. "Trust in the medical profession: Conceptual and measurement issues." *Health Services Research* 37:1436–1439.

Hall, M. A., Dugan, E., Zheng, B., and Mishra, A. K. 2001. "Trust in physicians and medical institutions: What is it, can it be measured, and does it matter?" *Milbank Quarterly* 70:613–639.

Halpern, J. 2001. *From Detached Concern to Empathy*. New York: Oxford University Press.

Ham, C. 1998. "Retracing the Oregon trail: The experience of rationing and the Oregon health plan." *British Medical Journal* 316:1965–1969.

Hardin, R. 2002. *Trust and Trustworthiness*. New York: Russell Sage Foundation.

Hart, S. 1995. "Cultural sociology and social criticism." *Newsletter of the Sociology of Culture Section of the American Sociological Association* 9(3):1–6.

Harvan, R. A. 1993. "An assessment of ethical sensitivity: Implications for interdisciplinary education." *Journal of Allied Health* 22:353–362.

Hayry, M. 1991. "Measuring the quality of life: Why, how, and what?" *Theoretical Medicine* 12:97–116.

Herman, B. 1993. *The Practice of Moral Judgment*. Cambridge, MA: Harvard University Press.

Herr, S. S., Arons, S., and Wallace, R. E. 1983. *Legal Rights and Mental Health Care*. Ton, MA: Lexington Books.

Herzlinger, R. E. 1999. *Market-Drive Health Care: Who Wins, Who Loses in the Transformation of America's Largest Service Industry*. San Francisco: Perseus.

Herzlinger, R. E. 2003. *Consumer-Driven Health Care: Implications for Providers, Payers, and Policy Makers*. San Francisco: Jossey-Bass.

Hippocrates. 1923. *Hippocrates*. Vol. 2. Trans. W. H. S. Jones. Cambridge, MA: Harvard University Press.

Hollis, M. 1998. *Trust within Reason*. Cambridge: Cambridge University Press.

Holmes, O. W. [1881] 1963. *The Common Law*. Boston: Little, Brown.

Hook, S., ed. 1959. *Psychoanalysis, Scientific Medicine, and Philosophy*. New York: New York University Press.

Howe, D. W. 1997. *Making the American Self: Jonathan Edwards to Abraham Lincoln*. Cambridge, MA: Harvard University Press.

Hrobjartsson, A. and Brorson, S. 2002. "Interpreting results from randomized clinical trials of complementary/alternative interventions: The role of trial quality and pre-trial beliefs." In D. Callahan, ed., *The Role of Complementary and Alternative Medicine: Accommodating Pluralism*, 107–121. Washington, DC: Georgetown University Press.

Hrobjartsson, A. and Gotzsche, P. C. 2001. "Is the placebo powerless?—An analysis of clinical trials comparing placebo with no treatment." *New England Journal of Medicine* 344:1594–1602.

Hufford, D. J. 2002. "CAM and cultural diversity: Ethics and epistemology converge." In D. Callahan, ed., *The Role of Complementary and Alternative Medicine: Accommodating Pluralism*, 15–35. Washington, DC: Georgetown University Press.

Hughes, H. S. 1974. *Consciousness and Society: The Reorientation of European Social Thought 1890–1930*. Frogmore, St. Albans: Paladin.

Huyler, J. 1995. *Locke in America: The Moral Philosophy of the Founding Era*. Lawrence: University Press of Kansas.

Hume, D. [1739] 1978. *A Treatise of Human Nature*. Oxford: Clarendon Press.

Hume, D. [1748] 1975. *Enquiry Concerning Human Understanding*. Ed. P. H. Nidditch. Oxford: Oxford University Press.

Hunter, K. M. 1994. *Doctors' Stories: The Narrative Structure of Medical Knowledge*. Princeton, NJ: Princeton University Press.

Illich, I. 1976. *Medical Nemesis*. New York: Random House.

Illingworth, P. 2000. "Bluffing, puffing, and spinning in managed-care organizations." *Journal of Medicine and Philosophy* 25:62–76.

Institute of Medicine. 1999. *To Err Is Human: Building a Safer Health System.* Ed. L. T. Kohn, J. N. Corrigan, and M. S. Donaldson. Washington, DC: National Academy Press.

Irwin, W., ed. 2002. *The Matrix and Philosophy: Welcome to the Desert of the Real.* Chicago: Open Court.

Jacob, M. C. 1976. *The Newtonians and the English Revolution, 1689–1720.* Ithaca, NY: Cornell University Press.

Jacobson, P. D. 2002. *Strangers in the Night: Law and Medicine in the Managed Care Era.* New York: Oxford University Press.

Jacobson, P. D. and Cahill, M. T. 2000. "Applying fiduciary responsibilities in the managed care context." *American Journal of Law and Medicine* 26:155–173.

Jakobovits, I. 1959. *Jewish Medical Ethics: Comparative and Historical Study of the Jewish Religious Attitude to Medicine and Its Practice.* New York: Bloch.

James, W. [1902] 1987. *The Varieties of Religious Experience.* New York: Library of America.

James, W. [1909] 1987. *A Pluralistic Universe,* 625–819. New York: Library of America.

Johnson, A. G. 1983. "Teaching medical ethics as a practical subject: Observations from experience." *Journal of Medical Ethics* 9:5–7.

Jonas, W. B. 2002. "Evidence, ethics, and the evaluation of global medicine." In D. Callahan, ed., *The Role of Complementary and Alternative Medicine: Accommodating Pluralism,* 122–147. Washington, DC: Georgetown University Press.

Jones, H. 1910. *The Working Faith of the Social Reformer and Other Essays.* London: Macmillan.

Jones, J. H. 1981. *Bad Blood: The Tuskegee Syphilis Experiment.* New York: Free Press.

Jones, K. 1996. "Trust as an affective attitude." *Ethics* 107:4–25.

Jonsen, A. 1983. "The therapeutic relationship: Is moral conduct a necessary condition?" In E. E. Shelp, ed., *The Clinical Encounter: The Moral Fabric of the Patient-Physician Relationship,* 267–287. Dordrecht: D. Reidel.

Jonsen, A. 1998. *The Birth of Bioethics.* New York: Oxford University Press.

Jonsen, A., Siegler, M., and Winslade, W. J. 1998. *Clinical Ethics: A Practical Approach to Ethical Decisions in Clinical Medicine.* 4th ed. New York: McGraw-Hill.

Jonsen, A. and Toulmin, S. 1988. *The Abuse of Casuistry: A History of Moral Reasoning.* Berkeley: University of California Press.

Kahneman, D. and Tversky, A. 1984. "Choices, values, and frames." *American Psychologist* 39:341–350.

Kahneman D. and Tversky, A., eds. 2000. *Choices, Values, and Frames.* Cambridge: Cambridge University Press.

Kant, I. [1781, 1787] 1998. *Critique of Pure Reason*. Trans. P. Guyer and A. W. Wood. Cambridge: Cambridge University Press.

Kant, I. [1785] 1996. *Groundwork of the Metaphysic of Morals*. In I. Kant, *Practical Philosophy*, trans. M. J. Gregor, 49–108. Cambridge: Cambridge University Press.

Kant, I. [1788] 1996. *Critique of Practical Reason*. In I. Kant, *Practical Philosophy*, trans. M. J. Gregor, 153–271. Cambridge: Cambridge University Press.

Kant, I. [1798] 1996. *The Conflict of the Faculties*. In I. Kant, *Religion and Rational Theology*, ed. A. W. Wood and G. di Giovanni, trans. M. J. Gregor and R. Anchor, 239–327. Cambridge: Cambridge University Press.

Kao, A. C., Green, D. C., Davis, N. A., Koplan, J. P., and Cleary, P. D. 1998a. "Patients' trust in their physicians: Effects of choice, continuity, and payment method." *Journal of General Internal Medicine* 13:681–686.

Kao, A. C., Green, D. C., Davis, N. A., Zaslavsky, A. M., Koplan, J. P., and Cleary, P. D. 1998b. "The relationship between method of physician payment and patient trust." *JAMA* 280:1708–1714.

Karlawish, J., Quill, T., and Meier, D. E. 1999. "A consensus-based approach to providing palliative care to patients who lack decision-making capacity." *Annals of Internal Medicine* 130:835–840.

Katz, J. 1984. *The Silent World of Doctor and Patient*. New York: Free Press.

Kelly, D. F. 1979. *The Emergence of Roman Catholic Medical Ethics in North America: A Historical-Methodological-Bibliographical Study*. New York: Edwin Mellen Press.

Kierkegaard, S. [1849] 1955. *The Sickness unto Death*. Trans. W. Lorrie. Garden City, NY: Doubleday.

Kircher, T. and David, A., eds. 2003. *The Self in Neuroscience and Psychiatry*. Cambridge: Cambridge University Press.

Kirmayer, L. J. 1988. "Mind and body as metaphors: Hidden values in biomedicine." In M. Lock and D. Gordon, eds., *Biomedicine Examined*, 57–93. Dordrecht: Kluwer Academic Publishers.

Kirschner, S. R. 1996. *The Religious and Romantic Origins of Psychoanalysis*. Cambridge: Cambridge University Press.

Kleinman, A. 1988. *The Illness Narratives: Suffering, Healing, and the Human Condition*. New York: Basic Books.

Kohlberg, L. 1984. *Essays on Moral Development, Vol. 2: The Nature and Validity of Moral Stages*. San Francisco: Harper & Row.

Kolakowski, L. 1968. *The Alienation of Reason: History of Positivist Thought*. Garden City, NY: Doubleday.

Kopelman, L. M. 1995. "Philosophy and medical education." *Academic Medicine* 70:795–805.

Kopelman, L. M. 1999. "Values and virtues? How should they be taught?" *Academic Medicine* 74:1307–1310.

Kopelman, L. M. 2002. "The role of science in assessing conventional, complementary, and alternative medicines." In D. Callahan, ed., *The Role of Complementary and Alternative Medicine: Accommodating Pluralism*, 36–53. Washington, DC: Georgetown University Press.

Korsgaard, C. M. 1996. *The Sources of Normativity*. Cambridge: Cambridge University Press.

Kultgen, J. 1995. *Autonomy and Intervention: Parentalism in the Caring Life*. New York: Oxford University Press.

Kurtz, P. W. 1958. "Need reduction and normal value." *Journal of Philosophy* 55:555–568.

LaFond, J. Q. and Durham, M. L. 1992. *Back to the Asylum: The Future of Mental Health Law and Policy in the United States*. Oxford: Oxford University Press.

Lagerspetz, O. 1998. *Trust: The Tacit Demand*. Dordrecht: Kluwer Academic Publishers.

Lahno, B. 2001. "On the emotional character of trust." *Ethical Theories and Moral Practice* 4:171–189.

Laine, C. and Davidoff, F. 1996. "Patient-centered medicine." *JAMA* 275:152–156.

Lammers, S. E. and Verhey, A., eds. 1987. *On Moral Medicine: Theological Perspectives in Medical Ethics*. Grand Rapids, MI: William B. Erdmans.

Landau, R. L. 1993. ". . . And the least of these is empathy." In H. Spiro, M. G. M. Curran, and D. St. James, eds., *Empathy and the Practice of Medicine: Beyond Pills and the Scalpel*, 103–109. New Haven, CT: Yale University Press.

Langewitz, W., Denz, M., Keller, A., Kiss, A., Ruttimann, S., and Wossmer, B. 2002. "Spontaneous talking at start of consultation in outpatient clinic: Cohort study." *British Medical Journal* 325:682–683.

Lasagna, L. 1977. "Discussion of do no harm." In S. Spicker and H. T. Engelhardt, Jr., eds., *Philosophical Medical Ethics: Its Nature and Significance*. Dordrecht: D. Reidel.

LaTour, K. 2002. "Lost in the fog." *Cancer Updates, Research & Education* 1:40–45.

Lawrence, C. and Weisz, G. 1998. "Medical holism: The context." In C. Lawrence and G. Weisz, eds., *Greater Than the Parts: Holism in Biomedicine 1920–1950*, 1–22. Oxford: Oxford University Press.

Layman, E. 1996. "Ethics education: Curricular considerations for the allied health disciplines." *Journal of Allied Health* 25:149–160.

Lehmann, L. S., Kasoff, W. S., Koch, P., and Federman, D. D. 2004. "A survey of medical ethics education at U.S., and Canadian medical schools." *Academic Medicine* 79:682–689.

Leitch, V. B., ed. 2001. *The Norton Anthology of Theory and Criticism*. New York: Norton.

Levi, B. H. 1999. *Respecting Patient Autonomy*. Urbana: University of Illinois Press.

Levinson, W., Gorawara-Bhat, R., and Lamb, J. 2000. "A study of patient clues and physician responses in primary care and surgical settings." *JAMA* 284:1021–1027.

Lindley, R. 1986. *Autonomy*. Atlantic Highlands, NJ: Humanities Press International.

Lo, B. 1995. *Resolving Ethical Dilemmas: A Guide for Clinicians*. Baltimore: Williams & Wilkins.

Lo, B., Quill, T., and Tulsky, J. 1999. "Discussing palliative care with patients." *Annals of Internal Medicine* 130:744–749.

Lo, B. and Schroeder, S. A. 1981. "Frequency of ethical dilemmas on an inpatient medical service." *Archives of Internal Medicine* 141:1062–1064.

Locke, J. [1690] 1980. *The Second Treatise of Government*. Indianapolis: Hackett.

Locke, J. [1700] 1975. *An Essay Concerning Human Understanding*. Ed. P. H. Nidditch. Oxford: Clarendon Press.

Løgstrup, K. E. 1971. *The Ethical Demand*. Trans. T. I. Jensen. Philadelphia: Fortress Press.

Luhmann, N. 1979. *Trust and Power*. New York: Wiley.

Lukes, S. 1973. *Individualism*. Oxford: Blackwell.

Macfarlane, A. 1978. *The Origins of English Individualism*. Oxford: Blackwell.

MacIntyre, A. 1979. "Medicine aims at the care of persons rather than what ...?" In E. E. Shelp, ed., *The Clinical Encounter: The Moral Fabric of the Patient-Physician Relationship*, 83–96. Dordrecht: D. Reidel.

MacIntyre, A. 1984. *After Virtue*. 2nd ed. Notre Dame, IN: University of Notre Dame Press.

Mackenzie, C. and Stoljar, N. 2000. "Introduction." In C. Mackenzie and N. Stoljar, eds., *Relational Autonomy: Feminist Perspectives on Autonomy, Agency, and the Social Self*, 3–31. New York: Oxford University Press.

MacPherson, C. B. 1962. *The Political Theory of Possessive Individualism: Hobbes to Locke*. Oxford: Clarendon Press.

Mariner, W. 1995. "Business vs. business ethics: Conflicting standards for managed care." *Journal of Law, Medicine and Ethics* 23:236–246.

Marvel, M. K., Epstein, R. M., Flowers, K., and Beckman, H. B. 1999. "Soliciting the patient's agenda: Have we improved?" *JAMA* 281:283–287.

Matthews, D. A., Suchman, A. L., and Branch, W. T., Jr. 1993. "Making 'connexions'; Enhancing the therapeutic potential of patient-clinician relationships." *Annals of Internal Medicine* 118:973–977.

Mauss, M. 1985. "A category of the human mind: The notion of person; the notion of self." In M. Carrithers, S. Collins, and S. Lukes, eds., *The Category of the Person: Anthropology, Philosophy, History*, 1–25. Cambridge: Cambridge University Press.

May, W. F. 1972. "Code, covenant, contract, or philanthropy." *Hastings Center Report* 5:29–38.

May, W. F. 1983. *The Physician's Covenant: Images of the Healer in Medical Ethics*. Philadelphia: Westminster Press.

McCullough, L. B. 1985. "Virtue, etiquette and Anglo-American medical ethics in the eighteenth and nineteenth centuries." In E. E. Shelp, ed., *Virtues and Medicine: Explorations in the Character of Medicine*, 81–92. Dordrecht: D. Reidel.

McCullough, L. B. 1993. "John Gregory's medical ethics and Humean sympathy." In R. Baker, D. Porter, and R. Porter, eds., *The Codification of Medical Morality*, 145–160. Dordrecht: Kluwer Academic Publishers.

McDonald, C. J. 1996. "Medical heuristics: The silent adjudicators of clinical practice." *Annals of Internal Medicine* 124:56–62.

McKinlay, J. B. and Marceau, L. D. 2002. "The end of the Golden Age of doctoring." *International Journal of Health Services* 32:379–416.

McNeil, B. J., Pauker, S. G., Sox, H. C., Jr., and Tversky, A. 1982. "On the elicitation of preferences for alternative therapies." *New England Journal of Medicine* 306:1259–1262.

Mead, G. H. 1934. "A contrast of individualistic and social theories of the self." In C. W. Morris, ed., *Mind, Self, and Society*, 222–226. Chicago: University of Chicago Press.

Mechanic, D. 1996. "Changing medical organization and the erosion of trust." *Milbank Quarterly* 74:171–189.

Mechanic, D. and Schlesinger, M. 1996. "The impact of managed care on patients' trust in medical care and their physicians." *JAMA* 275:1693–1697.

Menand, L. 2001. *The Metaphysical Club: A story of ideas in America*. New York: Farrar, Straus, and Giroux.

Merton, R. K. [1938] 1970. *Science, Technology, and Society in Seventeenth-Century England*. New York: Harper & Row.

Metzinger, T. 2003. *Being No One: The Self-Model of Subjectivity*. Cambridge, MA: MIT Press.

Meyers, D. T. 1989. *Self, Society and Personal Choice*. New York: Columbia University Press.

Miles, S. H., Lane, L. W., Bickel, J., Walker, R. M., and Cassell, C. K. 1989. "Medical ethics education: Coming of age." *Academic Medicine* 64:705–714.

Mill, J. S. [1859] 1972. *On Liberty*. In H. B. Acton, ed., *Utilitarianism, On Liberty, and Considerations on Representative Government*, 69–185. London: Dent.

Mill, J. S. [1861] 1972. *Utilitarianism*. In H. B. Acton, ed., *Utilitarianism, On Liberty, and Considerations on Representative Government*, 1–67. London: Dent.

Misztal, B. A. 1996. *Trust in Modern Societies: The Search for the Bases of Social Order*. Cambridge: Polity Press.

Moore, F. D. 1959. *Metabolic Care of the Surgical Patient*. Philadelphia: W. B. Saunders.

Morreim, E. H. 1995. *Balancing Act: The New Medical Ethics of Medicine's New Economics*. Washington, DC: Georgetown University Press.

Morris, D. 2002. "Narrative, ethics, and pain: Thinking *with* stories." In R. Charon and M. Montello, eds., *Stories Matter: The Role of Narrative in Medical Ethics*, 196–218. New York: Routledge.

Morson, G. S. 1988. "Prosaics: An approach to the humanities." *The American Scholar* 57:515–528.

Morson, G. S. 1991. "Bakhtin and the present moment." *The American Scholar* 60:201–222.

Morson, G. S. and Emerson, C. 1990. *Mikhail Bakhtin: Creation of a Prosaics*. Palo Alto, CA: Stanford University Press.

Mulhall, S. and Swift, A. 1992. *Liberals and Communitarians*. Oxford: Blackwell.

Murphy, E. A. 1997. *The Logic of Medicine*. 2nd ed. Baltimore: Johns Hopkins University Press.

Murphy, E. A., Butzow, J. J., and Suarez-Murias, E. L. 1997. *Underpinnings of Medical Ethics*. Baltimore: Johns Hopkins University Press.

Murphy, J., Chang, H., Montgomery, J. E., Rogers, W. H., and Safran, D. G. 2001. "The quality of physician-patient relationships: Patients' experiences 1996–1999." *Journal of Family Practice* 50:123–129.

Myser, C., Kerridge, I. H., and Mitchell, K. R. 1995. "Teaching clinical ethics as a professional skill: Bridging the gap between knowledge about ethics and its use in clinical practice." *Journal of Medical Ethics* 21:97–103.

Nagel, T. 1986. *The View from Nowhere*. Oxford: Oxford University Press.

Najder, Z. 1975. *Values and Evaluations*. London: Clarendon Press.

Nelson, H. C., ed. 1997. *Stories and Their Limits: Narrative Approaches to Bioethics*. New York: Routledge.

Nelson, J. L. 1992. "The rights and responsibilities of potential organ donors: A communitarian approach." *Communitarian Position Paper*. Washington, DC: Communitarian Network.

Nietzsche, F. [1887] 1967. *On the Genealogy of Morals*. Trans. W. Kaufmann and R. J. Holingdale. New York: Vintage.

Noddings, N. 1984. *Caring: A Feminist Approach to Ethics and Moral Education*. Berkeley: University of California Press.

Normand, C. 1991. Economics, health, and the economics of health. *British Medical Journal* 303:1572–1575.

Nordenfelt, L. 1995. *On the Nature of Health: An Action-Theoretic Approach.* 2nd ed. Dordrecht: Kluwer Academic Publishers.

Novack, D. H., Volk, G., Drossman, D. A., and Lipkin, M. 1993. "Medical interviewing and interpersonal skills teaching in US medical schools: Progress, problems, and promise." *JAMA* 269:2101–2105.

Nozick, R. 1974. *Anarchy, State, and Utopia.* New York: Basic Books.

Nussbaum, M. 2001. *Upheavals of Thought: The Intelligence of Emotions.* Cambridge: Cambridge University Press.

Olafson, F. A. 1998. *Heidegger and the Ground of Ethics: A Study of Mitsein.* Cambridge: Cambridge University Press.

Oliver, J. 1939. "An ancient poem on the duties of a physician, part I." 7 *Bulletin of the History of Medicine* 315. Reprinted in C. Burns, ed., *Legacies in Ethics and Medicine.* New York: Science History Publications, 1977.

O'Neill, O. 2002. *Autonomy and Trust in Bioethics.* Cambridge: Cambridge University Press.

Parfit, D. 1984. *Reasons and Persons.* Oxford: Oxford University Press.

Parks, T. 2000. "In the locked ward." *New York Review of Books*, February 24, 2000, pp. 14–15.

Patenaude, J., Niyonsenga, T., and Fafard, D. 2003. "Changes in students' moral development during medical school: A cohort study." *Canadian Medical Association Journal* 168:840–844.

Payer, L. 1988. *Medicine and Culture: Varieties of Treatment in the United States, England, West Germany, and France.* New York: Henry Holt.

Peabody, F. W. 1927. *The Care of the Patient.* Cambridge, MA: Harvard University Press.

Pearson, S. D. and Raeke, L. H. 2000. "Patients' trust in physicians: Many theories, few measures, and little data." *Journal of General Internal Medicine* 15:509–513.

Peirce, C. S. [1871] 1984. "Fraser's *The Works of George Berkeley*." In E. C. Moore, ed., *Writings of Charles S. Peirce: A Chronological Edition, Vol. 2, 1867–1871.* Bloomington: Indiana University Press.

Pellegrino, E. D. 1979a. *Humanism and the Physician.* Knoxville: University of Tennessee Press.

Pellegrino, E. D. 1979b. "Philosophical grounding for treating the patient as a person: A commentary on Alasdair McIntyre." In E. J. Cassell and M. Siegler, eds., *Changing Values in Medicine*, 97–104. Frederick, MD: University Publications of America.

Pellegrino, E. D. and Harvey, J. C. 2001. "Whom should the patient trust? A friendly reply to Kevin Wildes." *America* 185:19–22.

Pellegrino, E. D. and McElhinney, T. K. 1982. *Teaching Ethics, the Humanities, and Human Values in Medical Schools: A Ten-Year Overview.* Washington, DC: Institute on Human Values in Medicine.

Pellegrino, E. D. and Thomasma, D. C. 1981. *A Philosophical Basis of Medical Practice: Toward a Philosophy and Ethic of the Healing Professions.* New York: Oxford University Press.

Pellegrino, E. D. and Thomasma, D. C. 1988. *For the Patient's Good: The Restoration of Beneficence in Health Care.* New York: Oxford University Press.

Pellegrino, E. D. and Thomasma, D. C. 1993. *The Virtues in Medical Practice.* New York: Oxford University Press.

Percival, T. [1803] 1927. *Percival's Medical Ethics.* Ed. C. D. Leake. Baltimore: Williams & Wilkins.

Pernick, M. S. 1982. "The patient's role in medical decisionmaking: A social history of informed consent in medical therapy." In *President's Commission for the Study of Ethical Problems in Medicine and Biomedical and Behavioral Research, Making Health Care Decisions.* 1–35. Washington, DC: U.S. Government Printing Office.

Pickstone, J. 1993. "Thomas Percival and the production of *Medical Ethics.*" In R. Baker, D. Porter, and R. Porter, eds., *The Codification of Medical Morality,* 161–178. Dordrecht: Kluwer Academic Publishers.

Porn, I. 1984. "An equilibrium model of health." In L. Nordenfelt and B. I. B. Lindhal, eds., *Health, Disease, and Causal Explanations in Medicine,* 3–9. Boston: D. Reidel.

Preston, T. 1981. *The Clay Pedestal: A Re-Examination of the Doctor-Patient Relationship.* Seattle: Madrona.

Proctor, R. N. 1991. *Value-Free Science? Purity and Power in Modern Knowledge.* Cambridge, MA: Harvard University Press.

Psaty, B. M., Heckbert, S. R., Koepsell, T. D., Sisscovick, D. S., Raghunathan, T. E., Weiss, N. S., Rosendaal, F. R., et al. 1995. The risk of myocardial infarction associated with anti-hypertensive drug therapies. *JAMA* 274:620–625.

Putnam, H. 1990. Beyond the fact/value dichotomy. In J. Conant, *Realism with a Human Face,* 135–141. Cambridge, MA: Harvard University Press.

Putnam, H. 2002. *The Collapse of the Fact/Value Dichotomy and Other Essays.* Cambridge, MA: Harvard University Press.

Putnam, R. A. 1985. "Creating facts and values." *Philosophy* 60, 187–204.

Putnam, R. D. 2000. *Bowling Alone: The Collapse and Revival of American Community.* New York: Simon and Schuster.

Quine, W. V. O. 1963. "Two dogmas of empiricism." In *From a Logical Point of View,* 2nd ed., 20–46. New York: Harper & Row.

In re Quinlan, 70 N.J. 10, 355 A.2d 647 (1976).

Railton, P. 2003. *Facts, Values, and Norms: Essays towards a Morality of Consequence*. Cambridge: Cambridge University Press.

Ramsey, P. 1970. *The Patient as Person: Medical and Legal Intersections*. New Haven, CT: Yale University Press.

Rawls, J. [1971] 1999. *A Theory of Justice*. Cambridge, MA: Harvard University Press.

Rawls, J. 1993. *Political Liberalism*. New York: Columbia University Press.

Regehr, G. 2004. "Trends in medical education research." *Academic Medicine* 79:939–947.

Reinhardt, U. E. 1997. "Hippocrates and the 'securitization' of patients." *JAMA* 277:1850–1851.

Reiser, S. J. and Banner, R. S. 2003. "The charter on medical professionalization and the limits of medical power." *Annals of Internal Medicine* 138:844–846.

Richards, J. R. 1980. *The Skeptical Feminist*. Boston: Routledge and Kegan Paul.

Richardson, R. D., Jr. 1995. *Emerson: The Mind on Fire*. Berkeley: University of California Press.

Richman, K. A. 2004. *Ethics and the Metaphysics of Medicine: Reflections on Health and Beneficence*. Cambridge, MA: MIT Press.

Robinson, R. V. and Jackson, E. F. 2001. "Is trust in others declining in America? An age-period-cohort analysis." *Social Science Research* 30:117–145.

Rodwin, M. A. 1995. "Strains in the fiduciary metaphor: Divided physician loyalties and the obligations in a changing health care system." *American Journal of Law and Medicine* 21:241–257.

Romanell, P. 1984. *John Locke and Medicine: A New Key to Locke*. Buffalo, NY: Prometheus Books.

Roochnik, D. 1987. "Applied ethics: Some Platonic questions." *Philosophy in Context* 17:40–51.

Rorty, R. 1989. "The philosophy of the oddball." *New Republic*, June 19, 1989, pp. 38–41.

Rorty, R. 1999. *Philosophy and Social Hope*. London: Penguin Books.

Rose, N. 1990. *Governing the Soul: Shaping the Private Self*. London: Routledge.

Rose, S. 1998. *Inventing Ourselves: Psychology, Power, and Personhood*. Cambridge: Cambridge University Press.

Rosen, S. 2002. *The Elusiveness of the Ordinary: Studies in the Possibility of Philosophy*. New Haven, CT: Yale University Press.

Rosenberg, C. 1998. "Holism in twentieth-century medicine." In C. Lawrence and G. Weisz, eds., *Greater Than the Parts: Holism in Biomedicine 1920–1950*, 335–355. New York: Oxford University Press.

Rosenhan, D. L. 1973. "On being sane in insane places." *Science* 179:250–258.

Roter, D. L., Stewart, M., Putnam, S. M., Lipkin, M., Jr., Stiles, W., and Inui, T. S. 1997. "Communication patterns of primary care physicians." *JAMA* 277:350–356.

Rothman, D. J. 1991. *Strangers at the Bedside: A History of How Law and Bioethics Transformed Medical Decision Making*. New York: Basic Books.

Rothman, D. J. 2001. "The origins and consequences of patient autonomy: A 25-year retrospective." *Health Care Analysis* 9:255–264.

Sadler, J. Z. 1997. "Recognizing values: A descriptive-causal method for medical/scientific discourses." *Journal of Medicine and Philosophy* 22:541–565.

Sandel, M. 1982. *Liberalism and the Limits of Justice*. Cambridge: Cambridge University Press.

Sandel, M. 1996. *Democracy's Discontent: America in Search of a Public Philosophy*. Cambridge, MA: Harvard University Press.

Savulescu, J. 2000. "Rational non-interventional paternalism: Why doctors ought to make judgments of what is best for their patients." In M. Boylan, ed., *Medical Ethics*, 72–79. Upper Saddle River, NJ: Prentice Hall.

Savulescu, J., Crisp, R., Fulford, K. W. M., and Hope, T. E. 1999. "Evaluating ethics competence in medical education." *Journal of Medical Ethics* 25:367–374.

Savulescu, J. and Monmeyer, R. W. 2000. Should informed consent be based on rational beliefs?" In M. Boylan, ed., *Medical Ethics*, 128–140. Upper Saddle River, NJ: Prentice Hall.

Sayers, G. M., Barratt, D., Gothard, C., Onnie, C., Perera, S., and Schulman, D. 2001. "The value of taking an ethics history." *Journal of Medical Ethics* 27:114–117.

Sayre-McCord, G. 1988. "Introduction: The many moral realisms." In G. Sayre-McCord, ed., *Essays on Moral Realism*, 1–23. Ithaca, NY: Cornell University Press.

Schaffner, K. F. 2002. "Assessments of efficacy in biomedicine: The turn toward methodological pluralism." In D. Callahan, ed., *The Role of Complementary and Alternative Medicine: Accommodating Pluralism*. Washington, DC: Georgetown University Press.

Schagen, S. B., van Dam, F. S., Muller, M. J., Boogerd, W., Lindeboom, J., and Bruning, P. F. 1999. "Cognitive defects after postoperative adjuvant chemotherapy for breast cancer." *Cancer* 85:640–650.

Schneewind, J. B. 1992. "Autonomy, obligation, and virtue: An overview of Kant's moral philosophy." In P. Guyer, ed., *The Cambridge Companion to Kant*, 309–341. Cambridge: Cambridge University Press.

Schneewind, J. B. 1998. *The Invention of Autonomy: A History of Modern Moral Philosophy*. New York: Cambridge University Press.

Schneider, C. E. 1998. *The Practice of Autonomy: Patients, Doctors, and Medical Decisions*. New York: Oxford University Press.

Schmidt, H. 1998. "Integrating the teaching of basic sciences, clinical sciences, and biopsychosocial issues." *Academic Medicine* 73:S24–S31.

Schultz, M. M. 1985. "From informed consent to patient choice: A new protected right." *Yale Law Review* 95:219–295.

Sedgwick, P. 1982. *Psycho Politics: Laing, Foucault, Goffman, Szasz, and the Future of Psychiatry.* New York: Harper & Row.

Seedhouse, D. 1986. *Health: The Foundations for Achievement.* New York: Wiley.

Self, D. J. 1993. "The moral development of medical students: A pilot study of the possible influence of medical education." *Medical Education* 27:26–34.

Self, D. J., Wolinsky, F. D., and Baldwin, D. C. 1989. "The effect of teaching medical ethics on medical students' moral reasoning." *Academic Medicine* 64:755–759.

Seligman, A. B. 1992. *The Idea of Civil Society.* New York: Free Press.

Seligman, A. B. 1997. *The Problem of Trust.* Princeton, NJ: Princeton University Press.

Seligman, A. B. 2000. *Modernity's Wager: Authority, the Self, and Transcendence.* Princeton, NJ: Princeton University Press.

Shain, B. A. 1994. *The Myth of American Individualism: The Protestant Origins of American Political Thought.* Princeton, NJ: Princeton University Press.

Shaw, G. B. [1906] 1985. *The Doctor's Dilemma.* In *George Bernard Shaw: Three Plays*, 257–424. New York: Signet.

Sheehan, T. J., Husted, S. D. R., Candee, D., Cook, C. D., and Bargen, M. 1980. "Moral judgment as a predictor of clinical performance." *Evaluation and the Health Professional* 3:393–404.

Shem, S. 2002. "Fiction as resistance." *Annals of Internal Medicine* 137:934–937.

Shils, E. 1968. "The sanctity of life." In D. H. Labby, ed., *Life or Death: Ethics and Options*, 2–38. Seattle: University of Washington Press.

Shortell, S. M., Waters, T. M., Clarke, K. W. B., and Budetti, P. P. 1998. "Physicians as double agents: Maintaining trust in an era of multiple accountabilities." *JAMA* 280:1102–1108.

Shorter, E. 1992. *From Paralysis to Fatigue: A History of Psychosomatic Illness in the Modern Era.* New York: Free Press.

Shue, H. 1996. *Basic Rights.* 2nd ed. Princeton, NJ: Princeton University Press.

Simon, W. M. 1963. *European Positivism in the Nineteenth Century.* Ithaca, NY: Cornell University Press.

Singer, P. A. 2000. "Recent advances: Medical ethics." *British Medical Journal* 321:282–285.

Singer, P. A., Pellegrino, E. D., and Siegler, M. 2001. "Clinical ethics revisited." *BMC Medical Ethics* 2:1. http://www.biomedicalcentral.com/1472–6939/2/1.

Skoyles, J. R. and Sagan, D. 2002. *Up from Dragons: The Evolution of Human Intelligence.* New York: McGraw-Hill.

Smith, A. [1790] 1982. *The Theory of Moral Sentiments.* Indianapolis: Liberty Classics.

Smith, R. 1997. *The Norton History of the Human Sciences.* New York: Norton.

Smuts, J. C. 1926. *Holism and Evolution.* New York: Macmillan.

Sober, E. and Wilson, D. S. 1999. *Unto Others: The Evolution and Psychology of Unselfish Behavior.* Cambridge, MA: Harvard University Press.

Spector, J. 2003. "Value in fact: Naturalism and normativity in Hume's moral psychology." *Journal of the History of Philosophy* 41:145–163.

Sperry, L. 1991. "Teaching the biopsychosocial perspective: A comparison of two approaches." *Psychological Reports* 68:99–102.

Spiro, H. 1993. "What is empathy and can it be taught?" In H. Spiro, M. G. M. Curran, and D. St. James, eds., *Empathy and the Practice of Medicine: Beyond Pills and the Scalpel,* 7–14. New Haven, CT: Yale University Press.

Spiro, H., Curran, M. G. M., and St. James, D., eds. 1993. *Empathy and the Practice of Medicine: Beyond Pills and the Scalpel.* New Haven, CT: Yale University Press.

Spiro, H. and Norton, P. W. 2003. Dean Milton C. Winternitz at Yale. *Perspectives in Biology and Medicine* 46, 403–412.

Stack, G. J. 1992. *Nietzsche and Emerson: An Elective Affinity.* Athens: Ohio University Press.

Starr, P. 1983. *The Social Transformation of American Medicine.* New York: Basic Books.

Stein, H. F. 1985. *The Psychodynamics of Medical Practice: Unconscious Factors in Patient Care.* Berkeley: University of California Press.

Stempsey, W. E. 1999. *Disease and Diagnosis: Value-Dependent Realism.* Dordrecht: Kluwer Academic Publishers.

Stern, D. 1998. "Practicing what we preach? An analysis of the curriculum of values in medical education." *American Journal of Medicine* 104:569–575.

Stoeckle, J. D. 1987 "Introduction." In J. D. Stoeckle, ed., *Encounters between Patients and Doctors.* Cambridge, MA: MIT Press.

Stokstad, E. 2000. "Stephen Straus's impossible job." *Science* 288:1568–1570.

Sulmasy, D. P., Geller, G., Levine, D. M., and Faden, R. R. 1990. "Medical house officers' knowledge, attitudes, and confidence regarding medical ethics." *Archives of Internal Medicine* 150:2509–2513.

Szasz, T. S. 1961. *The Myth of Mental Illness: Foundations of a Theory of Personal Conduct.* New York: Dell.

Szasz, T. S. and Hollender, M. H. 1956. "A contribution to the philosophy of medicine: The basic models of the doctor-patient relationship." *Archives of Internal Medicine* 97:585–592.

Sztompka, P. 1999. *Trust: A Sociological Theory.* New York: Cambridge University Press.

Talbot, M. 2000. "The placebo prescription." *New York Times Magazine,* January 9, 2000, pp. 34–39, 44, 58–60.

Tam, H. 1998. *Communitarianism: A New Agenda for Politics and Citizenship.* New York: New York University Press.

Tauber, A. I. 1971. "The Last Puritan." Letter. *New England Journal of Medicine* 284:922–923.

Tauber, A. I. 1992. "The two faces of medical education: Flexner and Osler revisited." *Journal of the Royal Society of Medicine* 85:598–602.

Tauber, A. I. 1993. "Goethe's philosophy of science: Modern resonances." *Perspectives in Biology and Medicine* 36, 244–257.

Tauber, A. I. 1994. *The Immune Self: Theory or Metaphor?* Cambridge: Cambridge University Press.

Tauber, A. I. 1996. "From Descartes' dream to Husserl's nightmare." In: A. I. Tauber, *The Elusive Synthesis: Aesthetics and Science,* 289–312. Dordrecht: Kluwer Academic Publishers.

Tauber, A. I. 1997. "Introduction." In A. I. Tauber, ed., *Science and the Quest for Reality,* 1–49. London: Macmillan and New York: New York University Press.

Tauber, A. I. 1999a. *Confessions of a Medicine Man: An Essay in Popular Philosophy.* Cambridge, MA: MIT Press.

Tauber, A. I. 1999b. "Is biology a political science?" *BioScience* 49:479–486.

Tauber, A. I. 2001. *Henry David Thoreau and the Moral Agency of Knowing.* Berkeley: University of California Press.

Tauber, A. I. 2002a. "Medicine, public health and the ethics of rationing." *Perspectives in Biology and Medicine* 45:16–30.

Tauber, A. I. 2002b. "The quest for holism in medicine." In D. Callahan, ed., *The Role of Complementary and Alternative Medicine: Accommodating Pluralism,* 172–189. Washington, D.C.: Georgetown University Press.

Tauber, A. I. 2003a. "Autonomy gone mad." *Philosophy in the Contemporary World* 10:75–80.

Tauber, A. I. 2003b. "The philosopher as prophet: The case of Emerson and Thoreau." *Philosophy in the Contemporary World* 10:89–103.

Tauber, A. I. 2003c. "A philosophical approach to rationing." *Medical Journal of Australia* 178:454–456.

Tauber A. I. and Sarkar, S. 1993. "The ideological basis of the Human Genome Project." *Journal of the Royal Society of Medicine* 86:537–540.

Taylor, C. 1985. *Philosophy and the Human Sciences.* Cambridge: Cambridge University Press.

Taylor, C. 1989. *The Sources of the Self*. Cambridge, MA: Harvard University Press.

Thagard, P. 1999. *How Scientists Explain Disease*. Princeton, NJ: Princeton University Press.

Thalberg, I. 1978. "Hierarchical analyses of unfree action." *Canadian Journal of Philosophy* 8:211–225.

Thom, D. H. and Campbell, B. 1997. "Patient-physician trust: An exploratory study." *Journal of Family Practice* 44:169–176.

Thomas, J. E. and Waluchow, W. J. 1998. *Well and Good: A Case Study Approach to Biomedical Ethics*, 3rd ed. Peterborough, Ontario: Broadview Press.

Thomasma, D. C. 1978. "Training in medical ethics: An ethical workup." *Forum on Medicine* 1:33–36.

Thomasma, D. C. 1981. "'Capstone' Conference Workshops: Reflections on the State of the Art." In E. D. Pellegrino and T. K. McElhinney, eds., *Teaching Ethics, the Humanities, and Human Values in Medical Schools: A Ten-Year Overview*. Washington, DC: Institute on Human Values in Medicine; Society for Health and Human Values.

Thomasma, D. C. 1984. "The basis of medicine and religion: Respect for persons." *Linacre Quarterly* 47:142–150.

Thoreau, H. D. [1854] 1971. *Walden*. Princeton, NJ: Princeton University Press.

de Tocqueville, A. [1840] 2000. *Democracy in America*. H. C. Mansfield and D. Winthrop, trans. and ed. Chicago: University of Chicago Press.

Toombs, S. K. 1992. *The Meaning of Illness: A Phenomenological Account of the Different Perspectives of Physician and Patient*. Dordrecht: Kluwer Academic Publishers.

Toulmin, S. 1981. "The tyranny of principles." *Hastings Center Report* 11:31–39.

Toulmin, S. 1982. "How medicine saved the life of ethics." *Perspectives in Biology and Medicine* 25:736–750.

Toulmin, S. 1988. "The recovery of practical philosophy." *The American Scholar* 57:337–352.

Toulmin, S. 1993. "Knowledge and art in the practice of medicine: Clinical judgment and historical reconstruction." In C. Delkeskamp-Hayes and M. A. G. Cutter, eds., *Science, Technology, and the Art of Medicine*, 231–250. Dordrecht: Kluwer Academic Publishers.

Tversky, A. and Kahneman, D. 1981. "The framing of decisions and the psychology of choice." *Science* 211:453–458.

Twain, M. [1867] 1992. "Official physic." In L. J. Budd, ed., *Mark Twain: Collected Tales,Sketches, Speeches, and Essays 1852–1890*, 228–230. New York: Library of America.

Twain, M. [1899] 1992. "Christian Science and the book of Mrs. Eddy." In L. J. Budd, ed., *Mark Twain: Collected Tales, Sketches, Speeches, and Essays 1891–1910*, 371–389. New York: Library of America.

Twain, M. [1901] 1976. "Remarks on Osteopathy." In P. Fatout, ed., *Mark Twain Speaking*, 384–388. Iowa City: University of Iowa Press.

Veatch, R. M. 1972. "Models for ethical medicine in a revolutionary age." *Hastings Center Report* 2:5–7.

Veatch, R. M. 1981. *A Theory of Medical Ethics*. New York: Basic Books.

Veatch, R. M. 1983a. "The case for contract in medical ethics." In E. E. Shelp, ed., *The Clinical Encounter: The Moral Fabric of the Patient-Physician Relationship*, 105–112. Dordrecht: D. Reidel.

Veatch, R. M. 1983b. "The physician as stranger: The ethics of the anonymous patient-physician relationship." In E. E. Shelp, ed., *The Clinical Encounter: The Moral Fabric of the Patient-Physician Relationship*, 187–207. Dordrecht: D. Reidel.

Veatch, R. M. 1996. "Which grounds for overriding autonomy are legitimate?" *Hastings Center Report* 26:42–43.

Verhey, A. and Lammers, S. E., eds. 1993. *Theological Voices in Medical Ethics*. Grand Rapids, MI: William B. Erdmans.

Verkerk, M., Lindemann, H., Maeckelberghe, E., Feenstra, E., Hartoungh, R., and de Bree, M. 2004. "Enhancing reflection. An interpersonal exercise in ethics education." *Hastings Center Report* 34:31–38.

Veterans Administration Cooperative Study Group. 1970. Effects of treatment on morbidity in hypertension. II. Results in patients with diastolic blood pressure averaging 90 through 115 mm Hg. *JAMA* 213:1143–1152.

Wallace, R. J. 1998. "Moral sentiments." In E. Craig, ed., *Routledge Encyclopedia of Philosophy*, vol. 6, 548–550. New York: Routledge.

Walsh, D. 1983. *The Mysticism of Innerworldly Fulfillment: A Study of Jacob Boehme*. Gainsville: University Presses of Florida.

Walton, M. 1998. *The Trouble with Medicine: Preserving the Trust between Patients and Doctors*. St. Leonards, NSW: Allen & Unwin.

Walzer, M. 1983. *Spheres of Justice*. New York: Basic Books.

Walzer, M. 1994. *Thick and Thin*. Notre Dame: University of Notre Dame Press.

Watson, G. 1975. "Free agency." *Journal of Philosophy* 72:205–220.

Wear, D. 1998. "On white coats and professional development: The formal and the hidden curricula." *Annals of Internal Medicine* 129:734–737.

Weber, M. [1904–1905] 1958. *The Protestant Ethic and the Spirit of Capitalism*. Trans. T. Parsons. New York: Scribners.

Weber, M. [1915] 1946. "Religious rejections of the world and their directions." In H. H. Gerth and C. W. Mills, ed. and trans., *From Max Weber: Essays in Sociology*, 323–359. New York: Oxford University Press.

Weed, L. L. 1969. *Medical Records, Medical Education, and Patient Care: The Problem-Oriented Record as a Basic Tool.* Cleveland: The Press of Case Western Reserve University.

Weed, L. L. 2004. "Shedding our illusions: A better way of medicine." *Sexuality, Reproduction & Menopause* 2:45–52.

Weed, L. L. and Weed, L., Jr. 1994. "Reengineering medicine." *Federation Bulletin: The Journal of Medical Licensure and Discipline* 81:149–183.

Weinstein, M. C. and Fineberg, H. V. 1980. *Clinical Decision Analysis.* Philadelphia: Saunders.

Weinstein, M. M. 1999. "Managed care's other problem: It's not what you think." *New York Times*, February 28, 1999, section 4, pp. 1, 4.

Whitbeck, C. 1981. "A theory of health." In A. L. Caplan, H. T. Engelhardt Jr., and J. J. McCartney, eds., *Concepts of Health and Disease: Interdisciplinary Perspectives*, 611–626. Reading, MA: Addison-Wesley.

Wieneke, M. H. and Dienst, E. R. 1995. "Neuropsychological assessment of cognitive functioning following chemotherapy for breast cancer." *Psycho-Oncology* 4:61–66.

Wildes, K. W. 2001. "Patient no more: Why did the golden age of medicine collapse?" *America* 185:8–11.

Williams, B. 1985. *Ethics and the Limits of Philosophy.* Cambridge, MA: Harvard University Press.

Williams, B. 1988. "Formal structures and social reality." In D. Gambetta, ed., *Trust: Making and Breaking Cooperative Relations*, 3–13. Oxford: Blackwell.

Wills, G. 1999. *A Necessary Evil: A History of American Distrust of Government.* New York: Simon and Schuster.

Wilson, A. N. 1999. *God's Funeral: A Biography of Faith and Doubt in Western Civilization.* New York: Ballantine Books.

Wilson, T. D. 2002. *Strangers to Ourselves: Discovering the Adaptive Unconscious.* Cambridge, MA: Harvard University Press.

Winick, B. J. 1997. *The Right to Refuse Mental Health Treatment.* Washington, DC: American Psychological Association.

Wispe, L. 1986. "The distinction between sympathy and empathy: To call forth a concept, a word is needed." *Journal of Personality and Social Psychology* 50:314–321.

Wittgenstein, L. [1921] 1961. *Tractatus Logico-Philosophicus.* Trans. D. F. Pears and B. McGuinness. London: Routledge.

Wittgenstein, L. 1958. *Philosophical Investigations.* New York: Macmillan.

Wolf, S. M., ed. 1996. *Feminism and Bioethics: Beyond Reproduction.* New York: Oxford University Press.

Wolfe, A., ed. 1991. *America at Century's End.* Berkeley: University of California Press.

Wolpe, P. 1998. "The triumph of autonomy in American bioethics: A sociological view." In R. DeVries and J. Subedi, eds., *Bioethics and Society: Constructing the Ethical Enterprise*, 38–59. Englewood Cliffs, NJ: Prentice-Hall.

Wood, A. W. 1999. *Kant's Ethical Thought*. Cambridge: Cambridge University Press.

Wynia, M. K., Cummins, D. S., Van Geest, J. B., and Wilson, I. B. 2000. "Physician manipulation of reimbursement rules for patients: Between a rock and a hard place." *JAMA* 283:1858–1865.

Wynia, M. K., Van Geest, J. B., Cummins, D. S., and Wilson, I. B. 2003. "Do physicians not offer useful services because of coverage restriction?" *Health Affairs* 22:190–197.

Young, R. 1980. "Autonomy and socialization." *Mind* 89:565–576.

Zuckert, M. P. 1994. *Natural Rights and the New Republicanism*. Princeton, NJ: Princeton University Press.

Zussman, R. 1992. *Intensive Care: Medical Ethics and the Medical Profession*. Chicago: University of Chicago Press.

Index

Abolitionists, 71
Accountability, 5–6
Activism, 4
Addams, Jane, 255n1
Administrative issues
  cost and, 162–163
  time and, 3
*Advice to a Young Physician
  Respecting the Way in Which He is
  to Conduct Himself in the Practice
  of Medicine, in View of the
  Indifference of the Public to the
  Subject, and Considering the
  Complaints That Are Made about
  Physicians* (De Sorbière), 67
Allison, Henry, 102
Alterity, 261n14
American dream, 89–90
American Medical Association
  (AMA), 72–77
"American Scholar, The" (Emerson),
  90
Ameriks, Karl, 98
Analytical philosophy, 235
Anderson, L. A., 164
Annas, George, 77–78, 80, 244n6
Annison, M. H., 161
Anthropology, 30
Antirealism, 235
Antonovsky, A., 218
Appelbaum, P. S., 75, 77, 264n7
Aristotle, 86, 240–241, 249n6
Arnold, R. M., 206

Art, 30
Atomistic self, 86, 117
  choice and, 87–88
  Kant and, 100
  Locke and, 88–92
  Transcendentalism and, 90–95
Austin, John, 235, 237
Autonomous authorization, 135–136,
  152
Autonomy, 4–5, 20–21, 157–158,
  251n1, 263n2
  American Medical Association and,
  72–74
  atomistic self and, 86–95, 100,
  117
  beneficence and, 18–19, 24–25,
  59–60
  chemo-brain effects and, 143–144
  choice and, 83–84, 97–98, 100, 112
  (*see also* Choice)
  commercialism and, 90
  communitarianism and, 259n12
  competence and, 142–143
  definition of, 83–85, 127
  desire for, 14–15
  dignity and, 16, 57, 76–82m,
  189–202, 219–231
  disease identifiers and, 43, 62
  doctor-patient relationship and,
  62–82
  dominant desires and, 128–132
  employee health plans and, 163
  enhancement of, 160–161

Autonomy (cont.)
  Enlightenment and, 58, 68, 70,
    112–113
  fiduciary expansion and, 151–155
  Frankfurt-Dworkin model and, 121,
    129–131, 133, 142, 144
  government and, 60
  independence and, 89–90, 94–95,
    98, 112–123
  informed consent and, 59–60,
    65–68, 74–78 (*see also* Informed
    consent)
  integrity view of, 149
  Kant and, 97–98, 100–101,
    105–107, 260n12
  legal issues and, 15–16, 137–145
    (*see also* Legal issues)
  Locke and, 88–92
  loss of, 47
  mandatory, 140
  Master-Slave schema and, 115–116
  Mill and, 108–112
  minimalism and, 103–104
  moral space and, 17, 75
  optional, 140
  paternalism and, 25, 57–58, 65–67,
    139–140
  philosophy and, 68–69
  physical fitness and, 15
  physician authority and, 60
  plasticity of, 126
  pluralism and, 60–61
  politics and, 60
  post–World War II era and, 16
  principled, 105–107
  prophylaxis argument and, 140–141
  protection of, 15
  Ramsey and, 79
  rational self and, 95–100
  relationship and, 94–95, 115–117,
    120–123
  religion and, 16–17, 93–94
  requirements of, 160–161
  responsibility and, 16–19
  salvaging of, 127–133
  sanctity of life and, 16

  schizophrenia and, 47–48
  self-examination and, 128
  selfhood and, 86–88 (*see also*
    Selfhood)
  socialization and, 128
  standards for, 125–127
  technology and, 14–15
  trust and, 160–161 (*see also*
    Trust)
  utilitarianism and, 108–112
  varying degrees of, 125

Bacon, Francis, 36, 38, 252n6
Baier, Annette, 122, 168, 170,
    179–180, 212
Baier, Kurt, 122
Baker, R., 68–70
Bakhtin, Mikhail, 241
Baldwin, D. C., 206
Balint, M., 57, 81
Barbour, Allen, 193, 195, 198
Bar codes, 49
Barondess, J., 191
Barzansky, B., 207
Bayesian inference, 52–53
Beauchamp, Tom, 153–154, 238
  doctor-patient relationship and,
    65–66, 75–77
  moral epistemology and, 24, 158,
    181
  patient rights and, 135–136, 152
Beckman, H. B., 196, 200
Beecher, Henry, 80
Bellah, Robert N., 91
Belmont Report, 80
Benbassat, J., 214
Bender, C. M., 143
Beneficence, 21, 24–25, 140, 245n8
  competence and, 264n7
  proactive role and, 191–202
  selfhood and, 59–60
Beneficence-in-trust, 18–19
Ben Gurion University, 270n4
Benn, S. I., 128
Benson, J., 164, 167
Berkeley, George, 36

Berlin, Isaiah, 127
Bernstein, J., 206
Berwick, Donald M., 161
Beyond Good and Evil (Nietzsche),
    94
Biopsychosocial model
  vs. biomedical model, 193–202
  description of, 193–194
  empathy and, 199–200
  Engel and, 193–194
  moral elements of, 194–197
  pathography and, 197–198
  selfhood and, 200–202
Bissonette, R., 204
Blank, L., 163
Blendon, R., 163–164, 167
Bodenheimer, T., 163
Boorse, Christopher, 31, 33, 35
Branch, W. T., Jr., 200
Brock, Daniel, 149–151
Brody, Howard, 28, 81, 149
Brook, B., 32
Brown, T. M., 194
Bryullov, 240
Buchanan, A., 162
Burkemper, J., 211
Burns, C., 74
Bush, George W., 232
Butler, J., 104
Butzow, J. J., 225

Cabot, Richard C., 74–75
Cadavers, 203
Cahill, M. T., 6, 155, 162
Callahan, Daniel, 16–17, 32, 53
Calvinism, 257n5
Camenisch, P. E., 16
Campbell, A. T., 164
Canguilhem, George, 14, 33, 131
Canterbury v. Spence, 76
Caplan, A. L., 33
Carlton, W., 214, 218
Carmel, J., 206
Cartesianism, 38–40
Cartwright, Nancy, 45
Cassell, Eric, 11–12, 49, 191, 198

Causal-network description, 35
Cavell, Stanley, 235, 237
Chambers, Todd, 271n5
Chance, 102–103
Chapman H. H., 194
Chapman, J. E., 194
Character, 241, 275n2
Charon, Rita, 197
Charter on Medical Professionalism,
    163, 254n15
Chemo-brain effects, 143–144
Chevalier, Michel, 90
Childress, James, 24, 151–154, 238
Choice, 201, 224–225, 243n2
  chemo-brain effects and, 143–144
  coercion and, 136
  competence and, 142–144
  context and, 143–145
  delegation of, 142–143
  deliberative model and, 134
  doctors' expertise and, 125
  dominant desires and, 128–132
  drug effects and, 143
  employee health plans and, 163
  enlistment and, 129–130
  Frankfurt-Dworkin model and, 121,
    129–131, 133, 142, 144
  Hume and, 101–105
  informed consent and, 74–76,
    135–136, 152, 159, 254n14 (*see
    also* Informed consent)
  interpretative model and, 134
  Kant and, 97–98, 100, 102–103
  Mill and, 108–112
  passions and, 101–102
  prophylaxis argument and, 140–141
  propositional attitude and, 153–154
  Protestantism and, 93–94
  psychological factors and, 138–139
  risk and, 139, 176–177
  selfhood and, 87–88, 112
  socialization process and, 128
Christman, J., 129
"Circles" (Emerson), 93, 256n4
Citizenship, 88–89
Civil disobedience, 92

Civil rights advocates, 71
Clement, Grace, 119–120, 122
Code, Lorraine, 118
Code of Medical Ethics, 72–74
Cody, J., 205, 214
Coercion, 63, 136
Cognitive science, 127–128
Coleridge, Samuel Taylor, 90
Collegial model, 177
Commercialism, 90
Communitarianism, 5, 16, 60,
    259n12
  civil society and, 183–184
  moral categories and, 181–185
  republicanism and, 182
  trust and, 181–188
Competence, 133–134, 142–144,
    152–154, 264n7
Complementary and alternative
    medicine (CAM), 247n5
Complimentary identities, 87–88
Compulsion, 102–103
Confessions of a Medicine Man
    (Tauber), 7–8, 16, 17, 18, 59, 148,
    175, 176, 228, 229, 238, 241,
    270n2
Confidence, 166–167
Consent-seeking, 59–60, 65–66
Contract model, 7, 163, 170,
    177–179
"Contrast of Individualistic and
    Social Theories of the Self, A"
    (Mead), 86
Cooper, Richard A., 216–217
Core self. *See* Atomistic self
Coulehan, J. L., 199–200
Cousins, Norman, 198
Covenant model, 178–181
Critique of Pure Reason (Kant),
    258n9
Cuff, P. A., 29, 216
Cull, A., 143
Culver, C. M., 209
*Current Opinions of the Judicial
    Council* (AMA), 77
Cutter, M. A. G., 53

Darwin, Charles, 68
Daston, Lorraine, 30, 40
Davidoff, F., 193
Davis, K., 163
Decision-analysis programs, 52–53
Decision theory, 210–211
Dedrick, R. F., 164
Defining Issues Test, 212
Delbanco, Thomas L., 57, 200
Deliberative model, 134
Delkeskamp-Haycs, C., 53
Democracy, 4, 165–166
Descartes, René, 38–39, 86–87, 92
Desensitization, 203–205
De Sorbière, 67
Detachment, 2, 202–203
Determinism, 44–45, 94, 102–103,
    127–128
Dewey, John, 109, 235, 255n1
Diagnosis
  biomedical vs. biopsychosocial
    models, 193–202
  conceptual framework for, 191–202
  conversation and, 193–202
  economic issues and, 227–228
  empathy and, 199–200, 228–229
  healing mind and, 199
  likelihood ratios and, 52
  listening and, 196
  person-centered, 195–196
  QALY and, 250n10
  quality of life and, 53–54
  test interpretation and, 51–52
  underlying principles for, 217–218
  whole person and, 192–193
Dialectical synthesis, 114–115
Dienst, E. R., 144
Diggins, John P., 109, 255n1
Dignity, 16, 189
  bedside manner reform and,
    219–231
  conceptual framework for, 191–202
  doctor-patient relationship and, 57,
    76
  informed consent and, 77–78
  social context for, 78–82

Disease, 11–12
bar codes and, 49
biomedical vs. biopsychosocial
models, 193–202
character of, 31–32
choice delegation and, 142–143
defined, 49
diagnosis framework for, 191–202
human genome and, 246n3
vs. illness, 191–192
medical model and, 191–192
pathography and, 197–198
as patient identifier, 43, 62
positivism and, 31–32
psychosocial approach to, 22
social values and, 32
symptoms and, 49–50
value judgments and, 33–36
"Divinity School Address, The"
(Emerson), 90
Doctor-patient relationship, 158. *See
also* Physicians
ambivalence in, 61–62
American Medical Association and,
72–76
biomedical vs. biopsychosocial
models, 193–202
Code of Medical Ethics and, 72–74
collaboration and, 57
collegial model and, 177
commodity sharing and, 63–65
conceptions of, 65–78
contract model and, 177–179
conversation and, 193–202
covenant model and, 178–181
cultural context for, 72
decision making and, 71
dependency and, 57, 62–63
dialogue limits and, 191–192
dignity and, 57, 76
disclosure and, 65–67
educational effects on, 63–64, 68–69
engineering model and, 177
as equal partners, 62–63
game theory and, 172–176
Gregory and, 68–70

hearing the patient and, 192–193
hospital turf and, 63
informed consent and, 59–60,
65–68 (*see also* Informed consent)
knowledge issues and, 63–65
MacIntyre and, 57, 61–62
paternalism and, 25, 57–58, 65–67
priestly model and, 177
pro-active role and, 191–202
professionalization and, 64
provider-client relationship and, 62,
162
pseudo-identities and, 62
risk and, 176–177
social context for, 78–82
trust and, 59–62 (*see also* Trust)
Veatch-May study and, 177–178
Doctor's Dilemma, The (Shaw), 61
Donnelly, William, 271n5
Dowie, J., 31
Dualisms, 38–39
Dubler, N. N., 162
DuBois, J. M., 211
Duffy, J., 72, 74
Dugan, Daniel, 219, 272n7
Durkheim, Emil, 184–185
"Duties of Physicians to Their Patients"
(Code of Medical Ethics), 73
Duty, 73, 129–130
Dworkin, Gerald, 129. *See also*
Frankfurt-Dworkin model
Dworkin, Ronald, 149

Economic issues, 3, 126, 266n1
administration costs and, 162–163
alternative medicine and, 247n5
coverage restrictions and, 162
disease bar codes and, 49
employee health plans and, 163
game theory and, 172–176
insurance and, 6, 162–163,
173–174, 250n10
malpractice awards, 79–80
patient choice and, 6
reform and, 227–228
soft money, 48

Education, 22–24, 150, 270n4
  biopsychosocial model and,
    193–202
  content surveys and, 211–212
  current status of, 202–213
  Defining Issues Test and, 212
  desensitization and, 203–205
  detachment and, 2, 202–203
  doctor idolization and, 203
  doctor-patient relationship and,
    63–64, 68–69
  ethics and, 205–213
  evaluation of, 212–213
  faculty selection and, 212
  Hidden Curriculum and, 204–205
  informed consent and, 59–60,
    65–68
  laboratory-based approach and, 27
  motivating passion of, 206
  neutral standards for, 209–210
  objectivity and, 29, 202–203
  pathography and, 197–198
  pluralism and, 208–209
  positivism and, 29–46
  professional discipline and, 63–64
  prophylaxis argument and,
    140–141
  reform and, 4, 205–219, 229–231
  responsibility and, 198–199
  ripple effects in, 196
  Socratic method and, 211
  trust and, 4–5, 167
  underlying principles for, 217–218
  uniformity and, 211
Effective consent, 135–136
Egalitarianism, 95–100
Ego, 95–100
Ehrenreich, B., 32
Eisenberg, David, 247n5
Elliott, C., 24
Elstein, A., 3
Emanuel, E. J., 5–6, 134, 162
Emanuel, L. L., 5–6, 134
Emanuel Medical Center (EMC),
    272n7
Emerson, Caryl, 274n1

Emerson, Ralph Waldo, 111–114,
    256nn2–4
  selfhood and, 90–95
  Transcendentalism and, 90–95
Emotions, 30, 103–105, 263n1
  bedside manner and, 219–231
  case studies and, 146–148
  chemo-brain effects and, 143–144
  choice delegation and, 142–143
  desensitization and, 203–205
  dominant desires and, 128–132
  empathy, 27–31, 199–200, 228–229
  Frankfurt-Dworkin model and, 121,
    129–131
  healing mind and, 199
  Hume and, 101–102
  medical reform and, 213–231
  Mill and, 108–109
  psychosocial model and, 193–202
  sensitive approach and, 190
Empathy, 27–31, 199–200, 228–229
Empiricism, 235
Engel, George, 193–194
Engelhardt, Tristram, 16, 53, 110,
    142–143
Engineering model, 177
English, D., 32
Enlightenment, 58, 68, 70, 97, 183,
    252n6
  Hume and, 101
  objectivity and, 112–113
  principled autonomy and, 107
  selfhood and, 112–113
Enlistment, 129–130
*Essay on the History of Civil Society,
    An* (Ferguson), 183
Ethical Concerns record, 23,
    220–221, 231, 272n7
Ethics, 122–123, 232–233. *See also*
    Autonomy, Choice, *Confessions of
    a Medicine Man*, Moral
    epistemology, Patient rights,
    Philosophy, Responsibility
  action-based, 79
  American Medical Association and,
    72–74

Anglo-American, 68–72
Aristotle and, 240, 275n2
autonomy and, 14–15, 60–61, 85
  (*see also* Autonomy)
bedside manner and, 219–231
beneficence and, 21
care attitude and, 59
Charter on Medical Professionalism
  and, 163
Code of Medical Ethics and, 72–74
commitment and, 18
conceptual framework for, 191–202
conflict resolution and, 53–54
contract model and, 7, 163, 170,
  177–179
doctor-patient relationship and,
  57–58 (*see also* Doctor-patient
  relationship)
education and, 202–213
emergence of, 58–59
Enlightenment and, 58
European, 68
as formal discipline, 58
game theory and, 172–176
Gregory and, 68–70
groundwork for, 172–176
Hippocratic Oath and, 4
HMOs and, 81
human rights and, 4–5
informed consent and, 59–60,
  65–66, 77–78, 136–137 (*see also*
  Informed consent)
judicial-commercial context and, 61
justifications and, 13
Kant and, 84, 95–100, 105–107
Kennedy hearings and, 79
legal issues and, 16–17
medical records and, 221–226
medical reform and, 213–231
metaphysics for, 7
Mondale hearings and, 79
moral epistemology and, 7–8
ordinary, 235–238
paternalism and, 25, 57–58
Percival and, 68–73
pluralism and, 60–61

positivism and, 29–46
principlism, 24–25, 245n9
public relations and, 1–2
quality of life and, 53–54
Ramsey and, 79
religion and, 16–17, 58
responsibility and, 17–19
Rush and, 68–70
secularization of, 16–17
technology and, 58
theories of, 237–238
time and, 2–3
underlying principles for, 217–218
value judgments and, 33–36
Etzel, S., 207
Evans, J. H., 78
Existentialism, 235
"Experience" (Emerson), 114
Expressivist turn, 113

Fact-value distinction, 9–14, 19–20,
  36ff, 55. *See also* Knowledge
disease bar codes and, 49
Goethe and, 37
inductive method and, 36
interpretation and, 37–39
likelihood ratios and, 52
moral epistemology and, 36–42,
  46–53
need and, 53–54
observation and, 36–42
patient needs and, 53–56
positivism and, 36–42
processing and, 38
test interpretation and, 51–52
typology for, 46–53
worldview building and, 37–39
Faden, Ruth, 65–66, 75–77,
  135–136, 158
Fadiman, A., 32
Feinberg, Joel, 52, 127, 264n5
Feinstein, Alvan, 52
Feminism, 71, 237–238, 262n16
*Feminist Approach to Ethics and
  Moral Education, A* (Noddings),
  262n16

Ferguson, Adam, 183
Fiction of Bioethics, The (Chambers), 271n5
Filene, P. G., 76
Fineberg, Harvey V., 52
Fischbach, Ruth L., 57
Fischer, D. H., 93
Fissel, M. E., 69–70
Fletcher, Joseph, 16, 58
Flexner Report of 1910, 29
Foss, Laurence, 247n4
Foucault, Michel, 27, 32, 80
Fox, Renée C., 60
Frankel, R. M., 193, 196, 200, 222
Frankena, W. K., 238
Frankfurt, Harry, 129, 263n1. See also Frankfurt-Dworkin model
Frankfurt-Dworkin model, 121, 129–133, 142, 144, 201, 263n3
Freedom. *See also* Choice
  duty and, 129–130
  Hume and, 101–105
  Kant and, 95–105
Freeman, V. G., 6, 55, 162
Freud, Sigmund, 104, 127–128
Frost, N., 14
Fukuyama, Francis, 163, 165

Galaty, David H., 41
Galen, 24
Galileo, 252n6
Galison, Peter, 45
Gallup surveys, 167
Game theory, 172–176
Gauthier, David, 170
Gender, 51
Geyer-Kordesch, J., 68
Gilligan, Carol, 118–119, 212, 262n16
Glick, Shimon, 214, 230
God, 69, 92–95, 114, 256n4, 257n5
Goethe, Johann Wolfgang von, 37
Goldie, J., 206–211, 230
Good, 91, 100
Good, D. 32, 168
Goold, S. D., 163

Gorawara-Bhat, R., 200
Gougeon, Len, 91
Government, 4, 60
Govier, T., 170
Gray, T., 109
Great Society, 79
Gregory, John, 68–70, 253nn11, 12
Grisso, T., 264n7
Grodin, Michael A., 80
Grunbaum, Adolph, 194

Haakonssen, Knud, 269n11
Haakonssen, Lisbeth, 58, 68–70, 253nn11, 12,
Hall, Mark, 164, 169–170
Halpern, J., 199, 216
Hardin, Russell, 170–171, 187
Harvan, R. A., 206
Harvey, J. C., 154
Haskins v. Howard, 75
Hastings Center, 78
Hay, C., 143
Hayry, M., 53
Health care, 8
  administration costs and, 162–163
  biomedical vs. biopsychosocial models, 193–202
  bureaucratic effects and, 62
  Cabot and, 74–75
  as commodity, 126, 154–155
  context of care and, 43
  contract model and, 7, 163, 170, 177–179
  covenant model and, 178–181
  current state of, 1
  disease/illness dichotomy and, 49–50
  dyad of, 160–161
  employee health plans and, 163
  forced procedures and, 149
  HMOs and, 81, 162, 179
  humanist/technocrat dichotomy and, 48–49
  likelihood ratios and, 52
  medical records and, 23, 221–226, 231, 272n7
  mistrust and, 4–7

need and, 53–54
paternalism and, 57, 65–67
prophylaxis argument and, 140–141
psychosocial approach to, 22
reform of, 226–231 (*see also* Reform)
responsibility and, 17–19
sensitivity and, 3
success criteria and, 50–51
test interpretation and, 51–52
Health maintenance organizations
    (HMOs), 81, 162, 179
Hegel, Georg Wilhelm Friedrich,
    114–116
Heidegger, Martin, 172, 235
Helmholtz, Hermann, 41
Heraclitus, 236
Herman, Barbara, 99–100, 105, 112,
    171
Herzlinger, Regina, E. 155, 168
Hidden Curriculum, 204–205
Hippocrates, 4, 64–67, 251n4
Hippocratic Oath, 4
Holism, 11, 21–22, 42–44, 215,
    246n2
Hollender, M. H., 62–63
Hollis, M., 170
Holmes, Oliver Wendell, 264n7
Hook, Sidney, 194
Howell, J. D., 206
"How Medicine Saved the Life of
    Ethics" (Toulmin), 243n3
Human experimentation, 80–81
Humanists, 19, 30, 48–49, 58–59, 68
Human rights, 4–5, 71
  informed consent and, 59–60,
    65–66, 136–137 (*see also* Informed
    consent)
  insurance and, 6
  Japanese experiments and, 80
  Nazi experiments and, 80
  patient choice and, 6
  responsibilities and, 17–19
  Tuskegee syphilis study and, 80
Hume, David, 20, 130, 178–179
  autonomy and, 84, 114
  centrality of reason and, 101–102

compulsion and, 102–103
doctor-patient relationship and,
    68–69
Kant and, 101–105
liberty and, 102–103
Mill and, 108
moral epistemology and, 36–37
selfhood and, 95–96, 101–105
trust and, 171
Hume's law, 36–37
Hunter, K. M., 197
Hunt v. Bradshaw, 75
Husserl, Edmund, 235
Hyams, T. S., 167
Hypertension, 51

Idealism, 235
Identity. *See* Selfhood
Illich, Ivan, 80
Illingworth, P., 163
Illness
  biomedical vs. biopsychosocial
    models, 193–202
  conceptual framework for, 191–202
  defined, 49
  vs. disease, 191–192
  genetic determinism and, 44–45
  individualism and, 192
  pathography and, 197–198
  reductionism and, 41–45
  symptoms and, 49–50
  treatment framework for, 191–202
  value judgments and, 33–36
Impartial spectator, 184
In a Different Voice (Gilligan), 262n16
Independence, 89–90
  interdependence and, 121–123
  prevailing sense of, 112–120
  relationship and, 94–95, 120–123
  self-legislation and, 98
Individualism, 5, 118. *See also*
    Autonomy, Selfhood
  communitarianism and, 259n12
  Emerson and, 90–95
  illness treatment and, 192
  impartial spectator and, 184

Individualism (cont.)
Locke and, 88–92
Mill and, 108–112
relationship and, 94–95, 120–123
responsibility and, 119–120
Thoreau and, 92
Transcendentalism and, 90–95
trust and, 165–166
U.S. Constitution and, 89–90
Inductive method, 36
Informed consent, 159
autonomous authorization and,
135–136, 152
Cabot and, 74–75
Canterbury v. Spence and, 76
coercion and, 136
coining of term, 254n14
common law of torts and, 135
competence and, 133–134, 210,
264n7
constitutional protections of, 76–78
delegation of choice and, 141–142
deliberative model and, 134
De Sorbière and, 67–68
doctor-patient relationship and,
59–60, 65–68
effective consent and, 135–136
fiduciary expansion and, 151–155
Haskins v. Howard and, 75
Hunt v. Bradshaw and, 75
In re Quinlan and, 76–77
interpretative model and, 134
life decisions and, 140
presentation of, 146–149
as propositional attitude, 153–154
*Salgo v. Leland Stanford Jr.
University Board of Trustees* and,
76
*Schloendorff v. The Society of the
New York Hospital* and, 75
social context for, 77–82
as stopgap, 126
In Quest of the Ordinary (Cavell), 237
Institute of Medicine, 161
Institutio Orztoria (Quintilian),
268n8

Instrumentalism, 8–9
Insurance, 250n10
choice and, 6
coverage restrictions and, 162
employee health plans and, 163
game theory and, 173–174
Interpretative model, 134
Intimacy, 3
Intimidation, 63

Jacob, M. C., 87
Jacobson, P. D., 6, 155, 162, 179
Jakobovits, I., 58
James, William, 244n4, 247n5
Japanese experiments, 80
Jargon, 141–142
Johnson, A. G., 211
Johnson, Lyndon B., 5
Johnson, Tom, 272n7
Jones, H., 80, 170
Jonsen, Albert, 16, 24, 58, 75, 78,
272n7
Justice, 98–99, 118–119, 262n17,
264n7

Kahneman, Daniel, 138
Kant, Immanuel, 20, 130–131, 184,
237–238
autonomy and, 84, 105–107, 111,
114, 119
choice and, 97–98, 100
Good and, 100
Hume and, 101–105
moral epistemology and, 95–100
natural world and, 258n9
rational self and, 95–100
religion and, 97
selfhood and, 257n7
self-legislation and, 98
trust and, 171
Kao, A. C., 6, 55, 162
Karlawish, J., 225
Katz, Jay, 105
doctor-patient relationship and,
65–67, 71, 74–75, 81
reform and, 197–201

Kelly, D. F., 58
Kennedy hearings, 79
Kennedy Institute, 78
Kerridge, I. H., 11
Kierkegaard, Søren, 114, 261n13
Kirmayer, L. J., 32
Kirschner, Suzanne R., 93
Kleinman, Arthur, 32, 49
Knowledge, 210, 246n1
  Bayesian inference and, 52–53
  biopsychosocial model and,
    193–202
  Code of Medical Ethics and, 72–74
  coercion and, 136
  collaboration and, 57
  competence and, 64–65
  comprehension and, 136
  deliberative model and, 134
  disclosure and, 65–66
  discussion degrees and, 144
  disease/illness dichotomy and, 49–50
  doctor-patient relationship and,
    62–82
  doctors' expertise and, 125
  dualisms and, 38–40
  Goethe and, 37
  Gregory and, 68–70
  impartial spectator and, 184
  inductive method and, 36
  informed consent and, 59–60,
    65–68, 74–78
  interpretative model and, 134
  Kant and, 95–100
  medical jargon and, 141–142
  medical records and, 221–226
  objectivity and, 36–42
  observation and, 36–42
  pathography and, 197–198
  positivism and, 29–46
  presentation of, 146–149
  private mind and, 39
  professionalization and, 64
  prophylaxis argument and, 140–141
  QALY and, 250n10
  risk-aversion and, 138–139
  self, 201

sharing of, 63–65
success criteria and, 50–51
test interpretation and, 51–52
value effects and, 46–53
worldview building and, 37–39
Kohlberg, Lawrence, 206, 212
Kolakowski, Leszek, 29
Kopelman, Loretta M., 205, 208
Korsgaard, Christine, 99, 105, 112,
  171
Kramer, P. A., 143
Kurtz, P. W., 53

Labor, 71
Lagerspetz, O., 170
Lahno, B., 170
Laine, C., 193
Lamb, J., 200
Lammers, S. E., 16
Landau, Richard, 202–203
Langewitz, W., 196
Lasagna, Louis, 11–12
LaTour, K., 143
Layman, E., 211–213
Lectures (Gregory), 69
Legal issues, 4, 7, 25, 61, 125, 244n6
  autonomy and, 15–16
  Bill of Rights and, 244n6
  Canterbury v. Spence and, 76
  case studies and, 145–151
  common law of torts and, 135
  competence and, 264n7
  constitutional protections and,
    76–78
  Declaration of Independence and,
    244n6
  fiduciary expansion and, 151–155,
    245n7
  forced procedures and, 149
  Haskins v. Howard and, 75
  Hunt v. Bradshaw and, 75
  informed consent and, 59–60,
    65–68, 74–78, 136–137, 254n14
  Quinlan and, 76–77
  malpractice, 19–20, 58, 79–80, 126,
    134–136

Legal issues (cont.)
  paradigms in, 137–145
  Salgo v. Leland Stanford Jr.
    University Board of Trustees and,
    76
  Schloendorff v. The Society of the
    New York Hospital and, 75
  Tuskegee syphilis study and, 80
Lehmann, Lisa S., 211–212
Levi, B. H., 149, 208
Levinson, W., 200
Liberty, 102–103, 105, 122
Lidz, C. W., 75, 77
Life decisions, 76–77, 140, 143,
  146–148. *See also* Choice
Lindley, R., 37, 83, 102–103, 129
Lo, B., 225, 227
Locke, John, 20, 36–39, 68, 88–92,
  252n5
Løgstrup, Knud E., 157
Love, S. B., 143
Luhmann, Niklas, 166–168, 267n6
Lukes, S., 93

McCullough, Laurence, 68–69, 181
McDaniel, S. H., 193, 196, 222
McDonald, C. J., 51
McElhinney, T. K., 206–208
Macfarlane, A., 93
MacIntyre, Alsadair, 57, 61–62
Mackenzie, Catherine, 104, 132, 238,
  263n1
McKinlay, 161
McNeil, S. J., 61, 139
MacPherson, C. B., 89
Malpractice, 19–20, 126, 134
  doctor-patient relationship and,
    79–80
  effective consent and, 135–136
  ethics and, 58
  negligence and, 135
Marceau, L. D., 161
Mariner, Wendy, 163
Marvel, M. K., 196
Marx, Karl, 94
Massachusetts General Hospital, 74

Master-Slave schema, 115–116
Matthews, D. A., 200
May, William, 59, 73, 177–178
Mead, George Herbert, 86, 94, 104,
  255n1
Mechanic, David, 6, 162, 168
Medicaid, 250n10
Medical Ethics (Percival), 70, 72–73
Medical records, 222–226, 271n6
  ethical concerns and, 23, 220–221,
    231, 272n7
Medicine
  biomedical vs. biopsychosocial
    models, 193–202
  as caring art, 28
  context of care and, 43
  economic issues and, 3 (*see also*
    Economic issues)
  evidence-based, 249n8
  Flexner Report of 1910 and, 29
  Gregory and, 68–70
  holistic approach and, 11, 21–22,
    42–44, 215, 246n2
  human evaluation and, 33–34
  illness treatment and, 192
  as industry, 80–81
  interpretation and, 32
  laboratory-based approach and, 27
  mistrust and, 4–7
  as moral epistemology, 27–56 (*see*
    also Moral epistemology)
  need and, 53–54
  neutrality and, 34
  objectivity and, 36–42
  observation and, 36–42
  pathography and, 197–198
  positivism and, 29–46
  psychosocial approach to, 22
  reform of, 4 (*see also* Reform)
  scientific character of, 29–36
  selection argument and, 247n5
  social values and, 32
  test interpretation and, 51–52
  time and, 2–3
  value judgments and, 33–36
  Western development of, 27

Meier, D. E., 225
Meisel, A., 75, 77
Merleu-Ponty, Maurice, 235
Merton, Robert K., 87
Metaphysics, 235
  Transcendentalism and, 90–95
Meyers, D. T., 117, 125
Miaskowski, C. M., 143
Miles, S. H., 209–210
Mill, John Stuart, 20, 84, 108–112,
  131, 259n11
Misztal, Barbara, 165, 186–187,
  269n12
Mitchell, K. R., 211
Mitsein (Olefson), 239
Momeyer, R. W., 150
Mondale hearings, 79
Montello, M., 197
Moore, Francis D., 154
Moral epistemology, 3, 7–8, 20,
  55–56, 240–241
  atomistic self and, 86–95
  autonomous authorization and,
    135–136 (*see also* Autonomy)
  bedside manner reform and,
    219–231
  biopsychosocial model and,
    194–197
  caring arts and, 28
  Cartesianism and, 38–39
  competence and, 142–143
  Defining Issues Test and, 212
  disease model and, 11–12
  effective consent and, 135–136
  egalitarianism and, 95–100
  empathy and, 27–29
  Enlightenment and, 68
  fact-value distinction and, 9–14,
    36–42, 46–53
  hearing the patient and, 192–193
  Hidden Curriculum and, 204–205
  HMOs and, 81
  humanist/technocrat dichotomy and,
    48–49
  Hume and, 101–105
  impartial spectator and, 184

  informed consent and, 59–60,
    65–68, 76–78, 136–137
  interpretation and, 37–39
  justifications and, 13
  Kant and, 95–105
  Locke and, 88–89
  medicine's character and, 29–36
  need and, 53–54
  objectivity and, 12–14
  positivism and, 27, 36–46
  proactive role and, 191–202
  Rawls and, 98–99
  reciprocity and, 182
  reductionism and, 42–46
  sanctity of life and, 16
  secularization of, 16–17
  sensitive approach and, 190
  solitude and, 91–92
  Transcendentalism and, 90–95
  trust and, 181–185 (*see also* Trust)
  Tuskegee syphilis study and, 80
  value judgments and, 33–36
  World War II era and, 80
Morreim, Haavi, 140, 163
Morris, D., 197–198
Morson, Gary Soul, 241, 274n1
Murphy, Edmond A., 31, 34,
  167–168, 225
Myser, C., 211

Nagel, Thomas, 88
Natural philosophy, 88
Nature (Emerson), 90–91
Nazis, 80
Necessity, 102–103
Need, 53–56
Negligence, 135
Nelson, J. L., 197
Neo-Harringtonians, 182
New Jersey Supreme Court, 76
Newman, Mark, 270n2
Newton, Isaac, 88
Nietzsche, Friedrich Wilhelm, 94,
  110, 171, 241
Nixon, Richard M., 5
Niyonsenga, T., 204

Noddings, Nel, 262n16
Nonconformity, 112
Nordenfelt, L., 8, 35
Nurses, 139–140, 167, 204–205
Nussbaum, Martha, 199

Objectivity, 12–14, 81
  education and, 202–203
  Enlightenment and, 112–113
  Goethe and, 37
  managed-care surveillance and,
    55–56
  observation and, 36–42
  positivism and, 29–42
"Obligations of Patients to Their
  Physicians" (Code of Medical
  Ethics), 73
Observation, 36–42
Olafson, Frederick A., 172, 239
Oliver, James, 198–199
O'Neill, Onora, 17–18, 159, 171
  autonomy and, 105–107, 117
  patient rights and, 144, 151, 153
On Liberty (Mill), 108, 111
Oregon, 250n10
Osler, William, 59

Parmenides, 236
Patenaude, J., 204
Paternalism, 25, 57, 65, 139–140
  forced procedures and, 149
  Hippocrates and, 66–67
  Katz and, 66–67
Pathography, 197–198
Patient as Person, The (Ramsey),
  79
Patient rights, 157–158
  autonomous authorization and,
    135–136 (*see also* Autonomy)
  coercion and, 136
  competence and, 142–144, 149–152
  comprehension issues and, 136
  as conceit, 125
  effective consent and, 135–136
  forced procedures and, 149
  formal affirmation of, 79

informed consent and, 77–78, 126
  (*see also* Informed consent)
intention protection and, 135–136
physician dismissal, 140
prophylaxis argument and, 140–141
trust and, 147–149
Tuskegee syphilis study and, 80
Patients. *See also* Doctor-patient
  relationship, Physicians
alternative choices for, 47
autonomy and, 14–15 (*see also*
  Autonomy)
bedside manner reform and,
  219–231
biomedical vs. biopsychosocial
  models, 193–202
choice and, 6 (*see also* Choice)
as clients, 62, 162
clinical paternalism and, 25, 57
commitment to, 18
competence and, 210, 264n7
conceptions of, 60–65
as consumers, 60, 159
context of care and, 43
contract model and, 7
coverage restrictions and, 162
curing aspirations and, 158
decision making and, 71
dehumanization of, 141–142
dignity and, 1, 16, 25, 57, 76, 78
  (*see also* Dignity)
disease identifiers and, 62, 219
disease/illness dichotomy and, 49–50
employee health plans and, 163
healing facilitation and, 158
informed consent and, 59–60,
  65–68, 74–78
intimacy and, 3
listening to, 196
managed-care surveillance and,
  55–56
medical history of, 192, 271n5
medical jargon and, 141–142
medical model and, 191–192
moral space of, 17
need and, 53–56

positivism and, 27
quality of life and, 53–54
reassurance of, 160
risk and, 176–177
sanctity of life and, 16
values and, 47
whole person and, 192–193
Payer, Lynn, 32
Peabody, Francis, 59
Pearson, S. D., 164
Pellegrino, Edmund, 18–19, 154, 238
autonomy and, 117
doctor-patient relationship and, 65
moral epistemology and, 25, 50
reform and, 206–209, 224, 228
Percival, Thomas, 68–70, 253n12
Pernick, Martin, 65
Pharmacists, 167
Phenomenology, 115, 235
Phenomenology of Spirit, The
(Hegel), 115
Philosophy, 24, 114, 132–133. *See
also* Autonomy, Choice, Ethics,
Moral epistemology, Specific
philosophers
communitarianism, 259n12
defining, 235–241
determinism, 44–45, 94, 102–103,
127–128
dualism and, 38–40
egalitarianism and, 95–100
Enlightenment and, 58, 68, 70, 97,
101, 107, 112–113, 183, 252n6
facts vs. values, 9–14
impartial spectator and, 184
instrumentalism and, 8–9
language and, 235
liberal democracy and, 96
limits of, 42–46
ordinary, 235–238
pluralism and, 60–61, 95–100, 169,
208–209
positivism and, 10, 27–46 (*see also*
Positivism)
praxis and, 235–241
propositional attitude and, 153–154

reductionism, 27, 38–46, 247n4
selfhood and, 86–88 (*see also*
Selfhood)
Transcendentalism and, 90–95
truisms and, 32
utilitarianism and, 108–112
Physical fitness, 15
Physicians, 1. *See also* Patients
accountability and, 5–6, 163–164
admitting doubt and, 64–65
autonomy and, 16 (*see also*
Autonomy)
bedside manner reform and,
219–231
beneficence and, 18–19, 21
biomedical vs. biopsychosocial
models, 193–202
commitment of, 18
conflict resolution and, 53–54
context of care and, 43
deliberative model and, 134
demands upon, 5–6
desensitization of, 203–205
detachment and, 202–203
dismissal of, 140
empathy and, 199–200, 228–229
expertise of, 125
hearing the patient and, 192–193
Hidden Curriculum and, 204–205
Hippocratic Oath and, 4
as historian, 192
hospital turf and, 63
idolizing of, 203
informed consent and, 59–60,
65–68 (*see also* Informed consent)
intimacy and, 3
interpretative model and, 134
as knowledge providers, 138
listening and, 196
medical jargon and, 141–142
medical records and, 23, 220–226,
231, 272n7
motivating passion of, 206
normative theories and, 33–34
paternalism and, 25, 57, 65–67,
139–140, 149

Physicians (cont.)
  as philosophers, 24 (*see also*
    Philosophy)
  proactive role of, 191–202
  as providers, 159, 162
  pseudo-identities of, 62
  sensitivity and, 3, 190
  technical competence and, 133–134
  time schedules and, 2–3
  value judgments and, 33–36
  virtues for, 70
Physics, 33–34
Physiologists, 41
Piaget, Jean, 262n16
Pickstone, J., 68
Pluralism, 60–61, 169
  education and, 208–209
  egalitarianism and, 95–100
Policy, 5–6
  Cabot and, 74–75
  Code of Medical Ethics and, 72–74
  common law of torts and, 135
  informed consent and, 77–78, 135
    (*see also* Informed consent)
  objectivity and, 12–13
  patient needs and, 53–56
  reform and, 189 (*see also* Reform)
Politics, 4–6, 27, 113, 127, 232, 239,
    250n10
  autonomy and, 60
  doctor-patient relationship and, 72
  egalitarianism and, 95–100
  Kant and, 84
  philosophy and, 96
  pluralism and, 60–61
  selfhood and, 90
  trust and, 165–166, 182–183,
    185–188
Porn, I., 8
Porter, D., 69
Porter, R., 69
Positivism, 10, 27
  classification and, 30
  disease character and, 31–32
  empathy and, 31
  experience and, 30

fact-value distinction and, 36–42,
    46–53
  Hume's law and, 36–37
  interpretation and, 37–39
  knowledge and, 29–30
  limits of, 29–30, 42–46
  medicine's character and, 29–36
  objectivity and, 29–30
  observation and, 36–42
  social values and, 32
  subjectivity and, 29–30
  technology and, 30
  value judgments and, 33–36
Povar, G. J., 206
Pragmatism, 109–110, 235, 255n1
Preston, T., 62–63, 251n3
Priestly model, 177
Principled autonomy, 105–107
Principles of Medical Ethics (AMA),
    73–76
Principlism, 24–25, 245n9
Proctor, Robert N., 34
Professionalism, 5, 251n2, 252n9.
    See also Doctor-patient relationship
  American Medical Association and,
    72–76
  Charter on Medical
    Professionalization and, 254n15
  coercion and, 63
  competence and, 64–65
  detachment and, 2
  disunity and, 45–46
  education and, 203–204 (*see also*
    Education)
  empathy and, 27–29
  focus splitting and, 6
  hospital turf and, 63
  informed consent and, 59–60,
    65–68, 74–78, 136–137
  interpersonal skills and, 1
  intimidation and, 63
  quality of life and, 53–54
  trust and, 161 (*see also* Trust)
  value judgments and, 33–36
Professionalization, 64
Prophylaxis argument, 140–141

Propositional attitude, 153–154
Protestant Ethic and the Spirit of Capitalism, The (Weber), 257n5
Protestantism, 93–94
Psaty, B. M., 51
Psychology, 30, 35, 158
  biopsychosocial model and, 193–202
  choice effects and, 138–139
  empathy and, 199–200
  listening and, 196
  success criteria and, 50–51
  trust and, 161
  unconscious mind and, 200–201
Public relations, 1–2
Puritanism, 93, 257n5
Putnam, Hilary, 10, 37, 47, 249n6
Putnam, Robert, 165–167
Putnam, Ruth Anna, 53

Quality Adjusted Life Year (QALY), 250n10
Quality of life, 53–54
Quill, T., 193, 196, 222, 225
Quine, W. V. O., 153
Quinlan, Karen, 76–77
Quintilian, 268n8

Raeke, L. H., 164
Ramsey, Paul, 16, 79
Randomness, 102–103
Rational self, 89, 95–100, 235–237
  expressivist turn and, 113
  Mill and, 108–112
  passions and, 101–102
  principled autonomy and, 105–107
Rawls, John, 98–99, 105, 112, 171, 238, 258n10, 259n12
Reciprocity, 182
Reductionism, 27, 247n4
  Cartesian, 38–40
  dualisms and, 38–39
  genetic determinism and, 44–45
  holism and, 42–44
  impact of, 41–42

limits of, 42–46
  observation and, 36–42
Reform, 232–233
  at bedside, 219–231
  biomedical vs. biopsychosocial models, 193–202
  conceptual framework for, 191–202
  economic issues and, 227–228
  education and, 205–219, 229–231
  empathy and, 199–200
  Hidden Curriculum and, 204–205
  opposition to, 213–215, 226–231, 270n1
  records and, 221–226
  underlying principles for, 217–218
Reid, Thomas, 69
Relationships, 94–95, 117, 120–123
  doctor-patient, 57–82 (*see also* Doctor-patient relationship)
  impartial spectator and, 184
  Master-Slave schema and, 115–116
  moral categories and, 181–185
  risk and, 176–177
  trust and, 171–172
Religion, 67, 69, 78, 114, 145–146, 257nn5, 6
  autonomy and, 16–17, 93–94
  Emerson and, 90–92
  Enlightenment and, 58
  ethics and, 58
  Kant and, 97
  Locke and, 89–90
  pragmatism and, 255n1
  Protestantism and, 93–94
  Transcendentalism and, 90–95
Republicanism, 182
Responsibility, 23–24, 123
  autonomy and, 16–19
  choice and, 132
  delegation of, 133–134
  education and, 205–213
  game theory and, 172–176
  Gregory and, 69–70
  groundwork for, 172–176
  individualism and, 119–120

Responsibility (cont.)
  informed consent and, 59–60,
    65–68, 126
  morality and, 170–172
  plasticity of, 126
  reform and, 198–199
  trust and, 171
Revolutionary War, 68, 82
Richards, J. R., 128
Richman, Kenneth A., 8, 34–35, 131,
  134
Risk, 139, 176–177
Robertson, William, 68
Rodwin, Mark A., 154
Romanticism, 30, 38
  Transcendentalism and, 90–95
Roochnik, David, 207
Rorty, Richard, 109–110, 235, 237
Rose, Nikolas S., 104
Rosen, Stanley, 235–236
Roter, D. L., 200
Rothenberg, Kenneth, 247n4
Rothman, David, 1, 58, 61, 66,
  76–78, 80, 251n2
Rousseau, Jean-Jacques, 91, 111, 182
Rush, Benjamin, 68–70, 253n12

Salgo, Martin, 76, 254n14
Salgo v. Leland Stanford Jr.
  University Board of Trustees, 76
Sanctity of life, 16, 78, 80
Sandel, Michael, 4, 16, 86
Sarkar, Sahotra, 44
Savulescu, Julian, 139, 150, 206
Schaffner, Kenneth F., 45
Schagen, S. B., 144
Schizophrenia, 47–48
Schlesinger, M., 6, 162
Schloendorff v. The Society of the
  New York Hospital, 75
Schmidt, H., 196
Schneewind, Jerry, 84, 100
Schneider, Carl, 18, 125, 138,
  140–143, 157, 263n3, 264nn4, 6
Schroeder, S. A., 227
Schultz, M. M., 77

Science, 10
  aesthetic elegance and, 33
  cognitive, 127–128, 143–144
  empathy and, 27–28
  Flexner Report of 1910 and, 29
  holistic approach and, 11
  humanism and, 58–59, 68
  illness treatment and, 192
  inductive method and, 36
  Locke and, 88–89
  medicine's character and, 29–36
  natural philosophy and, 33, 68
  neutrality and, 34
  objectivity and, 29, 36–42
  observation and, 36–42
  physical, 33
  positivism and, 29–46
  theory types of, 33
  unity of, 45
  value judgment and, 33–36
  Western development of, 27
Seedhouse, D., 8
Self-determination, 118
Self, D. J., 2, 204, 206
Selfhood, 54–55, 157–158. See also
  Patients
  alterity and, 261n14
  atomistic self and, 86–95, 100,
    117
  beneficence and, 60
  biopsychosocial model and,
    200–202
  characterization of, 85
  choice and, 87–88, 93–94, 112 (see
    also Choice)
  commercialism and, 90
  community and, 60, 181–188
  complex nature and, 110–111
  complimentary identities and,
    87–88
  Descartes and, 86–87
  dialectical synthesis and, 114–115
  disease identifiers and, 43, 62
  dominant desires and, 128–132
  dualism and, 39–40
  egalitarianism and, 95–100

Emerson and, 90–95, 113–114
expressivist turn and, 113
as forensic term, 89
fulfillment and, 114
good and, 91
Hume and, 95–96, 101–105, 257n7, 258n8
independence and, 89–90, 117–118
inner ego and, 95–100
Kant and, 95–105, 257n7
Locke and, 88–92
managed-care surveillance and, 55–56
Master-Slave schema and, 115–116
Mill and, 108–112
nature-nurture dichotomy and, 44–45
as object, 115–116
passions and, 101–105 (*see also* Emotions)
pluralism and, 60–61
pragmatism and, 255n1
principled autonomy and, 105–107
process and, 115
rational self and, 89, 95–100, 113, 235–237
Rawls and, 98–99
social self and, 86–88
Thoreau and, 92
thought and, 86–87
Transcendentalism and, 90–95
trust and, 112–113
two modalities of, 86–88
utilitarianism and, 108–112
worldview and, 37–39
Self-legislation, 98
"Self-Reliance" (Emerson), 90
Seligman, Adam, 94, 107, 168–169, 182–184, 267n6
Sensitivity, 3
Shain, Barry A., 90
Shaw, George Bernard, 61
Sheehan, T. J., 206
Shem, S., 121
Shortell, S. M., 6, 162–163
Shorter, E., 32

Sickle cell patients, 49–50
Siegler, M., 272n7
Simon, W. M., 29
Singer, Peter, 244n4
Slave, 115
Smith, Adam, 68, 184, 269n11
Smith, R., 30
Sober, E., 170
Social capital, 166–167, 267n3
Social contract, 92
  Rawls and, 98–99
  trust and, 176–181
Social self, 86–88
Society for Health and Human Values, 78
Sociology, 125, 128, 158, 268n7
  doctor-patient relationship and, 62–82
  egalitarianism and, 95–100
  ethics and, 58 (*see also* Ethics)
  impartial spectator and, 184
  informed consent and, 77–78
  Locke and, 88–92
  moral epistemology and, 27, 30, 32, 35, 45–46, 181–185
  pluralism and, 208–209
  positivism and, 29–46
  private mind and, 39
  socialization effects and, 128
  success criteria and, 50–51
  Transcendentalism and, 90–95
  Tuskegee syphilis study and, 80
Socrates, 211, 236
Soft money, 48
Solitude, 91–92
Spector, J., 37
Sperry, L., 196
"Spirit" (Emerson), 93
Spiro, Howard, 2
Stack, George, J., 94
Standards
  Charter on Medical Professionalization and, 254n15
  common law of torts and, 135
  Frankfurt-Dworkin model and, 121, 129–131, 133

Standards (cont.)
  medical records and, 221–226
  neutral educational, 209–210
  trust and, 164 (*see also* Trust)
Starr, Paul, 27, 64, 73
Stephen, Leslie, 240
Stern, D., 204
Stoeckle, J. D., 62–63
Stoljar, Natalie, 104, 132, 238,
  263n1
Stump, D. J., 45
Suarez-Murias, E. L., 225
Subjectivity, 10. *See also* Selfhood
  managed-care surveillance and,
  55–56
  symptoms and, 49–50, 54
Suchman, A. L., 200
Suicide (Durkheim), 185
Sulmasy, D. P., 206
Sympathy, 200, 269n11
Symptoms, 49–50
Szasz, Thomas, 33, 62–63, 80
Sztompka, Piotr, 168, 181–182,
  268n7

Taylor, Charles, 86, 88, 113,
  115–116
Technocrats, 48–49
Technology, 1, 239
  anxiety over, 80–81
  autonomy and, 14–15
  decision-analysis programs, 52–53
  disease bar codes and, 49
  efficacy debates over, 161
  ethics and, 58
  medical jargon and, 141–142
  pathography and, 198
  positivism and, 30
Thagard, Paul, 35
Thalberg, Irving, 263n2
Theory of Justice, A (Rawls), 98–99
Theory of Moral Sentiments (Smith),
  184, 269n11
Thom, D. H., 164
Thomasma, David, 16, 18–19, 238,
  272n7

doctor-patient relationship and, 65
moral epistemology and, 25, 50
patient rights and, 154
reform and, 206, 209, 224, 228
Thoreau, Henry David, 27, 92, 111,
  235, 240, 256n3
Time, 2–3
Titchener, 199
Tocqueville, Alexis de, 90, 165–166,
  259n12
Tolstoy, Leo, 240
Toombs, S. K., 198
Torts, 135
Toulmin, Stephen, 24, 192–193, 195,
  243n3, 245n8
Transcendentalism, 90–95
Treatise of Human Nature, A
  (Hume), 36–37, 101, 179
Treatment. *See* Diagnosis
Truisms, 32
Trust, 158, 243n1
  American Medical Association and,
  72–74
  behavior regulation and, 160
  beneficence and, 18–19, 21,
  24–25
  biopyschosocial model and,
  193–202
  characterization of, 160–165
  communication and, 167–168
  community and, 181–188
  confidence and, 166–167
  contract model and, 7, 163, 170,
  177–179
  covenant model and, 178–181
  defining, 168–172
  democracy and, 165–166
  education and, 167
  employee health plans and, 163
  enhancement of, 160–161
  erosion of, 4–7, 61–62, 159,
  165–168, 267n4
  game theory and, 172–176
  groundwork for, 172–176
  HMOs and, 81, 162
  individualism and, 165–166

informed consent and, 59–60,
  65–66, 74–75, 159 (*see also*
  Informed consent)
insurance and, 162
knowledge sharing and, 63–65
modernity effects and, 185–188
moral interpretations of, 161–162,
  181–185
organic, 59–60
paradoxes in, 160–161
paternalism and, 66–67
patient rights and, 147–149
politics of, 165–166, 182–188
predicated stance and, 170
problem of, 160–165
professional confidence and, 161
psychological response and, 161
reassurance measures and, 160
relationships and, 169–172
responsibility and, 17–19, 171
risk and, 176–177
selfhood and, 112–113
skeptical stance and, 170
social capital and, 166–167
social contract and, 176–181
supportive stance and, 170
survey results of, 61–62, 167
systemic, 164
Tuskegee syphilis study and, 80
Trust and Power (Luhmann), 168
Tulsky, J., 225
Tuskegee syphilis study, 80
Tversky, Amos, 138
Twain, Mark, 74, 254n13

United States, 1
  alternative medicine and, 247n5
  American dream and, 89–90
  American Medical Association and,
    72–74
  autonomy and, 15
  commercialism and, 90
  Constitution and, 72, 89
  Declaration of Independence and,
    89, 244n6
  democracy and, 165–166

independence and, 89–90
legal issues and, 140
Locke and, 89–90
medical school surveys in, 211
optimism of, 91, 93
pluralism and, 60–61
Revolutionary War era and, 68
Transcendentalism and, 90–95
World War II era, 166
University of California at Los
  Angeles (UCLA), 1
University of Edinburgh, 68
Utilitarianism, 108–112

Values, 189, 239. *See also* Fact-value
  distinction
balance and, 9–14
Bayesian inference and, 52–53
Cabot and, 74–75
decision-analysis programs, 52–53
defining, 250n9
doctor-patient relationship and,
  57–58 (*see also* Doctor-patient
  relationship)
empathy and, 27–29
informed consent and, 59–60,
  65–68, 74–78
intimacy and, 3
judgment and, 10, 33–36
knowledge effects and, 46–53
need and, 53–54
patient choice and, 47
positivism and, 29–47
psychosocial model and, 193–202
reform and, 213–219, 226–231
science and, 10–11, 47
symptoms and, 54
test interpretation and, 51–52
typography of, 27
underlying principles for, 217–218
Vanselow, N. A., 29, 216
Veatch, Robert, 59, 149, 177–178,
  181
Verhey, A., 16
Verkerk, M., 202
Veterans Administration, 51

Veterinarians, 167
Vietnam War era, 4, 79

Wallace, R. J., 252n7
Walsh, David, 257n6
Walton, M., 189
Wartman, Steven, 149–151
Watson, Gary, 263n2
Weber, Max, 94, 257n5
Weed, Lawrence, 223–224, 271n6
Weinstein, M. C., 52
Whitbeck, Carol, 8
Wieneke, M. H., 144
Wildes, K. W., 154, 181
Wilford, D. S., 161
Williams, Bernard, 101, 110,
    170–171
Wills, G., 82
Will to Power (Nietzsche), 94
Wilson, A. N., 94
Wilson, D. S., 170
Wilson, T. D., 127, 170
Winick, B. J., 264n7
Winslade, W. J., 272n7
Winternitz, Milton, 270n1
Wispe, L., 200
Wittgenstein, Ludwig, 173, 235, 237
Wolfe, Alan,, 165
Wolinsky, F. D., 206
Wolpe, P., 58, 60–61, 159, 245n9,
    251n1
Wood, Allen, 106
Worldview, 37–39
World War II era, 80, 166, 247n5,
    251n2
Wynia, M. K., 6, 55, 162

Young, R., 128

Zuckert, Michael, P., 89
Zussman, R., 137